...XBR... ...LEGE LIBRARY

D0433289

EXERCISE PHYSIOLOGY

FOURTH EDITION

STUDY GUIDE

VICTOR L.
KATCH

Professor, Department of Movement Science
Division of Kinesiology
Associate Professor, Pediatrics
School of Medicine
University of Michigan
Ann Arbor, Michigan

FRANK I.
KATCH

Professor, Department of Exercise Science
University of Massachusetts
Amherst, Massachusetts

WILLIAM D.
McARDLE

Professor, Department of Health and Physical Education
Queens College of the City University of New York
Flushing, New York

EXERCISE PHYSIOLOGY

FOURTH EDITION

STUDY GUIDE

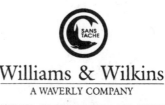

Williams & Wilkins

A WAVERLY COMPANY

BALTIMORE • PHILADELPHIA • LONDON • PARIS • BANGKOK
BUENOS AIRES • HONG KONG • MUNICH • SYDNEY • TOKYO • WROCLAW

Editor: Donna Balado
Managing Editor: Victoria M. Vaughn
Production Coordinator: Carol Eckhart
Copy Editor: Thomas Lehr
Designer: Ashley Pound Design
Typesetter: Peirce Graphic Services
Printer & Binder: Vicks Litho

Copyright © 1996, Williams & Wilkins

351 West Camden Street
Baltimore, Maryland 21201-2436 USA

Rose Tree Corporate Center
1400 North Providence Road
Building II, Suite 5025
Media, Pennsylvania 19063–2043 USA

All rights reserved. This book is protected by copyright. No part of this book may be reproduced in any form or by any means, including photocopying, or utilized by any information
storage and retrieval system without written permission from the copyright owner.

Crossword puzzles, Self-Assessment Tests (Section 2), Energy Expenditure Tables
(Section 4 A), and the Nutritive Values for Common Foods (Section 4 B) Copyright © 1993
by Frank I. Katch, Victor L. Katch, William D. McArdle, and Fitness Technologies, Inc., P.O.
Box 430, Amherst, MA 01004, fax (313) 662-8153. No part of these materials may be reproduced in any manner without written permission from the copyright holders.

Printed in the United States of America

ISBN 0-683-0-0103-3

The publishers have made every effort to trace the copyright holders for borrowed mate-
rial. If they have inadvertently overlooked any, they will be pleased to make the necessary
arrangements at the first opportunity.

Call our customer service department at **(800) 638–0672** for catalog information or fax
orders to **(800) 447–8438.** For other book services, including chapter reprints and large
quantity sales, ask for the Special Sales department.

To purchase additional copies of this book or for information concerning American College
of Sports Medicine certification and suggested preparatory materials, call **(800) 486–5643.**

Canadian customers should call **(800) 268–4178,** or fax **(905) 470–6780.** For all other calls
originating outside of the United States, please call **(410) 528–4223** or fax us at **(410)
528–8550.**

Visit Williams & Wilkins on the Internet: http://www.wwilkins.com or contact our customer service department at **custserv@wwilkins.com.** Williams & Wilkins customer service representatives are available from 8:30 am to 6:00 pm, EST, Monday through Friday,
for telephone access.

96 97 98 99 00
1 2 3 4 5 6 7 8 9 10

BLACKBURN COLLEGE
LIBRARY
Acc.No. 83914
Class No. 612·044 KAT
Date Jul '99

PREFACE

This *Study Guide* is a resource companion to the fourth edition of the textbook *Exercise Physiology: Energy, Nutrition, and Human Performance*. Its purpose is to help you better understand the text content by focusing on key terms and concepts and on specific questions within each chapter. The addition of sample quizzes and crossword puzzles should also make studying easier.

The *Study Guide* has four sections. The first section asks you to define key terms and concepts. Also included are study questions for each major topic heading, a sample quiz, and a crossword puzzle. For the study questions we have followed the sequence of each chapter. This means you should be able to easily locate the answers to each of the questions by referring back to the appropriate section heading within each chapter. Crossword puzzles, in our experience, have always been an entertaining yet challenging way to study.

Section 2 includes practical self-assessment tests. We encourage you to use these tests and think carefully about how to apply the results to enhance your own health and wellness, as well as the health and wellness of those with whom you come in professional contact. The purpose of presenting these assessment tools is to bring to life some of the text material and to show how much of the material can be practical.

Section 3 provides answers to the chapter quizzes and crossword puzzles.

Section 4 of the *Study Guide* presents material on the nutritive value of common foods, and a listing of the energy cost values for a variety of physical activities. These materials should help to complete several of the practical assessment tests in Section 2, and they should be useful in other applications.

In addition to this workbook as an accompanying study guide to our textbook, we are introducing a new concept related to both the textbook and the field itself. This project came about because of student and professor requests for ancillary information. To meet these needs, we have created a site on the World Wide Web of the Internet, called **The Exercise Physiology Club (ExPC).**

ExPC is a cyberspace kiosk for students, professors, professionals, and others interested in exercise physiology and related areas. The major purpose of the **ExPC** is to provide information that can catalyze and sustain interest in the diverse aspects of exercise physiology and its professional dimensions. **ExPC** on the Internet is divided into six main areas: Student Resources, Professionals, Sports Nutrition, Exercise Science Resources, Products, and ExPC Interactive (e-mail and bulletin board).

Point your browser to:

htpp://www.exer-phys-club.com

Since you are a user of our textbook and/or workbook, you are entitled to special offers through the ExPC. Use the following password to access this information:

EXPC1PR

As always, we wish to thank our wives, Heather, Kerry, and Kathy, for their support and patience.

Victor L. Katch • Ann Arbor, MI
Frank I. Katch • Amherst, MA
William D. McArdle • Sound Beach, NY

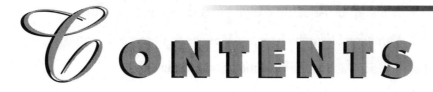

CONTENTS

SECTION 1

Define Key Terms and Concepts
Study Questions
Practice Quizzes
Crossword Puzzles

continued

SECTION 2

Self-Assessment Tests

SECTION 3

Answers to Chapter Quizzes
Crossword Puzzle Solutions

SECTION 4

Appendixes

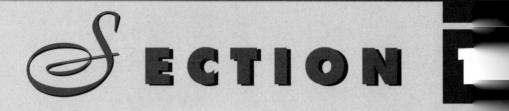

SECTION 1

DEFINE KEY TERMS AND CONCEPTS

STUDY QUESTIONS

PRACTICE QUIZZES

CROSSWORD PUZZLES

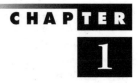
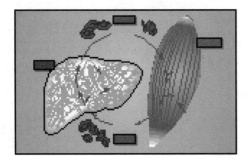

Carbohydrates, Lipids, and Proteins

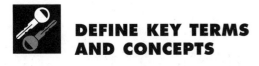 **DEFINE KEY TERMS AND CONCEPTS**

1. **Macronutrients**

2. **Carbohydrates**

3. **Glucose**

4. **Fructose**

5. **Galactose**

6. **Monosaccharides**

7. **Gluconeogenesis**

8. **Oligosaccharides**

9. **Disaccharides**

10. **Sucrose**

11. **Lactose**

12. **Maltose**

13. **Polysaccharides**

14. **Starch**

15. **Fiber**

16. **Cellulose**

17. **Glycogen**

18. **Glycogenolysis**

19. **Metabolic primer**

20. **Ketone bodies**

21. **Ketosis**

22. **Hypoglycemia**

23. **Glucose polymer**

24. **Triglycerides**

25. Glycerol

26. Fatty acid

27. Hydrolysis

28. Saturated fatty acid

29. Unsaturated fatty acid

30. *Trans* fatty acid

31. Monounsaturated fatty acids

32. Polyunsaturated fatty acids

33. Hydrogenation

34. Linoleic acid

35. Essential fatty acid

36. Compound fat

37. Phospholipids

38. Glycolipids

39. Lipoproteins

40. **High-density lipoproteins**

41. **Very low-density lipoproteins**

42. **Low-density lipoproteins**

43. **Derived fats**

44. **Cholesterol**

45. **Atherosclerosis**

46. **Proteins**

47. **Amino acids**

48. **Essential amino acids**

49. **Nonessential amino acids**

50. **RDA**

51. **Anabolism**

52. **Catabolism**

53. **Transamination**

54. **Nitrogen balance**

55.   **Alanine-glucose cycle** _____

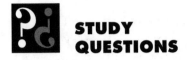

STUDY QUESTIONS

BASIC STRUCTURE OF NUTRIENTS

Atoms: Nature's Building Blocks

List four major atoms and the percentage of the body mass they represent.

1.

2.

3.

4.

THE NATURE OF CARBOHYDRATES

Give the chemical formula for glucose.

KINDS AND SOURCES OF CARBOHYDRATES

List three kinds of carbohydrates. Give an example of each.

            Kind   Example

1.

2.

3.

Polysaccharides

Plant Polysaccharides

List two types of plant polysaccharide.

1.

2.

List three advantages of including fiber in the diet.

1.

2.

3.

Give the recommended quantity of daily dietary fiber.

Animal Polysaccharides

Define gluconeogenesis and glycogenolysis.

• Gluconeogenesis

• Glycogenolysis

Indicate the average quantity of glycogen stored in liver and muscle.

• Liver

• Muscle

RECOMMENDED DIETARY INTAKE OF CARBOHYDRATES

List three carbohydrate-rich foods.

1.

2.

3.

Give the current percentage of carbohydrate in the typical American diet and the recommended percentage.

• Current

• Recommended

ROLE OF CARBOHYDRATE IN THE BODY

Energy Source

What is the main function of carbohydrate in the body?

Protein Sparing

List two ways in which carbohydrates spare protein.

1.

2.

Metabolic Primer

What compound is produced from incomplete lipid breakdown?

Fuel for the Central Nervous System

List three symptoms of hypoglycemia.

1.

2.

3.

CARBOHYDRATE BALANCE IN EXERCISE

What laboratory measure is used to determine carbohydrate use during exercise?

Intense Exercise

Which macronutrient is used almost exclusively during intense exercise?

Moderate and Prolonged Exercise

Detail the utilization of carbohydrate during the initial, middle, and end stages of moderate- to high-intensity, prolonged aerobic exercise.

Effect of Diet on Muscle Glycogen Stores and Endurance

How does depletion of carbohydrate affect (1) all-out short-term and (2) prolonged endurance exercise?

1.

2.

THE NATURE OF LIPIDS

Kinds and Sources of Lipids

List three main groups of lipids.

1.

2.

3.

What is a typical hydrogen-to-oxygen ratio for a common lipid?

Simple Lipids

List two kinds of fatty acid molecules and the differences between them.

1.

2.

Differences:

Lipids in the Diet

Give the current percentage of lipid in the typical American diet and the percentage currently recommended.

• Current

• Recommended

Compound Lipids

List three groups of compound lipids.

1.

2.

3.

List three types of lipoproteins.

1.

2.

3.

Derived Lipids

Indicate the most common derived lipid and its main function.

List three food sources high in cholesterol.

1.

2.

3.

Cholesterol–Heart Disease Controversy

List two reasons why a diet high in cholesterol and saturated fatty acids is a risk for coronary heart disease.

1.

2.

What is the recommended daily dietary intake of cholesterol?

ROLE OF LIPID IN THE BODY

List three major functions of lipids in the body.

1.

2.

3.

List three reasons why lipids are the "ideal cellular fuel."

1.

2.

3.

LIPID BALANCE IN EXERCISE

Lipid provides approximately what percentage of the total energy during prolonged, light to moderate exercise?

PROTEINS

The Nature of Proteins

What are the two building block constituents of protein, and how are they linked together?

Kinds of Protein

Name two categories of amino acids in the diet.

1.

2.

What is meant by the "biologic value" of a food?

Recommended Dietary Protein Intake

The RDA: A Liberal Standard

What is the RDA for protein?

Preparations of Simple Amino Acids

What is the rationale for the use of simple amino acid preparations?

Do simple amino acid preparations improve strength, power, muscle mass, and/or endurance?

Role of Protein in the Body

Approximately what percentage of the body mass consists of protein?

Dynamics of Protein Metabolism

Describe the broad steps in the use of protein for catabolic processes.

Protein Balance in Exercise and Training: Is the RDA Really Adequate?

Why is the maintenance of adequate carbohydrate and energy intake important for conserving the body's protein during heavy training?

The Alanine-Glucose Cycle

Of the total exercise energy requirement, approximately how much may be supplied by the alanine-glucose cycle?

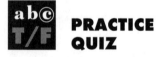 **PRACTICE QUIZ**

MULTIPLE CHOICE

1. **Which of the following is <u>not</u> a metabolic pathway for glucose after its absorption by the small intestine?**
    a. converted to lipids for energy storage
    b. stored as glycogen in the muscles and liver
    c. converted to protein in the kidneys
    d. used directly by the cell for energy
    e. b and c

2. **Disaccharides are:**
    a. double sugars
    b. composed of sucrose, fructose, and alanine
    c. composed of starch and fiber
    d. most common in the form of glucose
    e. none of the above

3. **Reconversion of glycogen to glucose is the process of:**
   a. deamination
   b. gluconeogenesis
   c. glycogenolysis
   d. transamination
   e. none of the above

4. **The main function of carbohydrates is to:**
   a. spare proteins
   b. provide insulation and protection for the vital organs
   c. serve as an energy fuel
   d. prevent hypoglycemia
   e. none of the above

5. **Cholesterol:**
   a. is a derived lipid
   b. is classified into three types: HDL, MDL, and GDL
   c. is found in foods of plant and animal origin
   d. is necessary for the synthesis of vitamins A and B
   e. all of the above

6. **Two common forms of plant polysaccharide are:**
   a. starch and fiber
   b. fiber and glucose
   c. fiber and maltose
   d. cellulose
   e. none of the above

7. **Gluconeogenesis is related to the conversion of:**
   a. glycogen to glucose
   b. protein to glucose
   c. glucose to glycerol
   d. glucose to sugar
   e. none of the above

8. **The main animal polysaccharide is:**
   a. glucose
   b. glycogen
   c. fiber
   d. fructose
   e. none of the above

9. **The RDA for protein is:**
   a. greater than 2.5 g per kilogram body mass
   b. less than 0.5 g per kilogram body mass
   c. 4 oz per day
   d. 0.8 g per kilogram body mass
   e. 2.5 oz per day

10. Sucrose is:
  a. a polysaccharide
  b. a common starch
  c. not found naturally occurring in food
  d. the sweetest of the simple sugars
  e. none of the above

TRUE / FALSE

1. _____ In a prudent diet, lipid intake should not exceed 30% of the total energy content of the diet.

2. _____ Adequate carbohydrate intake has a sparing effect on the body's lean tissue.

3. _____ Most vegetable oils are relatively high in unsaturated fatty acids.

4. _____ Cholesterol cannot be synthesized by the body.

5. _____ Protein breakdown during exercise is less in lean than in obese individuals.

6. _____ Lipoproteins are primarily made up of unsaturated fatty acids.

7. _____ Sugar drinks consumed during exercise should be avoided if they contain monosaccharides.

8. _____ Most vegetable oils are relatively high in unsaturated fatty acids.

9. _____ Saturated fatty acids contain only single bonds between carbon atoms.

10. _____ Of the macronutrients, an amino group occurs only in protein.

CROSSWORD PUZZLE

ACROSS

2 Sugar component of triglycerides
3 Milk sugar
4 Complex plant carbohydrate
7 No double bonds in this type of fatty acid
9 Protein building block
11 Liberal standard for nutrient intake
12 Macronutrients insoluble in H_2O
14 Classification of macronutrient
16 Fatty deposits in arterial wall
19 Glucose + glucose
20 Nondigestible plant component
21 Gluconeogenic amino acid
24 Product of incomplete lipid breakdown
25 Simple sugar
27 Derived lipid synthesized by liver
28 Chemical breakdown by addition of water
29 Transport form for blood lipids
30 Chemical bonding linking amino acids
31 Low blood sugar

DOWN

1 Building block of lipids
5 Glycerol + 3 free fatty acids
6 Lipoprotein with largest amount of lipid (abbr.)
8 Sweetest of monosaccharides
10 Carbon-containing compounds
13 Glucose synthesis from noncarbohydrate sources
15 Animal polysaccharide
16 Chemical reactions of synthesis
17 Fructose + glucose
18 Fatty acids + phosphorus-containing compound
22 Abnormally high levels of ketones
23 Monosaccharide not found freely in nature
26 Good cholesterol (abbr.)

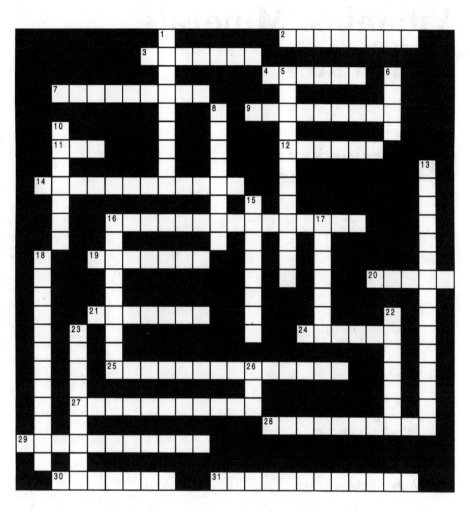

See page 367 for Crossword Puzzle Solution.

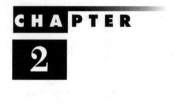

Vitamins, Minerals, and Water

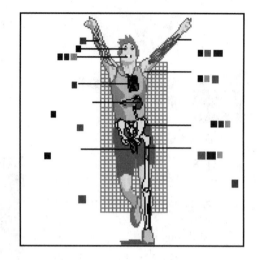

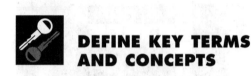 **DEFINE KEY TERMS AND CONCEPTS**

1. **Micronutrients**

2. **Vitamins**

3. **Provitamin**

4. **Carotenes**

5. **Fat-soluble vitamins**

6. **Water-soluble vitamins**

7. **Hypervitaminosis A**

8. **Free radicals**

9. **Oxidative stress**

10. **Lipid peroxidation**

11. **Antioxidants**

12. β-Carotene

13. **B-Complex vitamin**

14. **Megavitamins**

15. **Minerals**

16. **Major minerals**

17. **Trace minerals**

18. **Osteoporosis**

19. **Bone remodeling**

20. **Cortical bone**

21. **Trabecular bone**

22. **Calcitonin**

23. **Secondary amenorrhea**

24. **Hemoglobin**

25. **Myoglobin**

26. **Cytochromes**

27. **Transferrin**

28. **Non-heme iron**

29. **Heme iron**

30. **Iron deficiency anemia**

31. **Clinical anemia**

32. **Sports anemia**

33. **Electrolytes**

34. **Aldosterone**

35. **Sodium-induced hypertension**

36. **Intracellular fluid**

37. **Extracellular fluid**

38. **Metabolic water**

39. **Insensible perspiration**

40. **Relative humidity**

41. **Hyponatremia**

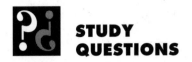

STUDY QUESTIONS

VITAMINS
The Nature of Vitamins

What was the first vitamin discovered?

Give the primary way the body acquires vitamins.

Kinds of Vitamins
Lipid-Soluble Vitamins

List the four lipid-soluble vitamins.

1.   3.

2.   4.

Water-Soluble Vitamins

List the nine water-soluble vitamins.

1.   6.

2.   7.

3.   8.

4.   9.

5.

Role of Vitamins in the Body

List three functions of vitamins in the body.

1.

2.

3.

List the two major functions of the lipid-soluble vitamins.

1.

2.

Do athletes require more vitamins than sedentary people? Explain.

Antioxidant Role of Specific Vitamins

List three vitamins that serve to protect against oxidative stress.

1.

2.

3.

Exercise, Free Radicals, and Antioxidants

List two ways free radicals are produced during exercise.

1.

2.

Are physically active individuals more prone to produce free radical damage? Explain.

Do physically active individuals require increased amounts of antioxidant substances? Explain.

Vitamin Supplements: The Competitive Edge?

Do vitamin supplements enhance physical performance? Explain.

Megavitamins

Is there any rationale for consuming megadoses of vitamins? Explain.

In what ways can megavitamins be harmful to the body?

MINERALS

The Nature of Minerals

What percent of the body's weight consists of minerals?

Kinds and Sources of Minerals

List four minerals and their function in the body.

Mineral   Function

1.

2.

3.

4.

What is the exception to the statement: "There is generally adequate mineral intake"?

Why is iodine important to bodily function?

Role of Minerals in the Body

What structural, functional, and regulatory roles do minerals play in the body?

• Structural

• Functional

• Regulatory

Calcium

List five functions of calcium in the body.

1.   4.

2.   5.

3.

Osteoporosis: Calcium, Estrogen, and Exercise

List two factors that can help prevent osteoporosis.

1.

2.

A Progressive Disease

Why is osteoporosis referred to as a "progressive disease"? Explain.

Prevention

What is the prime defense against bone loss with aging?

Exercise Is Helpful

What role does exercise have on skeletal aging?

Five Principles for Planning Exercise to Promote Bone Health

List five important principles that promote bone health.

1.

2.

3.

4.

5.

Is Too Much Training Harmful?

Explain how too much exercise might be counterproductive in preventing osteoporosis.

Phosphorus

Phosphorus is an essential component of what high-energy compounds?

Magnesium

Of what importance is magnesium to the body?

Iron

List four functions of iron in the body.

1.

2.

3.

4.

Females: A Population at Risk

Discuss the reasoning behind the reference to females as "a population at risk in terms of iron insufficiency."

Source of Iron Is Important

List two dietary sources of iron.

1.

2.

Exercise-Induced Anemia: Fact or Fiction?

List three factors that may be related to "sports anemia."

1.

2.

3.

Sodium, Potassium, and Chlorine

What role do sodium and chlorine play in the body's fluid regulation?

List two functions of sodium and potassium.

1.

2.

Sodium: How Much Is Enough?

What is the recommended daily intake of sodium?

List two possible negative effects of excess sodium intake.

1.

2.

Minerals and Exercise Performance

Discuss the magnitude of fluid and salt loss during exercise in hot weather.

What can be done to counteract this effect?

WATER

Water in the Body

Water constitutes what percentage of the weight of muscle tissue and what percentage of the weight of body fat?

- Weight of muscle
- Weight of body fat

Functions of Body Water

List five functions of water in the body.

1.

2.

3.

4.

5.

Water Balance: Intake versus Output

Water Intake

List and quantify three main sources of water intake.

	Source	Quantity
1.		
2.		
3.		

Water Output

List and quantify four primary ways in which water is lost from the body.

	Source	Amount
1.		
2.		
3.		
4.		

Water Loss Through the Skin

List two ways water is lost through the skin.

1.

2.

Discuss how evaporation of sweat provides the refrigeration mechanism to cool the body.

Water Requirement in Exercise

Discuss the effects of exercise on the body's water requirement.

Hyponatremia: Sweating + Water = Too Much of Two Good Things

Under what condition does hyponatremia occur?

Outline the dynamics for developing hyponatremia.

Factors That Predispose to Hyponatremia

List four factors that may predispose a person to hyponatremia.

1.

2.

3.

4.

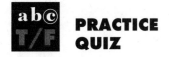

PRACTICE QUIZ

MULTIPLE CHOICE

1. **Vitamins are important components in physiologic processes related to:**
   a. fluid osmolality
   b. metabolic regulation
   c. temperature regulation
   d. insulation
   e. c and d

2. **Minerals:**
   a. function in both anabolic and catabolic metabolic process
   b. primarily come from animal dietary sources
   c. are of limited quantity in the plant kingdom
   d. alone can catalyze metabolic reactions
   e. a and d

3. **The water needs of the body are supplied from these three main sources:**
   a. liquids, fruits, vegetables
   b. foods, fluids, metabolism
   c. fruits, liquids, solids
   d. lipids, proteins, carbohydrates
   e. none of the above

4. **In extremely hot weather, the fluid needs of an active person increase by about:**
   a. 2 times normal
   b. 3 times normal
   c. 6 times normal
   d. 8 times normal
   e. 10 times normal

5. **Excess vitamin B_6 intake:**
   a. can lead to liver disease and nerve damage
   b. has no known side effects
   c. accelerates osteoporosis
   d. stunts growth if accompanied by excessive vitamin B_{12} intake
   e. can cause muscle atrophy

6. **Provitamins:**
   a. activate lipid clearing from the arterial walls
   b. are required to activate certain vitamins
   c. are composed primarily of lipid-soluble products
   d. are precursor substances found only in animals
   e. none of the above

7. **The two most plentiful minerals in the body are:**
   a. calcium and phosphorus
   b. iron and selenium
   c. calcium and magnesium
   d. chlorine and potassium
   e. calcium and iron

8. **Women on vegetarian-type diets:**
   a. are at a higher risk of developing iron insufficiency
   b. are at a lower risk of developing iron insufficiency
   c. need to decrease their intake of vitamin C–rich foods
   d. need to increase their intake of lipid-soluble vitamins to increase the availability of heme iron
   e. c and d

9. **Megadoses of Vitamin C:**
   a. can raise serum uric acid levels and precipitate gout in people predisposed to this disease
   b. are not dangerous, and the excess is eliminated during urination
   c. can lead to hypermetabolism during rest
   d. will enhance aerobic endurance performance
   e. none of the above

10. **The greatest loss of daily water is from:**
    a. urine
    b. feces
    c. skin
    d. pulmonary ventilation
    e. insensible perspiration

TRUE / FALSE

1. _____ The lipid-soluble vitamins are A, D, E, and K.

2. _____ Vitamin supplementation above the RDA improves exercise performance.

3. _____ Mineral intake is usually adequate when one consumes a well-balanced diet.

4. _____ Water makes up between 40 and 60% of the total body mass.

5. _____ The primary aim of fluid replacement is to maintain plasma volume.

6. _____ All vitamins can be synthesized in the body except vitamin E.

7. _____ Sports anemia occurs when hemoglobin in men decreases to about 14 g of hemoglobin per 100 mL of blood.

8. _____ Extracellular water volume exceeds the intracellular volume of water.

9. _____ Athletes require increased amounts of minerals above the RDA.

10. _____ Osteoporosis begins early in life due mainly to inadequate calcium intake.

CROSSWORD PUZZLE

ACROSS

1   Micronutrient for good health and growth
4   Disease typified by reduction in bone mass
7   Any substance such as a salt, acid, or base that ionizes and dissociates in water and is capable of conducting an electric current
10 Yellow vitamin precursors, found in carrots
12 Water vapor content of air
13 Ascorbic ____ is vitamin C
14 Number of fat-soluble vitamins
17 Outside the cell
21 Chemical abbr. for metallic element in electron transport
23 Oxygen-carrying group of hemoglobin
24 The body secretes 8 to 12 L during hot-weather exercise
25 Body's most abundant mineral (abbr.)
26 Low hemoglobin concentration
27 A substance that can be converted into a vitamin
28 Mostly metallic element that plays a vital role in metabolism
29 Inside the cell

DOWN

2   Iron-containing pigment in muscle
3   Iron-protein compound for O_2 transport
5   Minerals required in amounts less than 100 mg/day
6   A ____ vitamin is an inactive precursor form of a vitamin
8   Number of vitamins
9   Organic compound that neutralizes free radicals
11 Dietary component required in small quantities
12 Abnormally low concentration of sodium ions in blood plasma caused by consuming too much water after excessive sweating
15 Vitamin intake in excess of 10 times the RDA
16 Salt-regulating hormone of adrenal cortex
18 Type of bone; sponge bone
19 Hormone that regulates blood calcium level
20 A protein that transports iron in the blood
21 Chemical that has unshared electrons available for a reaction
22 Intramitochondrial iron protein compound

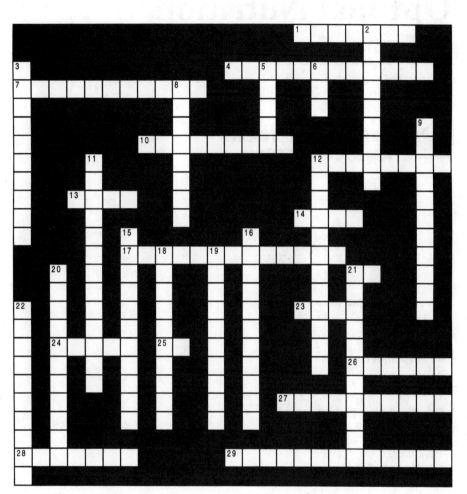

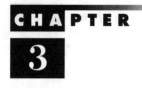

Optimal Nutrition for Exercise

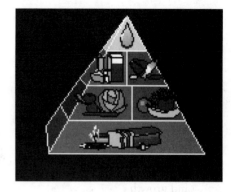

DEFINE KEY TERMS AND CONCEPTS

1. Optimal diet

2. Optimal protein intake

3. Optimal lipid intake

4. Optimal carbohydrate intake

5. The Eating-Right Pyramid

6. Tour de France

7. Ultramarathoner Kouros

8. Eat more, weigh less

9. Military Recommended Daily Allowances

10. Precompetition meal

11. **Liquid meals**

12. **Overshoot in insulin**

13. **Glycemic index**

14. **Athletes and calorie intake**

15. **Glycogen synthetase**

16. **Osmolality**

17. **Glucose-sodium cotransport**

18. **Ideal oral rehydration solution**

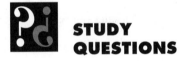

STUDY QUESTIONS

NUTRIENT REQUIREMENTS

"Sound nutrition for athletes is sound human nutrition." Explain.

Recommended Nutrient Intake

What is the approximate daily total energy requirement for men and women?

- Males

- Females

Protein

Give the protein RDA for both sedentary and physically active individuals.

- Sedentary

- Active

Lipids

To promote good health, lipid intake should probably not exceed what percent of the diet's energy content?

What is the optimal ratio of unsaturated to saturated fatty acid intake?

Carbohydrate

Discuss why adequate carbohydrate intake is crucial for an active person.

Carbohydrate Needs in Intense Training

What nutritional state may be related to the "staleness" experienced by certain athletes during heavy training?

Approximately how many days of rest or light exercise is needed to establish depleted muscle glycogen stores to pre-exercise levels?

The Eating-Right Pyramid: The Essentials of Good Nutrition

Outline the recommendations of the Eating-Right Pyramid and how they compare to the "basic four recommendation."

EXERCISE AND FOOD INTAKE

What would be the "extra" daily caloric expenditure per day for distance runners who train about 100 miles per week?

Tour de France

What is the approximate daily caloric intake for competitors in the Tour de France?

Ultraendurance Running Competition

What would be a recommended caloric intake for ultraendurance runners?

Other Athletic Groups

In what category of athletics do champion athletes sometimes need to upgrade the nutritional quality and quantity of their food?

Eat More, Weigh Less

How is it possible for physically active people to actually eat more than the average person, yet weigh less?

THE PRECOMPETITION MEAL

What is the main purpose of the pregame meal?

Is it beneficial for an athlete to fast prior to competition? Explain.

Protein or Carbohydrate?

List two reasons why it is important to reduce protein in the pre-event meal.

1.

2.

Give one reason why the pre-event meal should consist mainly of carbohydrate.

Liquid and Prepackaged Meals

List three reasons why a liquid pre-event meal may be beneficial.

1.

2.

3.

Application in the Military

What is the MRDA for food rations for military personnel?

Describe a self-heating individual meal module.

CARBOHYDRATE FEEDINGS BEFORE, DURING, AND IN RECOVERY FROM EXERCISE

What types of exercise can almost completely deplete muscle and liver glycogen?

During Exercise

Identify the macronutrient consumed during prolonged, high-intensity aerobic exercise that can benefit performance.

Before Exercise

What two negative effects might the intake of a high glycemic carbohydrate have if consumed within 1 hour before exercising?

1.

2.

Describe the "insulin overshoot" phenomenon.

Which of the monosaccharides is absorbed most slowly from the gut?

In Recovery

Outline the dietary procedure to speed carbohydrate replenishment after exhaustive exercise.

The Glycemic Index and Pre-exercise Feedings

How can the glycemic index be used to formulate the immediate pre-exercise feeding?

GLUCOSE FEEDINGS, ELECTROLYTES, AND WATER UPTAKE

Why is there no overshoot in the insulin response when consuming simple sugars during exercise?

Important Considerations

What two factors affect the rate of gastric emptying?

1.

2.

How can the negative effects of simple sugar molecules on gastric emptying be reduced?

Recommended Oral Rehydration Solution

What constitutes the "ideal" oral rehydration solution?

Practical Recommendations for Fluid and Carbohydrate Replacement

Give two practical recommendations for fluid and carbohydrate replacement.

1.

2.

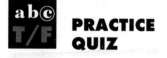 **PRACTICE QUIZ**

MULTIPLE CHOICE

1. **This activity is likely to burn the most total calories:**
   a. gymnastics practice
   b. triathlon
   c. daily swim practice for collegiate swimmers
   d. marathon
   e. one-mile run at maximal pace

2. **Fruits and vegetables are rich sources of:**
   a. lipids
   b. carbohydrates
   c. proteins
   d. lipoproteins
   e. none of the above

3. **Following prolonged exercise, at least how many hours are needed to restore muscle glycogen levels?**
   a. 48
   b. 24
   c. 12
   d. 2
   e. none of the above

4. **A high-protein pregame meal:**
   a. facilitates protein breakdown and subsequent dehydration
   b. is more difficult to digest than a high-carbohydrate pregame meal
   c. results in a decrease in total plasma cholesterol
   d. a and b
   e. a and c

5. **Liquid meals are beneficial for all of the following reasons <u>except</u>:**
   a. they are easily digested
   b. they are likely to provide sufficient energy without the feeling of fullness
   c. they contribute to fluid needs
   d. digestion is rapid and complete
   e. they decrease lactic acid production

6. **The major emphasis of the Eating-Right Pyramid is:**
   a. grains and vegetables
   b. fuits and meats
   c. dairy products and grains
   d. smaller portion sizes from plant sources
   e. equal portion sizes from each food group

7. **Which statement is <u>true</u> about the coefficient of digestibility for the macronutrients:**
   a. it is 97% for carbohydrates, 95% for lipids, and 92% for proteins
   b. it is 97% for lipids, 95% for carbohydrates, and 92% for proteins
   c. it is 97% for proteins, 95% for carbohydrates, and 92% for lipids
   d. it is 97% for lipids, 95% for proteins, and 92% for carbohydrates
   e. none of the above

8. **Which statement is <u>true</u> about a bomb calorimeter?**
   a. it produces Atwater factors
   b. it is used in direct calorimetry
   c. it is used in indirect calorimetry
   d. it is used to determine the digestive efficiency of food
   e. it is used to calculate the MET value of food

9. **Concerning the precompetition meal:**
   a. avoid foods high in lipid and protein
   b. avoid foods high in carbohydrate
   c. foods high in protein should be included
   d. include supplements of vitamins and minerals
   e. it should contain only polymerized vitamins and minerals

10. Carbohydrates in either liquid or solid form consumed during exercise:

a. benefit performance in relatively high-intensity, long-term aerobic exercise and repetitive short bouts of near-maximal effort

b. do not benefit endurance performance

c. benefit only short-duration submaximum effort

d. act to enhance aerobic performance by increasing the $\dot{V}O_2$max

e. a and d

TRUE/FALSE

1. _____ The glycemic index is a relative measure of how much blood glucose increases after ingesting a food containing 50 g of carbohydrate.

2. _____ Endurance athletes often experience "staleness" due to depletion of protein reserves.

3. _____ Fasting 24 hours prior to exercise is beneficial if you have "carbo-loaded" the week before competition.

4. _____ Timing of the pre-event meal is important due to the body's limited protein reserves.

5. _____ It is wise to consume carbohydrate-rich foods as soon as possible after heavy exercise to speed the replenishment process.

6. _____ A calorie expresses the heat or energy value of food.

7. _____ A "prudent diet" should contain about 60% of its calories in the form of high-quality protein.

8. _____ A 1-hour period is generally adequate for a meal to be digested and absorbed.

9. _____ The ideal oral rehydration solution contains a carbohydrate concentration between 5 and 8%.

10. _____ Drinking a strong sugar solution 30 minutes prior to exercise has been shown to improve endurance capacity.

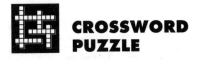

CROSSWORD PUZZLE

ACROSS

2   Index of carbohydrate absorption

4   International endurance bicycle race

6   Replenish water loss

8   Person weighing 77 kg requires this many grams of protein daily

10 Term for food consumed prior to competition

12 Famous living Greek marathoner

14 Concentration of particles in solution

16 Geometric-shaped system to classify food groups

18 One approach to weight loss

DOWN

1   Glycogen-synthesizing enzyme

3   Natives of Mexico who consume a diet high in complex carbohydrates

4   Minimum number of hours for glycogen replenishment

5   Fluid replacement should approach _____ percent of sweat rate

7   Animal polysaccharide

9   This intensity of aerobic exercise stresses glycogen reserves

10 Eating-Right _____

11 Many physically active people actually ___ ____ yet weigh less

13 Exaggerated insulin release in response to sugar challenge

15 Type of meal effective for pre-event feeding

17 Hormone secreted by beta cells of islets of Langerhans

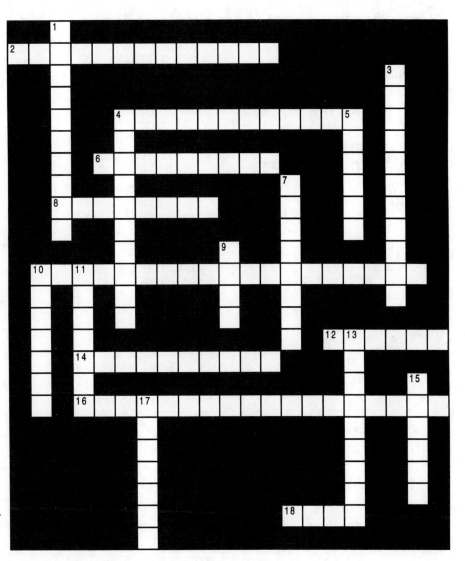

See page 367 for Crossword Puzzle Solution.

CHAPTER 4

Energy for Physical Activity

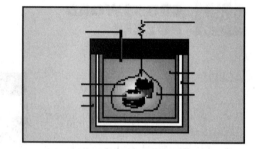

DEFINE KEY TERMS AND CONCEPTS

1. Energy

2. Calorie

3. Kilogram calorie

4. Joule

5. Bomb calorimeter

6. Direct calorimetry

7. Oxidation

8. Net energy value of food

9. Heat of combustion

10. 4.2 kcal·g^{-1}

36

11. **5.65 kcal·g^{-1}**

12. **9.4 kcal·g^{-1}**

13. **Net energy value of food**

14. **Coefficient of digestibility**

15. **USNDB**

16. **Atwater general factors**

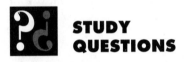

STUDY QUESTIONS

THE CALORIE AS A UNIT OF ENERGY MEASUREMENT

What is the difference between a calorie and a kilocalorie?

GROSS ENERGY VALUE OF FOODS

What instrument is used in direct calorimetry to measure a food's energy value?

Heat of Combustion

Lipid

What is the average heat of combustion per gram of lipid?

Carbohydrate

What is the average heat of combustion per gram of carbohydrate?

Protein

List two factors that affect the energy released during the combustion of protein.

1.

2.

What is the average heat of combustion per gram of protein?

Comparing the Energy Value of Nutrients

Which macronutrient has the most hydrogen atoms per molecule, allowing for the greatest energy release upon combustion?

NET ENERGY VALUE OF FOODS

Compare the heat of combustion of carbohydrates and lipids in the body with those determined by bomb calorimetry.

- In the body
- Bomb calorimetry

Coefficient of Digestibility

What is one effect that dietary fiber may have on the energy availability of ingested foods?

Caloric Value of a Meal

Calculate the caloric content of 100 grams of a food containing 5% protein, 14% lipid, and 20% carbohydrate. (*Hint: Use the Atwater general factors.*)

- kcal protein:
- kcal lipid:
- kcal carbohydrate:
- total kcal:

Is the caloric value of 150 kcal of cherry pie more or less than the caloric value of 150 kcal of sunflower seeds? Explain.

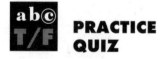

PRACTICE QUIZ

MULTIPLE CHOICE

1. **A kilogram calorie is the:**
   a. amount of heat necessary for metabolism
   b. amount of heat necessary to raise the temperature of 1 kg of water by 1°C
   c. same as the gross energy value of combustion
   d. amount of heat necessary to increase metabolism twofold
   e. amount of energy to produce 100 ft-lb of work

2. **A joule is:**
   a. a precious mineral
   b. another term for entropy
   c. an international standard for expressing energy
   d. the utilization of glucose in energy metabolism
   e. none of the above

3. **What are the average net energy values (kcal·g^{-1}) for the macronutrients carbohydrate, lipid, and protein?**
    a. 9, 9, 4
    b. 5, 9, 4
    c. 4, 4, 5
    d. 4, 9, 4
    e. none of the above

4. **The Atwater caloric values enable one to determine the:**
    a. energy cost of physical activity
    b. energy cost of breathing
    c. RDA for specific nutrients
    d. SDA for specific nutrients
    e. none of the above

5. **Proteins:**
    a. differ from lipids and carbohydrates because of nitrogen content
    b. contain only one amino acid per gram
    c. are easier to digest than lipids
    d. usually hydrogenate in water and donate electrons
    e. a and d

6. **The coefficient of digestibility is the:**
    a. ability to digest food
    b. proportion of ingested food actually digested and absorbed to serve the body's metabolic needs
    c. proportion of ingested food that remains undigested in the large intestine
    d. same for all the macronutrients
    e. none of the above

7. **The heat liberated by the burning or oxidation of a specific food is referred to as its:**
    a. metabolic equivalent
    b. energy cost factor
    c. heat of combustion
    d. Atwater factor
    e. oxidation coefficient

8. **The energy released from protein depends on the:**
    a. kind of protein and its relative proportions of protein and nonprotein nitrogenous substances
    b. number of amino acids and carbon atoms
    c. reducing power of coenzymes
    d. amount of oxygen and carbon dioxide in the protein molecule
    e. number of amino acids catabolized to hydrogen and oxygen

9. **Complete oxidation of lipid in the bomb calorimeter liberates ___ % more energy per gram than protein:**
    a. 65
    b. 25
    c. 90
    d. 50
    e. 100

10. **What would be the total kcal value for 1 gram of a substance that contains 5% protein, 20% lipid, and 30% carbohydrate?**
    a. 3.2 kcal
    b. 2.3 kcal
    c. 9.0 kcal
    d. 17.0 kcal
    e. none of the above

TRUE/FALSE

1. _____ To convert kcal to joules, multiply by 4.2.

2. _____ The basic principle of direct calorimetry is that energy can be evaluated by measuring heat changes.

3. _____ The energy content of lipid-rich food is greater than a food that is relatively lipid-free.

4. _____ The coefficient of digestibility for protein exceeds that of lipid and carbohydrate.

5. _____ Most common proteins contain approximately 16% nitrogen.

6. _____ The nitrogen content of most peanuts is about 19%.

7. _____ Because carbohydrates and lipids contain no nitrogen, their physiologic fuel value is identical to their heat of combustion determined by bomb calorimetry.

8. _____ The Atwater general factor for 200-proof alcohol is 7 kcal per gram.

9. _____ A calorie is a measure of food energy, regardless of its source.

10. _____ Fruits are generally digested more rapidly than eggs.

CROSSWORD PUZZLE

ACROSS

2 Heat to raise the temperature of 1 kg (1 L) of water 1°C, from 14.5° to 15.5°C

3 Chemical reaction involving addition of oxygen, removal of hydrogen, or loss of an electron

4 Heat of _____ is heat released when food is burned

7 Process of _____ calorimetry where food is burned

8 Heat to raise 1 kg water by 1°C

9 Energy determined by measuring heat production

13 ____ calorimeter measures energy value of food

14 One ____ of water weighs about 1 kg

15 Net energy value for macronutrients named after this chemist

16 Caloric value of one-half cup of apricot nectar

DOWN

1 One of these equals 4.2 kcal

5 Term describing food energy available to the body versus amount determined in bomb calorimeter

6 Digestive _____ must be considered when evaluating the net energy value of food

7 Coefficient representing food absorption in the body

8 2:1 is the ratio of H to O atoms in this nutrient

10 9.4 kcal = heat of combustion for this macronutrient

11 The capacity to do work

12 Accepted international standard for expressing energy

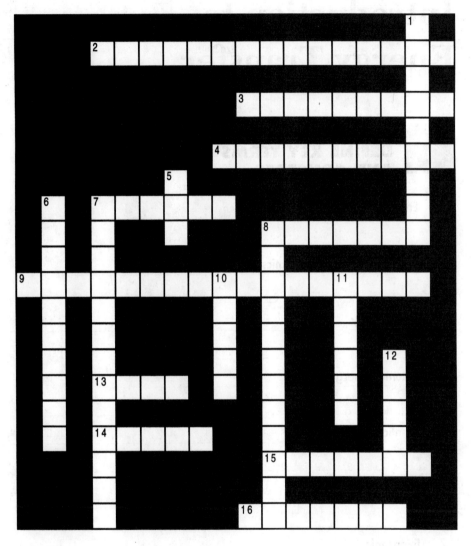

Introduction to Energy Transfer

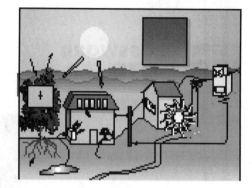

 DEFINE KEY TERMS AND CONCEPTS

1. Energy

2. First law of thermodynamics

3. Total energy

4. Potential energy

5. Kinetic energy

6. Biosynthesis

7. Exergonic

8. Free energy

9. Endergonic

10. Second law of thermodynamics

11.   **Entropy**

12.   **Photosynthesis**

13.   **Respiration**

14.   **Mechanical work**

15.   **Chemical work**

16.   **Diffusion**

17.   **Active transport**

18.   **Enzymes**

19.   **Substrate**

20.   **Coenzymes**

21.   **Lock and key mechanism**

22.   **Hydrolysis reactions**

23.   **Specificity**

24.   **Condensation reactions**

25.   **Reducing agent**

26. **Oxidizing agent**

27. **Redox**

28. **Mass action effect**

29. **Direct calorimetry**

30. **Indirect calorimetry**

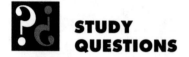 **STUDY QUESTIONS**

ENERGY: THE CAPACITY TO WORK
State the first law of thermodynamics.

Potential and Kinetic Energy
List two examples of potential energy.

1.

2.

Give one way in which potential energy is converted into kinetic energy.

Potential and kinetic energy have been compared to a waterfall. At which points of the waterfall would you find potential and kinetic energy?

• Potential energy

• Kinetic energy

Energy-Releasing and Energy-Conserving Processes
Give one reason why coupled reactions are important to the body.

Give one example each of an endergonic and an exergonic process.

• Endergonic

• Exergonic

All potential energy is ultimately degraded to what energy form?

INTERCONVERSION OF ENERGY

Complete the sentence: If the potential energy of a system decreases, the kinetic energy of that system _____.

Forms of Energy

List the six forms of energy.

1.   4.

2.   5.

3.   6.

Examples of Energy Conversions

List two fundamental examples of energy conversion.

1.

2.

Photosynthesis

What is the chemical formula for the process of photosynthesis?

What is the main function of solar energy when coupled with photosynthesis?

Cellular Respiration

What is the chemical formula for the process of cellular respiration?

Biologic Work in Humans

List the three forms of biologic work.

1.

2.

3.

Mechanical Work

What is the most important role of mechanical work in the body?

What part of the muscle converts chemical energy into mechanical energy?

Chemical Work

Give one example of chemical work in the body.

Transport Work

Give one example of transport work in the body.

FACTORS THAT AFFECT THE RATE OF BIOENERGETICS
Enzymes: Biologic Catalysts

How do enzymes function as catalysts?

Do enzymes make reactions occur? Discuss.

Coenzymes

Describe the main difference between an enzyme and a coenzyme.

Name one coenzyme and describe its role in metabolism.

HYDROLYSIS AND CONDENSATION: THE BASES FOR DIGESTION AND SYNTHESIS
Hydrolysis Reactions

Give two examples of hydrolysis reactions.

1.
2.

Condensation Reactions

Give one example of a condensation reaction.

Oxidation and Reduction Reactions

Give one example of a "redox" reaction during exercise.

What is a reducing agent? Give a biological example.

• Reducing agent

• Example

What is an oxidizing agent? Give a biological example.

• Oxidizing agent

• Example

The Mass Action Effect

Give one example of a mass action effect during cellular metabolism.

ab© T/F PRACTICE QUIZ

MULTIPLE CHOICE

1. **The first law of thermodynamics states that energy is:**
   a. consumed proportional to its use
   b. degraded to potential energy
   c. neither created nor destroyed, but transformed from one form to another
   d. transformed to other forms when heat is applied
   e. b and c

2. **There are ____ forms of energy:**
   a. 1
   b. 2
   c. 4
   d. 6
   e. 8

3. **Any substance acted on by an enzyme is called:**
   a. a coenzyme
   b. a catalyst
   c. an oxidizing agent
   d. a reducing agent
   e. a substrate

4. **$C_6H_{12}O_6 + 6O_2 \rightarrow 6CO_2 + 6H_2O$ is an:**
   a. expression of respiration
   b. expression of photosynthesis
   c. example of energy conservation
   d. example of an anaerobic reaction
   e. example of how carbohydrates and proteins are catabolized

5. **Energy metabolism in humans:**
   a. is only exergonic
   b. is both exergonic and endergonic
   c. only results in the release of kinetic energy
   d. is an expression of indirect calorimetry
   e. is only endergonic

6. Which of the following is an example of hydrolysis?
   a. AMP + ATP
   b. CP + ATP
   c. ATP + H_2O
   d. glucose + glucose
   e. CP + CP

7. The tendency for potential energy to degrade to kinetic energy with a lower capacity for work represents the:
   a. first law of thermodynamics
   b. law of specificity
   c. law of energy use and disuse
   d. second law of thermodynamics
   e. a and c

8. Some enzymes are totally inactive in the absence of additional substances termed:
   a. biological helpers
   b. hydrolytic substances
   c. catalysts
   d. coenzymes
   e. redox substances

9. Hydrolysis is a basic chemical process involving:
   a. catabolism
   b. anabolism
   c. redox reactions
   d. photosynthesis
   e. a and d

10. One example of an oxidizing agent is:
    a. oxygen
    b. hydrogen
    c. NAD^+
    d. ATP
    e. FAD

TRUE/FALSE

1. _____ Water is an example of a coenzyme.

2. _____ Photosynthesis is the opposite of respiration.

3. _____ Entropy is the process of energy conversion in which free energy increases.

4. _____ Direct calorimetry involves muscle biopsies.

5. _____ FAD is an example of a reducing agent.

6. _____ Ultimately, all of the potential energy in a biological system degrades to the nonusable form of kinetic energy or heat.

7. _____ The effect of the concentration of chemicals on the frequency of a particular chemical reaction reflects the law of mass action.

8. _____ $H_2 + O \rightarrow H_2O \ -68$ kcal per mole

9. _____ Basically there are only three forms of energy: heat, light, and nuclear.

10. _____ The first law of thermodynamics states that energy is neither created nor destroyed but is transformed from one form to another.

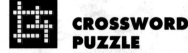

CROSSWORD PUZZLE

ACROSS

2 Measurement of energy
4 Effect of concentration of chemicals on the frequency of chemical reactions
5 Chemical reaction with simultaneous oxidation and reduction
8 Produces OH^- when ionized
9 Useful energy for work
10 Energy of motion
14 $6CO_2 + 6H_2O \rightarrow 6O_2 + C_6H_{12}O_2$
17 Organic, nonprotein cofactor needed for normal enzyme function
18 Degradation of large molecules by the addition of water
20 Process that results in an increase in free energy
22 Reactions that release free energy
23 Agent that adds an electron or H^+
24 Specific adaptations to imposed demands
25 Aerobic process of cellular energy release
27 Change of a gas to a liquid or a liquid to a solid

DOWN

1 696 kcal released when one mole of _____ is oxidized
3 Two laws related to energy
6 Passive movement of molecules down concentration gradient
7 Chemical compound acted on by an enzyme

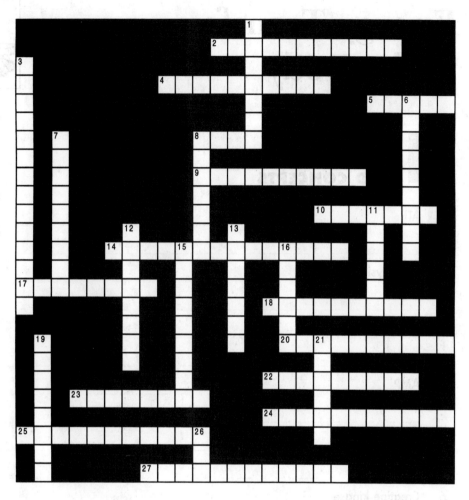

8 Compounds that minimize change in H^+
11 The capacity for work
12 This form of biologic work is required for growth and maintenance
13 Randomness in a system
15 Process involving removal of electrons

16 Biological catalyst
19 Type of calorimetry
21 Calorimetry that measures heat release
26 Hydrogen-accepting coenzyme that contains niacin

Energy Transfer in the Body

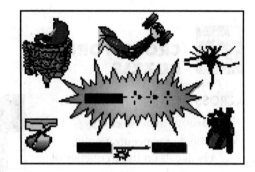

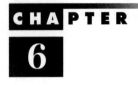 **DEFINE KEY TERMS AND CONCEPTS**

1. **ATP** _____

2. **Hydrolysis** _____

3. **ADP** _____

4. **AMP** _____

5. **CP** _____

6. **Creatine kinase** _____

7. **Phosphorylation** _____

8. **Mitochondria** _____

9. **Electron transport** _____

10. **NAD** _____

11. **FAD**

12. **Cytochromes**

13. **P/O ratio**

14. **Respiratory chain**

15. **Cytochrome oxidase**

16. **Oxidative phosphorylation**

17. **Chemiosmotic coupling**

18. **Phosphate bond energy**

19. **Anaerobic reaction**

20. **ATPase**

21. **Aerobic metabolism**

22. **Glycolysis**

23. **Glycogenolysis**

24. **Glucose 6-phosphate**

25. **Phosphatase**

26. Glycogen synthetase

_____

27. Phosphofructokinase

_____

28. Glycogen phosphorylase

_____

29. Substrate-level phosphorylation

_____

30. Malate-asparate shuttle

_____

31. Glycerol-phosphate shuttle

_____

32. Aerobic glycolysis

_____

33. Anaerobic glycolysis

_____

34. Lactic acid

_____

35. Lactic dehydrogenase

_____

36. Exchangeable lactate pool

_____

37. Cori cycle

_____

38. Acetyl-CoA

_____

39. Krebs cycle

_____

40. Coenzyme A

_____

41. **Oxaloacetate**

42. **Citrate**

43. **Lipolysis**

44. **Lipase**

45. **Adipocytes**

46. **Free fatty acids**

47. **Lipoprotein lipase**

48. **Cyclic AMP**

49. **Glycerol**

50. **β-Oxidation**

51. **Transamination**

52. **Deamination**

53. **The metabolic mill**

54. **Ketone bodies**

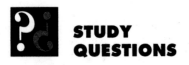

STUDY QUESTIONS

PHOSPHATE BOND ENERGY
Adenosine Triphosphate: The Energy Currency

List two major energy-transforming activities in the cell.

1.

2.

How much free energy (in kcal) is liberated per mole of ATP hydrolyzed to ADP?

Creatine Phosphate: The Energy Reservoir

What is the body's quantity of ATP and CP?

- ATP

- CP

What main function does CP play in energy transformation?

Cellular Oxidation

Where in the cell does the process of cellular oxidation occur?

What happens to most of the energy generated by cellular oxidation?

Electron Transport

List the two electron acceptors in the oxidation of food during energy metabolism.

1.

2.

Oxidative Phosphorylation

Describe the process of oxidative phosphorylation in 30 words or less.

Complete the following chemical reaction:

$$NADH + H^+ + 3\,ADP + 3\,P + \tfrac{1}{2}O_2 \rightarrow$$

Efficiency of Electron Transport and Oxidative Phosphorylation

How much energy (in kcal) is required to synthesize a mole of ATP?

What is the relative efficiency of electron transport-oxidative phosphorylation?

Role of Oxygen in Energy Metabolism

List three prerequisites for the continual aerobic resynthesis of ATP.

1.

2.

3.

List two functions of oxygen in energy metabolism.

1.

2.

ENERGY RELEASE FROM FOOD

Energy Release from Carbohydrates

Write the equation for the complete breakdown of one mole of glucose.

Give three reasons why the discussion of nutrient metabolism begins with carbohydrate.

1.

2.

3.

How much free energy (in kcal) is yielded by the complete breakdown of one mole of glucose to carbon dioxide and water?

Anaerobic versus Aerobic Metabolism

Give two differences between anaerobic and aerobic metabolic reactions.

1.

2.

Glycolysis Generates Anaerobic Energy from Glucose

Where in the cell does glycolysis take place?

Which enzyme is rate-limiting for glycolytic reactions?

Glycogen Catabolism

What is the ATP yield when carbohydrate catabolism begins with glycogen?

Substrate-Level Phosphorylation in Glycolysis

How many molecules of ATP (net gain) are formed during substrate-level phosphorylation in glycolysis?

Hydrogen Release in Glycolysis

In muscle, how many ATP molecules are formed when cytoplasmic NADH is oxidized by the respiratory chain?

How many molecules of ATP are generated from oxidizing the two moles of NADH formed in glycolysis?

Formation of Lactic Acid

Discuss why lactic acid does not accumulate during moderate-intensity exercise.

Discuss why lactic acid accumulates during high-intensity exercise.

Name the cycle that provides for lactic acid removal and subsequent reconversion to blood glucose and muscle glycogen.

The Krebs Cycle

How is pyruvic acid prepared for entrance into the Krebs cycle?

What is the most important function of the Krebs cycle?

Total Energy Transfer from Glucose Catabolism

What is the net ATP yield from the complete breakdown of one glucose molecule?

How many ATP molecules are formed from substrate-level phosphorylation, and how many are generated during oxidative phosphorylation?

• Substrate-level phosphorylation

• Oxidative phosphorylation

What Regulates Energy Metabolism?

What is the most important factor that provides regulatory control of the breakdown of carbohydrate, lipid, and amino acid for energy release?

Energy Release From Lipid

What function does the enzyme lipase have in lipid catabolism?

Sources for Lipid Catabolism

Name the three sources of lipids catabolized for energy.

1.

2.

3.

Adipocytes: The Site of Lipid Storage and Mobilization

Discuss the role of blood supply in the catabolism of lipids.

List three hormones that augment the activation of lipase and subsequent lipolysis and mobilization of FFA from adipose tissue.

1.

2.

3.

What role does cyclic AMP play in lipase activation?

Catabolism of Glycerol and Fatty Acids

How many molecules of ATP are synthesized in the breakdown of one glycerol molecule?

What is glycerol's important function in carbohydrate balance?

What is the importance of oxygen in the catabolism of fatty acids?

Total Energy Transfer from Lipid Catabolism

How many molecules of ATP are generated in the complete combustion of a neutral fat molecule?

Energy Release from Protein

Describe in a general sense the catabolism of an amino acid molecule.

The Metabolic Mill—Interrelationships among Carbohydrate, Lipid, and Protein Metabolism

What component of the triglyceride molecule cannot be used for gluconeogenesis ?

Lipids Burn in a Carbohydrate Flame

Explain why "lipids burn in a carbohydrate flame."

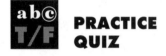 **PRACTICE QUIZ**

MULTIPLE CHOICE

1. **How much free energy is liberated per mole of ATP hydrolyzed to ADP?**
   a. 6.3 kcal
   b. 7.3 kcal
   c. 8.3 kcal
   d. 9.3 kcal
   e. none of the above

2. **The energy released from the breakdown of the high-energy phosphates ATP and CP can sustain all-out exercise for about:**
   a. 5 to 8 seconds
   b. 30 seconds
   c. 60 to 90 seconds
   d. 3 to 5 minutes
   e. longer than 5 minutes

3. **Which statement about oxidative phosphorylation is <u>false</u>?**
   a. it is a process whereby ATP becomes synthesized during the transfer of electrons from $NADH_2$ and $FADH_2$ to oxygen
   b. about 50% of ATP synthesis occurs in the respiratory chain by oxidative reactions coupled with phosphorylation
   c. three ATP molecules are formed for each $NADH_2$ molecule oxidized in the respiratory chain
   d. two ATP molecules are formed for each $FADH_2$ molecule oxidized in the respiratory chain
   e. b and c

4. **Which of the following is <u>not</u> a prerequisite for continual ATP resynthesis?**
   a. CP must be depleted in the cell
   b. $NADH_2$ or $FADH_2$ must be available
   c. oxygen must be present in the tissues
   d. cellular enzymes must be present in sufficient concentration
   e. a and c

5. **Which statement about carbohydrates is <u>true</u>?**
   a. it is the only nutrient whose stored energy generates ATP aerobically
   b. it supplies about half of the body's energy requirements during heavy exercise
   c. it functions as a metabolic primer for protein breakdown
   d. a continual breakdown of carbohydrate is required for lipid nutrients to be used for energy
   e. a and d

6. **The net ATP yield from the complete breakdown of glucose in skeletal muscle is:**
   a. 28 ATP
   b. 32 ATP
   c. 36 ATP
   d. 38 ATP
   e. none of the above

7. **Which statement concerning lactic acid is <u>false</u>?**
   a. it is formed during anaerobic glycolysis
   b. it is formed by hydrogens combining temporarily with pyruvic acid
   c. it is buffered to lactate in the blood and carried away from the site of energy metabolism
   d. it is a valuable source of chemical energy that accumulates during heavy exercise
   e. it is a by-product of excessive protein metabolism

8. **The most plentiful source of potential energy in the body is:**
   a. glucose
   b. proteins
   c. lipids
   d. minerals
   e. glucose plus glycogen

9. **Which statement about glycerol is <u>true</u>?**
   a. it is accepted into glycolysis during its catabolism
   b. it enters the Krebs cycle directly
   c. it is a precursor of fatty acids
   d. it aids in the removal of lactic acid from active muscle
   e. none of the above

10. **The liver removes nitrogen from amino acids in the process of:**
    a. deamination
    b. translocation
    c. gluconeogenesis
    d. glycogenolysis
    e. the Cori cycle

TRUE/FALSE

1. _____ The splitting of an ATP molecule requires oxygen.

2. _____ Cells store CP in larger quantities than ATP.

3. _____ NAD^+ and FAD accept hydrogens.

4. _____ The relative efficiency of electron transport-oxidative phosphorylation is approximately 90% for harnessing chemical energy.

5. _____ The activity level of glycogen synthetase places a limit on the rate of glycolysis during all-out exercise.

6. _____ Lactic acid accumulates when oxidation of NADH keeps pace with its formation.

7. _____ The main function of the Krebs cycle is to degrade acetyl-CoA substrate to carbon dioxide and nitrogen atoms within the mitochondria.

8. _____ As blood flow increases with exercise, more free fatty acids are removed from adipose tissue and delivered to active muscle.

9. _____ The breakdown of fatty acids is directly associated with oxygen uptake.

10. _____ Fats burn in the "flame" of carbohydrates.

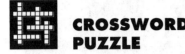

CROSSWORD PUZZLE

ACROSS

8 Heat energy is to an engine as
_____ _____ is to the cell

12 Cycle involved in glucose synthesis

13 Contains two high-energy phosphate bonds (abbr.)

15 _____ adenine dinucleotide

17 ATP and CP are rich in this form of energy

19 Fatty acids to acetyl compounds

20 Iron-protein electron carrier

22 Component of triglyceride molecule

23 Pyruvic acid + coenzyme A

DOWN

1 Breakdown of glycogen

2 "Powerhouses" of the cell

3 Removal of electrons

4 "____ ____ in a carbohydrate flame"

5 Removing nitrogen from amino acids

6 ____ energy is available for work

7 Water added during the breakdown process

9 Compounds that regulate rate of metabolism

10 Enzyme that catalyzes triglyceride breakdown

11 Mechanical, chemical, and transport are all forms of this broad category of work

14 Powers all biologic work (abbr.)

16 Pyruvic acid + 2 hydrogen

18 Breakdown of lipid

21 Electron transport ____

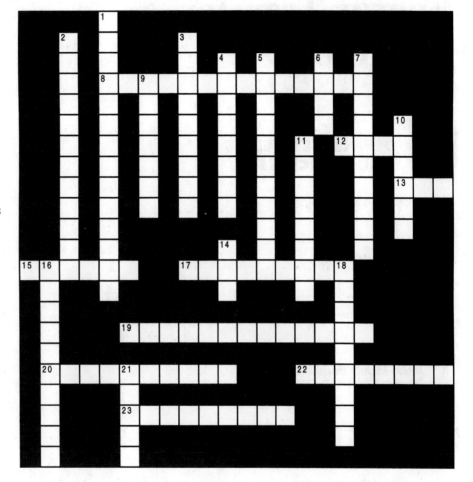

See page 368 for Crossword Puzzle Solution.

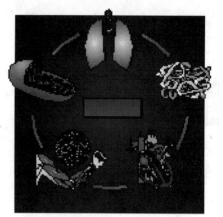

Energy Transfer
in Exercise

DEFINE KEY TERMS
AND CONCEPTS

1. Immediate energy system

2. NMR spectroscopy

3. Short-term energy system

4. Blood lactate threshold

5. Tissue hypoxia

6. Lactate dehydrogenase

7. Long-term energy system

8. Steady-rate aerobic metabolism

9. Oxygen deficit

10. Maximal oxygen uptake

11. Criteria for $\dot{V}O_2$max

12. Fast-twitch fiber

13. Slow-twitch fiber

14. Oxygen debt

15. A.V. Hill

16. Cori cycle

17. Alactacid oxygen debt

18. Lactacid oxygen debt

19. EPOC

20. Active recovery

21. Passive recovery

22. Lactate-using organs

23. Intermittent exercise

24. Interval training

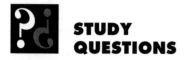

STUDY QUESTIONS

IMMEDIATE ENERGY: THE ATP-CP SYSTEM

How much ATP and CP are stored within the muscles of the body?

• ATP

• CP

Indicate the duration of a brisk walk, a slow run, and an all-out sprint that can be powered by the high-energy phosphates.

• Brisk walk

• Slow run

• All-out sprint

Nuclear Magnetic Resonance Spectroscopy to Study Exercise Muscle Metabolism

Indicate a primary function of NMR spectroscopy in energy metabolism studies.

SHORT-TERM ENERGY: THE LACTIC ACID SYSTEM

List three different activities that would be powered mainly by the lactic acid energy system.

1.

2.

3.

Blood Lactate Accumulation

At what percentage of the maximum oxygen uptake does blood lactate generally begin to rise?

Does the blood lactate threshold occur at a lower or higher percent of $\dot{V}O_2$max in trained than in untrained subjects?

Give a reasonable explanation of why blood lactate accumulates during exercise.

Lactate-Producing Capacity

How much more lactate can a sprint/power trained athlete accumulate compared to an untrained counterpart?

LONG-TERM ENERGY: THE AEROBIC SYSTEM

Oxygen Uptake during Exercise

Draw and label the curve for oxygen uptake during 10 minutes of moderate running exercise. Indicate the area of oxygen deficit and the area of steady-rate oxygen uptake. (*Hint: Refer to Figure 7.3 in your textbook.*)

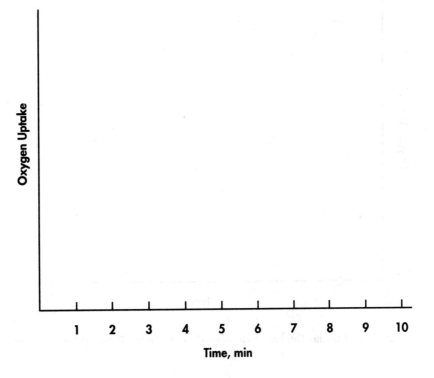

Express the oxygen uptake in relation to body mass for an individual who weighs 85 kg and consumes 2.0 L·min^{-1} of oxygen during jogging.

List two eventual fates of lactic acid.

1.

2.

Oxygen Deficit

What does the oxygen deficit most likely represent in terms of exercise metabolism?

Oxygen Deficit in the Trained and Untrained

Indicate how the previous graph of oxygen uptake during 10 minutes of moderate running would differ for an endurance-trained athlete.

Maximal Oxygen Uptake ($\dot{V}O_2$max)

Draw and label an oxygen uptake curve during exercise of progressively increasing work every 3 minutes until exhaustion. Indicate the $\dot{V}O_2$max (*Hint: Refer to Figure 7.5 in your textbook.*)

Oxygen Uptake

Time

Is it possible to exercise at a level greater than the level that elicited the $\dot{V}O_2$max? If so, explain how this exercise is accomplished.

FAST- AND SLOW-TWITCH MUSCLE FIBERS

Fast-Twitch Fiber

List two characteristics of fast-twitch (type II) muscle fibers.

1.

2.

What energy system most often supports fast-twitch muscle fiber activity?

Slow-Twitch Fiber

List two characteristics of slow-twitch (type I) muscle fibers.

1.

2.

What energy system most often supports slow-twitch muscle fiber activity?

THE ENERGY SPECTRUM OF EXERCISE

Explain how an understanding of the energy spectrum in exercise can help you to design a better training program for athletes in different sports.

Oxygen Uptake during Recovery: The "O₂ Debt"

Draw and label the oxygen uptake curves during recovery from light exercise, steady-rate exercise, and exhaustive exercise. Include the fast and slow components of the recovery where applicable. (*Hint: Refer to Figure 7.9 in your textbook.*)

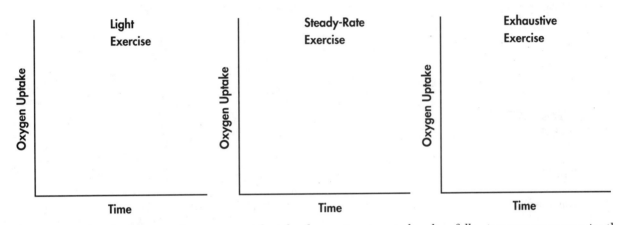

List four reasons that the postexercise oxygen uptake takes longer to return to baseline following strenuous exercise than following moderate exercise.

1.   3.

2.   4.

Traditional Concepts

Outline the traditional concepts to explain the recovery oxygen uptake.

• Steady-rate

• Non-steady-rate

Controversy with Traditional Explanation of Oxygen Debt

List two findings that do not support the traditional explanation of the "oxygen debt."

1.

2.

Contemporary Concepts

Outline the contemporary concepts to explain the recovery oxygen uptake from steady-rate and non-steady-rate exercise.

• Steady-rate

• Non-steady-rate

Implications of EPOC for Exercise and Recovery

List two ways in which knowledge of EPOC can influence strategies for sports training.

1.

2.

Intermittent Exercise

What is the major advantage of intermittent exercise for exercise performance and training?

Describe a practical application of the concept of intermittent exercise (interval training).

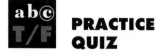

PRACTICE QUIZ

MULTIPLE CHOICE

1. **Blood lactate begins to rise at what percent of a healthy, untrained person's $\dot{V}O_2$max?**
    a. 45%
    b. 55%
    c. 65%
    d. 75%
    e. lactate does not accumulate in healthy individuals

2. **The oxygen uptake curve during constant-load submaximal exercise:**
    a. increases rapidly throughout the first 2 minutes of exercise
    b. reaches a plateau in the first 30 seconds
    c. never reaches a plateau
    d. only reaches a plateau if lipid is burned as the fuel
    e. none of the above are true

3. **Which statement is <u>true</u> about the oxygen deficit in the trained and untrained?**
    a. a trained person reaches a steady rate more rapidly and thus has a smaller oxygen deficit
    b. an untrained person reaches a steady rate more rapidly and thus has a smaller oxygen deficit
    c. a trained person reaches a steady rate more rapidly and thus has a larger oxygen deficit
    d. the trained and untrained reach a steady rate at the same time during exercise
    e. the oxygen deficit is always smaller in the untrained

4. **Fast-twitch muscle fibers:**
    a. are called type I fibers
    b. possess a high capacity for the aerobic production of ATP
    c. are resistant to fatigue
    d. predominate in short-term, sprint activities
    e. all of the above are true

5. **The recovery oxygen uptake reflects which of the following effects of exercise?**
    a. anaerobic metabolism
    b. respiratory adjustments
    c. thermal adjustments
    d. circulatory adjustments
    e. all of the above

6. **Recovery from steady-rate exercise is most rapid with:**
   a. active recovery
   b. passive recovery
   c. immersion in warm water
   d. immersion in cold water
   e. application of hot then cold packs

7. **The best way to train the aerobic energy system is:**
   a. sprint training
   b. strength training
   c. "super-maximal" exercise with brief rest intervals
   d. long-distance training
   e. combination of a and b

8. **The best indicator of one's ability to sustain high-intensity aerobic exercises is the:**
   a. $\dot{V}O_2$max
   b. maximal steady rate
   c. maximal oxygen debt
   d. maximal oxygen deficit
   e. maximal ventilation volume

9. **The alactacid debt:**
   a. represents the fast portion of the recovery oxygen uptake curve
   b. represents the slow portion of the recovery oxygen uptake curve
   c. indicates the quantity of protein used as a fuel
   d. "pays back" the oxygen deficit
   e. converts fatty acids to glycogen

10. **Success in sports such as 220-yd sprinting and weight lifting requires a highly trained:**
    a. aerobic energy system
    b. lactic acid energy system
    c. ATP-CP energy system
    d. b and c
    e. a and c

TRUE/FALSE

1. _____ The ability to generate high lactic acid levels can be increased with specific anaerobic training.

2. _____ The oxygen debt is the difference between the total oxygen consumed during exercise and the amount that would have been consumed had a steady rate been reached instantaneously.

3. _____ The recruitment of slow-twitch fibers favors lactic acid formation.

4. _____ The point when the oxygen uptake plateaus with increasing exercise intensity is called the maximal aerobic steady rate or the point of OBLA.

5. _____ The various means for energy transfer are considered to be on a continuum in exercise.

6. _____ The oxygen consumed in recovery from exercise is called the oxygen deficit.

7. _____ Lactic acid removal during recovery is accelerated by performing active aerobic exercise.

8. _____ Oxygen uptake during most forms of exercise does not depend on body size.

9. _____ OBLA occurs at a higher percent of $\dot{V}O_2$max for an untrained person than for a trained person.

10. _____ Slow-twitch muscle fibers have the capacity to generate more total ATP than fast-twitch fibers.

CROSSWORD PUZZLE

ACROSS

5 Marker enzyme for glycolytic capacity

10 Method of performing exercise with rest periods (abbr.)

11 High _____ phosphates provide the immediate energy for exercise

14 $\dot{V}o_2$ in $mL \cdot kg^{-1} \cdot min^{-1}$ adjusts for differences among individuals in ____ size

16 Approximately 5 mmol of ATP and 15 mmol of CP are _____ within each kilogram of muscle

17 Slow component of the "oxygen debt"

19 Nobel physiologist _____ Vivian Hill

20 Steady ____ is where exercise energy requirements are met by aerobic metabolism

21 This energy system relies on high-energy phosphates

DOWN

1 _____ recovery from heavy exercise requires steady-rate exercise

2 This energy system involves aerobic metabolism

3 These phosphates power all-out exercise for 6–8 seconds

4 _____-twitch fibers are activated in non-steady-rate exercise

6 Final electron acceptor in energy metabolism

7 The lactate _____ is that point in exercise where lactate rises above resting level

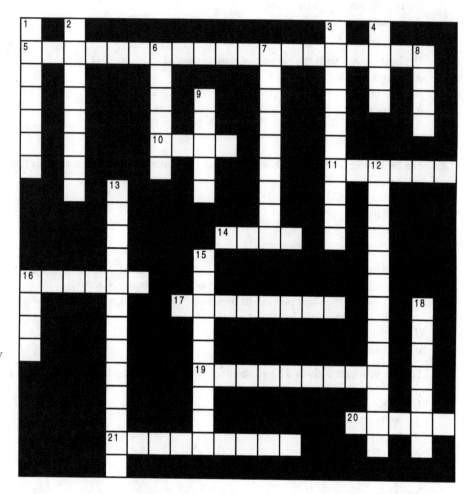

8 Recovery oxygen uptake (abbr.)

9 The _____-term energy system powers all-out exercise for about 90 seconds

12 Carbohydrate stores are likened to these in the traditional concept of "oxygen debt"

13 Start of exercise where energy expenditure is not matched by oxygen uptake

15 Rapid phase of recovery from exercise is the _____ portion of the oxygen debt

16 These fibers are activated in steady-rate exercise

18 The buffered form of lactic acid

See page 368 for Crossword Puzzle Solution.

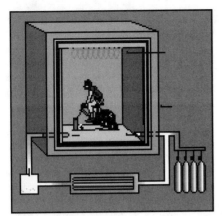

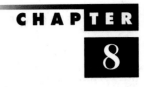

Measurement of Human Energy Expenditure

 DEFINE KEY TERMS AND CONCEPTS

1. Direct calorimetry

2. Atwater-Rosa human calorimeter

3. Indirect calorimetry

4. Micro-Scholander

5. Haldane method

6. Closed-circuit spirometry

7. Open-circuit spirometry

8. Portable spirometer

9. Douglas bag

10. Respiratory quotient

11. **Nonprotein RQ**

12. **Respiratory exchange ratio**

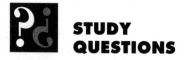

STUDY QUESTIONS

METHODS OF MEASURING THE BODY'S HEAT PRODUCTION

List the two methods used to determine heat production by the body.

1.

2.

Direct Calorimetry

List a piece of equipment used during human direct calorimetry.

Indirect Calorimetry

List the two methods of indirect calorimetry.

1.

2.

Closed-Circuit Spirometry

What is one disadvantage of closed-circuit spirometry during exercise studies?

Open-Circuit Spirometry

Give one positive aspect of each of the following procedures of indirect calorimetry during exercise studies.

- Portable spirometry

- Bag technique

- Computerized instrumentation

Methods of Calibration

Name two methods for analyzing the gas mixtures that are commonly used for calibrating electronic gas analyzers.

1.

2.

Direct versus Indirect Calorimetry

What is the degree of agreement between energy expenditure measured by direct calorimetry and that measured by indirect calorimetry?

THE RESPIRATORY QUOTIENT (RQ)

Write the formula for the RQ.

RQ for Carbohydrate

What is the RQ for carbohydrate?

RQ for Lipid

What is the RQ for lipid?

RQ for Protein

What is the generally accepted value for the RQ for protein?

RQ for a Mixed Diet

What is the RQ for a diet of approximately 40% carbohydrate and 60% lipid? What is the corresponding caloric equivalent?

- RQ

- Caloric equivalent

RESPIRATORY EXCHANGE RATIO (R)

What is the difference between the RQ and R?

How can exhaustive exercise cause the R to increase significantly above 1.00?

What may cause the respiratory exchange ratio to be less than 0.70?

METABOLIC CALCULATIONS

Write the formula for calculating $\dot{V}O_2$ from measures of open-circuit spirometry. (*Hint: See Appendix C in your textbook.*)

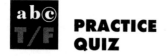

PRACTICE QUIZ

MULTIPLE CHOICE

1. **Which statement is *true* about direct and indirect calorimetry?**
   a. closed-circuit and open-circuit spirometry are methods of direct calorimetry
   b. a human calorimeter is used for indirect calorimetry
   c. indirect calorimetry is highly accurate and much less expensive than direct calorimetry
   d. direct calorimetry measures $\dot{V}O_2$ and $\dot{V}CO_2$ to estimate energy expenditure
   e. a and d

2. **Approximately this much heat energy is liberated when carbohydrate is burned to CO_2 and H_2O in 1 liter of oxygen:**
   a. 4 kcal
   b. 5 kcal
   c. 6 kcal
   d. 7 kcal
   e. none of the above

3. **Which of the following is <u>false</u>?**
   a. RQ for carbohydrate is 1.00.
   b. RQ for lipid is 0.90.
   c. RQ for protein is 0.82.
   d. RQ for a mixed diet is between 0.70 and 1.00.
   e. all of the above

4. **All energy metabolism ultimately depends on:**
   a. utilization of oxygen
   b. regeneration of STP
   c. SDA availability
   d. carbohydrate availability
   e. none of the above

5. **Two types of indirect calorimetry are _____ and _____ spirometry:**
   a. nitrogen analysis, oxygen analysis
   b. closed-circuit, direct
   c. open-circuit, Douglas bag
   d. bomb calorimetry, closed-circuit
   e. closed-circuit, open-circuit

6. **During closed-circuit spirometry:**
   a. the person rebreathes CO_2 with O_2 being absorbed
   b. oxygen uptake is measured using the respiratory exchange ratio
   c. CO_2 in exhaled air is absorbed by soda lime
   d. the respiratory exchange ratio is always determined
   e. none of the above

7. **In open-circuit spirometry, the subject:**
   a. inhales ambient air
   b. rebreathes from a spirometer containing pure oxygen
   c. inhales pure oxygen from a Douglas bag
   d. is always fully hydrated
   e. inhales and exhales approximately 100 times every 30 seconds

8. **To estimate the body's heat production it is necessary to know:**
   a. only the RQ
   b. only the RQ and the amount of oxygen consumed
   c. only the RQ and the amount carbon dioxide produced
   d. only the amount of oxygen consumed
   e. none of the above

9. **The nonprotein RQ:**
   a. can only be used during rest
   b. assumes that protein contributes 25% to the total energy production
   c. assumes that the contribution of protein to energy metabolism is relatively small
   d. can only be used during high-intensity exercise where there is excess CO_2 production
   e. none of the above

10. **The RQ for a mixed diet:**
    a. assumes combustion of 12% protein, 35% carbohydrate, and 25% lipid
    b. assumes combustion of 40% carbohydrate and 60% lipid
    c. is the same as the RQ for a high-carbohydrate diet at the same level of oxygen uptake
    d. assumes the combustion of an equal mixture of lipid and protein
    e. depends on the nutrient digestibility coefficient

TRUE/FALSE

1. _____ The open-circuit method is the most common technique to measure oxygen uptake.

2. _____ Portable spirometry, bag technique, and computerized instrumentation are direct calorimetry procedures.

3. _____ The ratio of metabolic gas exchange is termed the Weir factor.

4. _____ The ratio of CO_2 produced to O_2 consumed is termed the respiratory quotient.

5. _____ The RQ for lipid is about 0.70.

6. _____ The RQ for carbohydrate is about 1.00.

7. _____ The RQ for a mixed diet is about 0.82.

8. _____ The RQ is always greater than the R.

9. _____ R values in excess of 1.00 can reflect excess CO_2 "blow-off."

10. _____ The portable spirometer is commonly used in direct calorimetry.

CROSSWORD PUZZLE

ACROSS

1 Ventilatory maneuver that increases RQ

3 Spirometry in which the subject rebreathes from a prefilled container

4 Calorimetry that infers energy from O_2 uptake

5 Another term for KOH

7 $CO_2 \div O_2$ in exhaustive exercise is called the _____ _____ ratio

11 Scientists in this country developed the portable spirometer

12 Oxygen uptake is used to indirectly infer this

14 Collection device in open-circuit spirometry

15 Calorimetry that infers energy from change in water temperature

16 General RQ value for this macronutrient is 0.82

DOWN

2 Portion of RQ attributed to combustion of only carbohydrate and lipid

3 Measurement of heat production

6 Douglas bag method is an example of this type of spirometry

8 $CO_2 \div O_2$ in steady-rate exercise (abbr.)

9 4.84 kcal liberated when mixed diet is burned in this many liters of O_2

10 Recovery from this type of exercise is associated with RQ below 0.70

13 RQ is 0.70 for this macronutrient

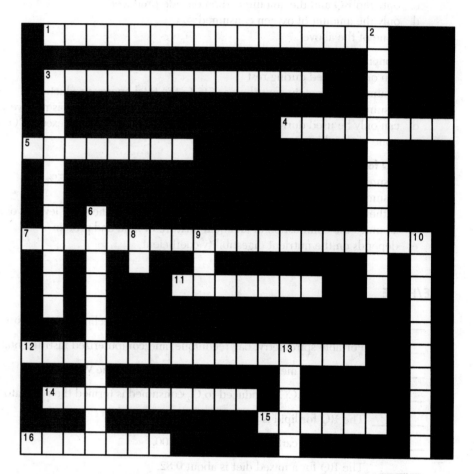

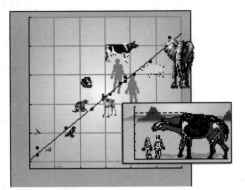

Human Energy Expenditure During Rest and Physical Activity

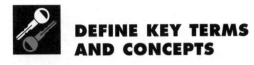

DEFINE KEY TERMS AND CONCEPTS

1. TDEE

2. Basal metabolic rate

3. Sex difference in BMR

4. Resting metabolic rate

5. Body surface area

6. FFM

7. Dietary-induced thermogenesis

8. Obligatory thermogenesis

9. Facultative thermogenesis

10. Specific dynamic action

11. **Physical activity ratio (PAR)**

12. **Calorigenic effects**

13. **Light work**

14. **Heavy work**

15. **Maximal work**

16. **MET**

17. **3.6 mL·kg^{-1}·min^{-1}**

18. **Weight-bearing exercise**

19. **Weight-supported exercise**

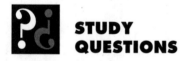 **STUDY QUESTIONS**

ENERGY EXPENDITURE AT REST

List three factors that influence the 24-hour energy expenditure.

1.

2.

3.

Basal Metabolic Rate

List three necessary conditions for measuring BMR.

1.

2.

3.

What is the average BMR for a college-age man and woman?

- Man

- Woman

Metabolism at Rest
By what percentage is the BMR for females lower than that for males?

Give one reason why a woman is likely to have a lower BMR than a man of similar age.

Estimating Daily Resting Energy Expenditure
Surface Area
Estimate the 24-hour basal energy expenditure (kcal) for a person with a BMR of 35 $kcal \cdot m^{-2} \cdot h^{-1}$.

Fat-Free Body Mass
Estimate the resting daily energy expenditure for a female who has a FFM of 43 kg.

Factors That Affect Energy Expenditure
List three factors that affect a person's total daily energy expenditure.

1.

2.

3.

Physical Activity
Physical activity normally accounts for what percentage of a person's daily energy expenditure?

Dietary-Induced Thermogenesis
How long after a meal will dietary-induced thermogenesis reach a maximum?

List two factors that affect the magnitude of dietary-induced thermogenesis.

1.

2.

Calorigenic Effect of Food on Exercise Metabolism

By what percentage does a breakfast meal increase the resting metabolic rate?

Is exercise likely to be more or less beneficial in terms of caloric expenditure when an individual eats prior to exercising? Explain.

Estimate the energy expended for 10 minutes of cycling at an oxygen uptake of 1.2 L·min^{-1}.

Climate

What two effects does exercising in the heat have on physiologic function that could elevate metabolism during exercise?

1.

2.

Give one factor that influences metabolic rate in a cold environment.

Pregnancy

List two ways women can take extra precautions to protect their fetus during exercise.

1.

2.

List two maternal metabolic and cardiorespiratory adaptations to pregnancy.

1.

2.

Effects of Exercise on Fetus

List three hypothetical risks of vigorous maternal exercise on the fetus.

1.

2.

3.

Status of Current Opinion

Summarize the current recommendations regarding exercise during pregnancy.

ENERGY EXPENDITURE DURING PHYSICAL ACTIVITY

Classification of Physical Activities by Energy Expenditure

Outline the PAR system for classifying the strenuousness of physical activity.

The MET

One MET is equivalent to how many liters of oxygen uptake per minute?

One MET is equivalent to _____ $mL \cdot kg^{-1} \cdot min^{-1}$.

Daily Rates of Average Energy Expenditure

What is the average daily caloric expenditure for men and women between the ages of 23 and 50 years?

- Men

- Women

Energy Cost of Household, Industrial, and Recreational Activities

The following equation computes the total cost of a physical activity:
Total caloric cost = _____ × _____

Effect of Body Mass

On the same graph, display the relationships between body mass and energy expenditure during weight-supported and

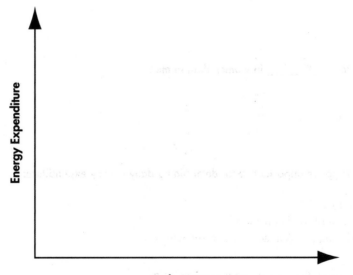

weight-bearing exercise.

Use of Heart Rate to Estimate Energy Expenditure

Heart rate is linearly related to what other factor during physical activity?

List two limitations of using heart rate to estimate $\dot{V}O_2$ (energy expenditure) during exercise.

1.

2.

List three factors, other than oxygen uptake, that influence exercise heart rate.

1.

2.

3.

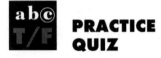

PRACTICE QUIZ

MULTIPLE CHOICE

1. **The three main factors that determine total daily energy expenditure are:**
   a. body composition, BMR, and hormone level
   b. thermogenic effect of food, body composition, and resting metabolic rate
   c. resting metabolic rate, thermogenic effect of food, and energy expended during physical activity and in recovery
   d. resting and exercise hormone levels, environmental conditions, and body composition
   e. none of the above

2. **For a typical person, the RMR accounts for about ____ % of the TDEE:**
   a. 20 to 30
   b. 60 to 70
   c. 15 to 30
   d. 40 to 50
   e. none of the above

3. **The BMR is about ____ to ___% _____ in women than in men:**
   a. 40, 60, higher
   b. 5, 10, lower
   c. 5, 10, higher
   d. 40, 60, lower
   e. none of the above

4. **Which of the following is <u>not</u> an important factor determining daily energy expenditure:**
   a. lean body mass
   b. resting metabolic rate
   c. thermogenic influence of food consumed
   d. energy expended during physical activity and recovery
   e. body stature

5. **Which statement is <u>true</u> about dietary-induced thermogenesis?**
   a. it reaches a maximum within 1 hour after a meal
   b. a meal of pure protein elicits the greatest thermic effect
   c. obese individuals often have a blunted thermic response to food
   d. it is variable among individuals
   e. all of the above are true

6. Which statement is <u>true</u> about average daily energy expenditure for men and women aged 23 to 50 years?
    a. it is 2000 kcal for men and 2700 for women
    b. it is 2500 kcal for men and 3000 for women
    c. it is 2700 kcal for men and 2000 for women
    d. it is 3000 kcal for men and 2500 for women.
    e. it accounts for up to 25% of total daily caloric expenditure

7. Which of the following best defines the term MET:
    a. maximum energy expenditure in training
    b. minimum level of energy expenditure
    c. a unit of the resting metabolism
    d. energy metabolism in training
    e. multiple of resting heart rate

8. What would be the daily resting energy expenditure (kcal) for a male weighing 90.2 kg with a FFM of 72.0 kg?
    a. 1925
    b. 1540
    c. 2200
    d. 4280
    e. 5000

9. Under normal conditions, physical activity accounts for between ____ and ____% of a person's total daily energy expenditure:
    a. 15, 30
    b. 5, 10
    c. 20, 30
    d. 40, 50
    e. none of the above

10. Facultative thermogenesis refers to:
    a. increase in energy expenditure due to exercise
    b. increase in energy expenditure due to digestion
    c. increase in energy expenditure due to body temperature
    d. increase in energy expenditure due to activation of the sympathetic nervous system and its stimulating effect on metabolism with food ingestion
    e. none of the above

TRUE/FALSE

1. _____ A meal of pure protein elicits a thermic effect that is nearly 25% of the meal's total calories.

2. _____ Body surface area is determined by FFM and stature.

3. _____ Values for $\dot{V}O_2$ during the BMR test usually range between 500 and 600 mL per minute.

4. _____ Percent body fat is the most important factor affecting the BMR.

5. _____ The BMR increases if FFM increases.

6. _____ Physical activity has the most profound effect on human energy expenditure.

7. _____ Moderate exercise after eating does not augment caloric expenditure.

8. _____ Pregnancy severely limits aerobic capacity.

9. _____ Thirty to 40 minutes of moderate aerobic exercise for a healthy, low-risk woman during an uncomplicated pregnancy does not compromise fetal oxygen supply.

10. _____ The RMR increases with age and is generally lower for men than for women.

CROSSWORD PUZZLE

ACROSS

2 Lowering of this blood macronutrient could adversely affect fetal development

7 ____-absorptive state is when no food is eaten for at least 12 hours

9 Body mass minus fat mass (abbr.)

10 External surface of the body (abbr.)

11 Stimulating effect of food ingestion on metabolism (abbr.)

14 Maternal "hyperventilation" in exercise attributed to effect of this hormone

18 Work requiring up to three times resting metabolism

19 Physical activity classification (abbr.)

20 Work requiring nine times or more the resting metabolism

21 Work requiring six to eight times the resting metabolism

22 Metabolism that is slightly higher than BMR (abbr.)

DOWN

1 Multiple of resting metabolic rate (abbr.)

3 Term meaning "heat producing"

4 Contributes about a 5–20% effect on metabolism

5 This bodily response to cold stress can easily double or triple the metabolic rate

6 Older term for increased metabolism with eating (abbr.)

8 Variations in body _____ largely explain sex difference in BMR

10 Minimum energy required to sustain body's vital functions in the waking state (abbr.)

12 Physiologic variable directly related to oxygen uptake throughout a large portion of the aerobic work range

13 Component of thermogenesis related to catecholamine release

14 This macronutrient elicits the highest thermic effect

15 These individuals often have a blunted thermic response to eating

16 Total energy expended during a day (abbr.)

17 Component of thermogenesis related to specific macronutrient ingested

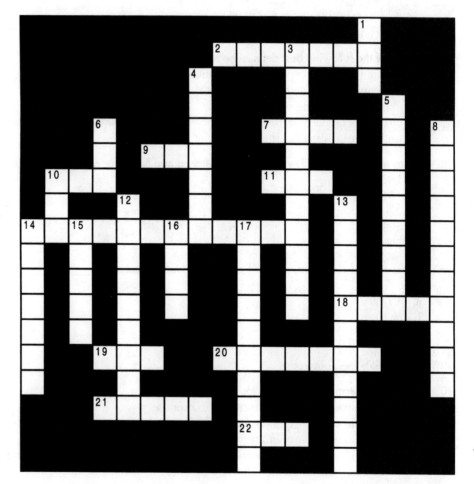

See page 369 for Crossword Puzzle Solution.

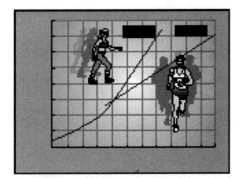

Energy Expenditure During Walking, Jogging, Running, and Swimming

DEFINE KEY TERMS AND CONCEPTS

1. Gross energy expenditure

2. Net energy expenditure

3. Economy of movement

4. Mechanical efficiency

5. $1 \text{ kcal·kg}^{-1}\text{·km}^{-1}$

6. Walking: sand versus hard surface

7. Negative work

8. Impact force in running

9. Running speed and stride length

10. **Running speed and stride frequency**

11. **Drafting**

12. **2 h: 06 min: 50 s**

13. **Wave drag**

14. **Skin friction drag**

15. **Viscous pressure drag**

16. **Swimming flume**

17. **Buoyancy**

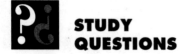 **STUDY QUESTIONS**

GROSS AND NET ENERGY EXPENDITURE

Net energy expenditure = _____ − _____

MOVEMENT ECONOMY AND MECHANICAL EFFICIENCY DURING EXERCISE

Discuss the concept of mechanical efficiency related to human movement.

What is the principal difference between movement economy and mechanical efficiency?

Economy of Movement

Is the running economy of a trained athlete higher or lower than that of an untrained person in the same exercise?

Mechanical Efficiency

Write the formula for calculating mechanical efficiency (%).

List two factors that affect the mechanical efficiency of human movement.

1.
2.

ENERGY EXPENDITURE DURING WALKING

Draw and label the relationship between speed of horizontal walking and running versus oxygen uptake.

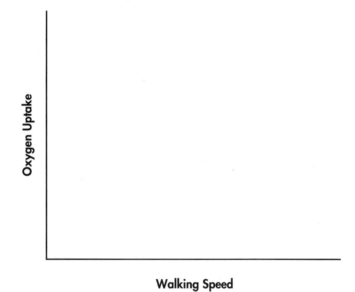

Influence of Body Mass

Calculate the total energy expenditure (kcal) for a person who weighs 54 kg and walks at 4.83 km·h^{-1} for 20 minutes. (*Hint: Refer to Table 10.5 in your textbook.*)

Effects of Terrain and Walking Surface

Of the walking surfaces discussed in the text, which results in the highest expenditure of energy at a given submaximum speed?

Downhill Walking

What is the decrease in the oxygen cost of walking downhill at −12% grade at a speed of 105 m·min^{-1} compared to walking on a level surface?

Effects of Footwear

What differences exist in energy expenditure between carrying weight on the torso, on the feet, and on the ankles?

- Torso

- Feet

- Ankles

Use of Hand-held and Ankle Weights

What effect do ankle weights have on the energy cost of walking?

Discuss the desirability of wearing ankle weights during running.

Competition Walkers

What is the difference in economy between walking and running at speeds faster than 8 $km \cdot h^{-1}$?

ENERGY EXPENDITURE DURING RUNNING

From an energy standpoint, at what speed does it become economical to begin to run?

The Economy of Running Fast or Slow

What effect does speed have on the energy cost of running a given distance?

What is the net energy cost of horizontal running?

Energy Cost Values

True or false? The energy requirement of running a given distance is independent of running speed.

Stride Length, Stride Frequency, and Speed

Running

In terms of stride frequency and length, running speed is increased mainly by _____.

At faster speeds, _____ becomes important when increasing running speed.

Competition Walking

What is the primary reason a person chooses to run rather than walk at speeds greater than 8 or 9 $km \cdot h^{-1}$?

Optimum Stride Length

What effect does shortening normal running stride and increasing the stride frequency have on running economy?

Running Economy: Children and Adults, Trained and Untrained

Give two reasons why running economy is lower for children than for adults.

1.

2.

Air Resistance

The effect of air resistance on the energy cost of running varies with what three factors?

1.

2.

3.

Are the negative effects of running into a headwind counterbalanced on one's return with the tailwind? Explain.

Drafting: Often a Wise Position

Quantify the performance and economy benefits of drafting.

Treadmill versus Track Running

What is the difference in energy cost between running on a track and running on a motorized treadmill?

Marathon Running

World-class marathon runners will run at about what percent of their $\dot{V}O_2max$?

SWIMMING

List two factors that contribute to the differences in energy expenditure between swimming and walking and running.

1.

2.

Methods of Measurement

Describe two methods for measuring energy expenditure during swimming.

1.

2.

Energy Cost and Drag

List the three components of the total drag force encountered during swimming.

1.

2.

3.

Ways to Reduce Effect of Drag Force

Describe one way to decrease the drag force during swimming.

Energy Cost, Swimming Velocity, and Skill

Is the steady-rate oxygen uptake at a given velocity of swimming higher or lower in trained than in untrained swimmers?

Effects of Water Temperature

Is more energy expended swimming in cold water or warm water? Discuss.

What is the optimal water temperature for competitive swimming?

Effects of Buoyancy: Men versus Women

Why can women achieve a lower energy expenditure than men while swimming at the same speed?

What is the percent difference in energy cost of swimming between males and females?

Endurance Swimmers

Are more calories expended swimming the English Channel or running a marathon? Explain.

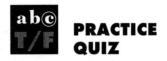 **PRACTICE QUIZ**

MULTIPLE CHOICE

1. The aerobic requirement of submaximal running (up to 286 m·min^{-1}) on the treadmill or track (either on level or up a grade), or the $\dot{V}O_2$max measured in both forms of exercise is:
    a. greater on the treadmill
    b. greater on the track
    c. the same on the track and on the treadmill
    d. lower on the treadmill
    e. none of the above

2. The three components of total drag force encountered during swimming are:
    a. wave, skin, viscous
    b. wave, temperature, pressure
    c. viscous, pressure, hydraulic
    d. hydraulic, pressure, internal
    e. wave, hydraulic, skin

3. Overcoming air resistance accounts for between ____ and ____ % of the cost of running in calm weather:
    a. 10, 15
    b. 3, 9
    c. 20, 30
    d. 1, 3
    e. none of the above

4. Which of the following influences daily energy expenditure?
    a. percent body fat
    b. resting metabolic rate
    c. thermogenic influence of food consumed
    d. energy expended during physical activity and recovery
    e. all of these factors

5. To establish differences among individuals in the economy of physical effort, one should primarily evaluate which of the following during steady-rate exercise?
    a. heart rate
    b. carbon dioxide production
    c. oxygen uptake
    d. blood pressure
    e. all of the above

6. Which statement is <u>true</u> about running economy?
    a. boys and girls are less economical in running than adults
    b. boys and girls are more economical in running than adults
    c. at the same speed, trained runners have a lower oxygen uptake than untrained runners
    d. at the same speed, trained runners have a higher oxygen uptake than untrained runners
    e. a and c

7. Which statement is <u>false</u> about running?
    a. the net energy cost for horizontal running per kilogram body mass per kilometer is approximately 1 kcal
    b. the relationship between oxygen uptake and speed of running is linear at normal running speeds
    c. it is more economical to run than to walk at speeds greater than 8 km/h
    d. using hand or ankle weights is highly desirable for increasing energy expenditure during running
    e. a and d

8. **Mechanical efficiency (%) is computed as:**
   a. actual work accomplished ÷ input of energy × 100
   b. input of energy ÷ actual work accomplished × 100
   c. actual work accomplished × input of energy × 100
   d. actual work accomplished × body mass ÷ input of energy
   e. none of the above

9. **Elite swimmers are able to swim a particular stroke at a given velocity at a _____ $\dot{V}O_2$ than untrained swimmers:**
   a. lower
   b. higher
   c. 5 to 10% higher
   d. 20 to 30% higher
   e. none of the above

10. **The energy cost of cutting through a headwind is:**
    a. counterbalanced on one's return with the tailwind
    b. the same as the energy cost of the tailwind
    c. less than the increase in the oxygen cost of drafting
    d. greater than the reduction in exercise $\dot{V}O_2$ observed with an equivalent wind velocity at one's back
    e. none of the above

TRUE/FALSE

1. _____ The total caloric cost of running a given distance at a steady-rate oxygen uptake is about the same whether the pace is fast or slow.

2. _____ For horizontal running, the net energy cost per kilogram of body mass per kilometer is approximately 1 kcal ($1\ kcal \cdot kg^{-1} \cdot km^{-1}$).

3. _____ Except at rapid speeds, running speed is increased mainly by increasing stride frequency.

4. _____ There is one "best" running style characteristic of elite runners.

5. _____ Children generally require significantly more oxygen to transport their body mass while running than adults.

6. _____ Heavier people expend more energy than lighter people performing the same activity.

7. _____ The economy of walking faster than $5\ km \cdot h^{-1}$ is one-half that of running at similar speeds.

8. _____ The energy cost of carrying weights on the feet or ankles is less than on the torso.

9. _____ The energy cost of swimming a given distance is four times greater than running the same distance.

10. _____ Untrained swimmers perform a particular stroke at a lower $\dot{V}O_2$ than trained swimmers.

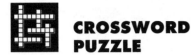

CROSSWORD PUZZLE

ACROSS

1 _____-bearing exercise occurs when the body weight is moved

3 Individuals with this CHD risk factor should probably not use hand-held weights

4 Walking or running downhill is a form of this type of work

6 Type of force on the leg while running; equal to three times body mass

13 Term for number of steps per minute

17 This factor is higher in adults than in children during running

18 This component of body composition contributes to sex difference in swimming economy

21 Force that impedes the body's movement through water

22 Drag force caused by waves that build up around swimmer

23 Term for distance between steps

DOWN

2 Gross energy _____ = rest + exercise

5 (Actual work accomplished ÷ Energy cost of the work) × 100

7 Because women possess more body fat they have a greater _____, and therefore float more easily than men

8 Type of drag force that counters the propulsive effort of swimming

9 "Swim-mill"

10 Rest + exercise energy expenditure

11 Form of swimming ergometry involving weight and pulley system

12 This type of feedback training may optimize stride length pattern in running

14 Following closely behind the lead athlete to increase economy

15 The economy of walking faster than 8 km per hour is about this percent lower than running at the same speed

16 Gross energy expenditure minus resting energy expenditure

19 It is considerably more costly to carry weight on this part of the lower body compared to weight attached to the torso

20 Walking in sand is this number of times more costly than walking on a paved surface

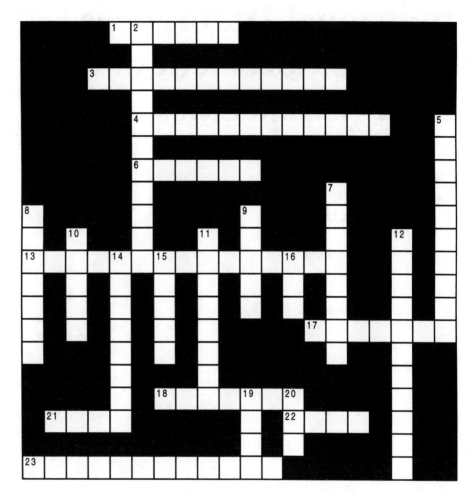

See page 369 for Crossword Puzzle Solution.

Individual Differences and Measurement of Energy Capacities

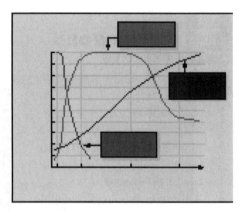

DEFINE KEY TERMS AND CONCEPTS

1. Individual differences

2. Specificity of metabolic capacity

3. Generality of metabolic capacity

4. Power

5. Watt

6. Stair sprinting power test

7. Jumping-power tests

8. Katch test

9. Anaerobic power

10. **Anaerobic capacity**

11. **Wingate test**

12. **Peak power**

13. **Average power**

14. **Rate of fatigue**

15. **Maximal lactate levels**

16. **Modalities for measuring $\dot{V}O_2$max**

17. **Peak oxygen uptake**

18. **Graded exercise**

19. **Ramp test**

20. **Genotype**

21. **Phenotype**

22. **Absolute $\dot{V}O_2$max**

23. **Relative $\dot{V}O_2$max**

24. **Cooper run**

25. HR-$\dot{V}O_2$ extrapolation procedure

26. **Queens College step test**

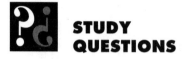
STUDY QUESTIONS

OVERVIEW OF ENERGY-TRANSFER CAPACITY DURING EXERCISE
Which energy system primarily supports the following activities:

- Standing vertical jump and reach

- 400-meter run

- 3-mile run

The formula for power is: _____ × _____ ÷ _____ .

ANAEROBIC ENERGY TRANSFER: THE IMMEDIATE AND SHORT-TERM ENERGY SYSTEMS
Evaluation of the Immediate Energy System
What type of tests typically measure the immediate anaerobic energy system?

What are the units of measurement for power?

Stair-Sprinting Power Tests
Compute the power output for a person who weighs 55 kg and traverses 9 steps in 0.75 second (each step is 0.175 meter).

Jumping-Power Tests
What is another name for the Sargent jump-and-reach test?

State one factor that might negatively influence power jumping test scores.

Other Power Tests
List two tests other than stair sprinting to estimate the power output capacity of the immediate energy system.

1.

2.

Interrelationships Among Power Tests

Explain why the relationship among power tests is not consistently strong.

Physiologic Evaluation of the ATP-PC Energy System

List three physiologic and biochemical measures used to estimate the capacity of the immediate energy system.

1.

2.

3.

Evaluation of the Short-Term Energy System

What type of test best estimates the power output of the short-term energy system?

Would tests of the short-term energy system exhibit task specificity? Explain.

Performance Tests for Anaerobic Power

List two tests to measure short-term energy capacity.

1.

2.

List three factors that affect anaerobic power performance.

1.

2.

3.

The Katch test and the Wingate test measure what aspect of energy-generating capacity?

What is the major difference between "peak power" and "average power"?

Lower in Children

Give one possible reason why children exhibit lower anaerobic power capacity compared to adults.

Sex Differences

Can sex differences in anaerobic power capacity be explained by differences in body composition? Discuss.

Blood Lactic Acid Levels

Draw and label the relationship between blood lactate levels and the duration of an all-out exercise test of short duration. (*Hint: Refer to Figure 11.5 in your textbook.*)

Glycogen Depletion

List two factors that determine the depletion patterns of muscle glycogen in different muscle fiber types within the same muscle.

1.

2.

Individual Differences in the Capacity for Anaerobic Energy Transfer

List three factors that differ among individuals in their capacity to generate short-term energy.

1.

2.

3.

Effects of Training

How does training affect the depletion pattern of anaerobic substrates and the capacity for lactic acid accumulation? (*Hint: Refer to Figure 11.7 in your textbook.*)

• Anaerobic substrate depletion

• Lactic acid accumulation

Buffering of Acid Metabolites

Do athletes have a better buffering capacity than non-athletes? Explain.

Motivation

What would you expect the relationship to be between "pain tolerance" and one's capacity for anaerobic exercise? Explain.

AEROBIC ENERGY: THE LONG-TERM ENERGY SYSTEM

List three categories of athletes that typically have high values for $\dot{V}O_2$max.

1.

2.

3.

Measurement of Maximal Oxygen Uptake

Criteria for $\dot{V}O_2$max

Describe the "gold standard" to indicate that a true $\dot{V}O_2$max has been attained.

List three additional criteria for establishing the $\dot{V}O_2$max.

1.

2.

3.

Tests of Maximal Oxygen Uptake

List two general criteria for a good test of maximal aerobic power.

1.

2.

Comparison of Tests

Give two examples of types of graded exercise tests to elicit the $\dot{V}O_2$max.

1.

2.

Commonly Used Treadmill Protocols

Treadmill tests for measuring $\dot{V}O_2$max generally vary with what three factors?

1.

2.

3.

Can Test Protocol Be Manipulated to Increase $\dot{V}O_2$max?

When two $\dot{V}O_2$max tests are administered to the same person in succession (2-minute recovery between tests), will there be differences between the test scores? Explain.

Factors that Affect Maximal Aerobic Power

List six factors that influence $\dot{V}O_2$max.

1.   4.

2.   5.

3.   6.

Mode of Exercise

What is the most common piece of exercise equipment used to test for the $\dot{V}O_2$max?

Heredity

What is the estimated magnitude of the heredity factor in determining $\dot{V}O_2$max?

Trainability and Genes

Are training-induced changes in functional capacity "genotype dependent?" Explain.

State of Training

In general, how much can $\dot{V}O_2$max be increased with training?

Sex

Give two reasons for sex-related differences in $\dot{V}O_2$max.

1.

2.

Body Size and Composition

What is the influence of body size and composition on $\dot{V}O_2$max?

What is the "best" way to express $\dot{V}O_2$max? Explain.

An Argument for Biological Differences Between Sexes

List two points that support the existence of real biological differences in $\dot{V}O_2max$ between sexes.

1.

2.

Age

After age 25, the $\dot{V}O_2max$ is likely to decrease by approximately what percent per year?

Children

Describe the trend in $\dot{V}O_2max$ ($L \cdot min^{-1}$) between ages 6 and 16 years. (*Hint: Refer to Figure 11.14A in your textbook.*)

Adults

Describe the trend in $\dot{V}O_2max$ ($mL \cdot kg^{-1} \cdot min^{-1}$) after age 25 years. (*Hint: Refer to Figure 11.14C in your textbook.*)

TESTS TO PREDICT AEROBIC CAPACITY

Walking Tests

What variable(s) are used to predict $\dot{V}O_2max$ during walking?

Endurance Runs

State one criticism of using distance runs to predict $\dot{V}O_2max$.

Predictions Based on Heart Rate

What four assumptions underlie the use of heart rate to predict $\dot{V}O_2max$?

1.

2.

3.

4.

The Step Test

Give one benefit of using a step test to predict $\dot{V}O_2max$.

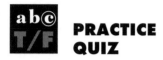

**PRACTICE
QUIZ**

MULTIPLE CHOICE

1. After age 25, the $\dot{V}O_2$max declines approximately ____% per year:
   a. 1
   b. 3
   c. 5
   d. 10
   e. 0

2. During exercise to approximately 80% of maximum intensity, $\dot{V}O_2$ and heart rate are:
   a. inversely proportional to each other
   b. linearly related to each other
   c. not related to each other
   d. curvilinearly related to each other
   e. inversely related to cardiac output

3. Which of the following is <u>not</u> a necessary assumption for accurately predicting $\dot{V}O_2$max from HR:
   a. linearity of the heart rate-$\dot{V}O_2$ relationship
   b. similar maximal heart rate for all subjects of the same age
   c. no day-to-day variation in exercise heart rate
   d. significant sex differences in maximal heart rate
   e. none of the above

4. Differences among individuals in short-term energy capacity are affected by all of the following <u>except</u>:
   a. training
   b. motivation
   c. distribution of fast-twitch fibers
   d. buffering of acid metabolites
   e. aerobic capacity

5. Which energy system predominantly powers 60 to 90 seconds of high-intensity all-out exercise?
   a. immediate system
   b. short-term system
   c. long-term system
   d. all contribute equally
   e. a and b

6. Which is a criterion for $\dot{V}O_2$max?
   a. when $\dot{V}O_2$ fails to increase with increasing exercise intensity
   b. blood lactic acid levels should reach 70 or 80 mg per 100 mL of blood or higher
   c. attainment of near age-predicted maximum heart rate
   d. respiratory exchange ratio (R) in excess of 1.00.
   e. each can be used as a criterion

7. Which is <u>true</u> about the relative $\dot{V}O_2$max values for men and women?
   a. values for women are 15–30% below values for men
   b. values for women are 15–30% above values for men
   c. values for women are 0–15% below values for men
   d. values for women are 0–15% above values for men
   e. none of the above

8. The relative contributions of anaerobic and aerobic energy transfer largely depend on:
   a. intensity of exercise
   b. duration of exercise
   c. mode of exercise
   d. a and c
   e. a and b

9. Which of the following <u>cannot</u> be evaluated using the Wingate test?
   a. peak power output
   b. average power output
   c. maximal oxygen uptake
   d. rate of fatigue
   e. a and c

10. Which energy system is evaluated by the stair-sprinting power test?
   a. immediate system
   b. short-term system
   c. long-term system
   d. a and c
   e. all of the above

TRUE/FALSE

1. _____ Men tend to have a higher $\dot{V}O_2$max than women because of their higher hemoglobin levels.

2. _____ Improvements in aerobic capacity with training usually range between 30 and 65%.

3. _____ Peak power is defined as "total power generated during a 30-second, all-out exercise period."

4. _____ Peak $\dot{V}O_2$ is usually nearly the same as $\dot{V}O_2$max.

5. _____ Jumping tests and stair-stepping tests are commonly used to predict maximal aerobic power.

6. _____ For each energy system, there is more specificity than generality.

7. _____ Depending on exercise intensity and duration, glycogen depletion occurs selectively in fast- and slow-twitch fibers.

8. _____ Short-term, high-intensity exercise performance can be enhanced by altering acid-base balance in the direction of alkalosis prior to exercising.

9. _____ Heredity has only a small effect on an individual's $\dot{V}O_2$max.

10. _____ Seventy percent of the differences in $\dot{V}O_2$max ($L \cdot min^{-1}$) among individuals can be explained by differences in body mass.

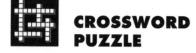

CROSSWORD PUZZLE

ACROSS

3 Genetic constitution of an individual

6 Oxygen uptake expressed in $L \cdot min^{-1}$

9 Intramuscular energy nutrient depleted in anaerobic exercise

12 Account for about 40% of the variability among people in $\dot{V}O_2max$

13 Test in increments of effort up to maximum is a _____ _____ test

17 The _____ treadmill test is an example of a ramp test

18 SI unit equal to $1 J \cdot s^{-1}$

20 Fundamental measure of aerobic power

21 Name of common vertical jump test (begins with letter S)

24 All-out 30-s test (named for university) on cycle ergometer with resistance equal to 0.075 kg per kilogram body mass

25 $\dot{V}O_2max$ is lower than running in this form of treadmill test

26 GXT in which work rate is progressively increased each minute

DOWN

1 Psychological component required for high levels of anaerobic exercise

2 Accounts for about 40% of the variability among people in $\dot{V}O_2max$

4 Opposite of specificity

5 The buffered by-product of anaerobic carbohydrate metabolism

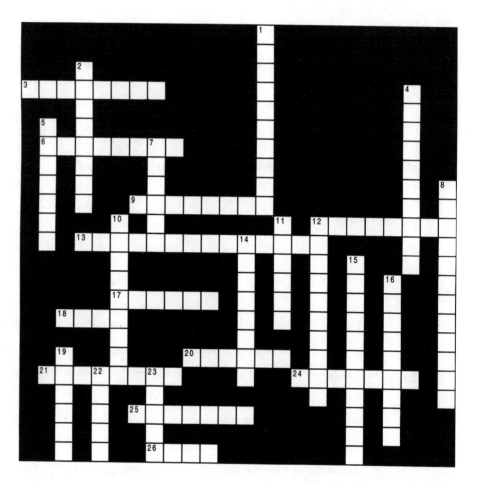

7 Minutes run during Air Force test to predict $\dot{V}O_2max$

8 Marathon runners possess a high maximum level of this

10 Name of all-out sprint cycling test of short duration (2 words)

11 Assumed relationship between HR and $\dot{V}O_2$

12 Blood component that contributes to sex differences in $\dot{V}O_2max$

14 Oxygen uptake expressed per unit body mass

15 Generally accepted criterion for reaching $\dot{V}O_2max$

16 Observable characteristics of an individual determined by genotype and environment

19 College for which step test is named

22 ____ = $F \times D \div T$

23 ____ sprinting test is used to evaluate anaerobic capacity

See page 369 for Crossword Puzzle Solution.

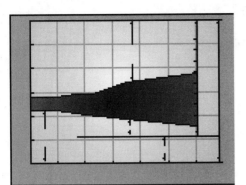

Pulmonary Structure and Function

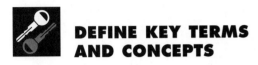

DEFINE KEY TERMS AND CONCEPTS

1. Pulmonary ventilation

2. Trachea

3. Bronchi

4. Bronchioles

5. Alveoli

6. Inspiratory muscles

7. Intrapulmonic pressure

8. Expiratory muscles

9. Valsalva maneuver

10. Glottis

11. **Intrathoracic pressure**

12. **Spirometer**

13. **Tidal volume**

14. **Inspiratory reserve volume**

15. **Expiratory reserve volume**

16. **Forced vital capacity**

17. **Residual lung volume**

18. **Total lung capacity**

19. **Helium method**

20. **Functional residual capacity**

21. **Oxygen dilution method**

22. **$FEV_{1.0}$ / FVC**

23. **Maximum voluntary ventilation**

24. **Asthma**

25. **Exercise-induced bronchospasm**

26. **Bronchodilators**

27. **Anti-inflammatory agents**

28. **Minute ventilation**

29. **Anatomic dead space**

30. **Alveolar ventilation**

31. **Physiologic dead space**

32. **Ventilation-perfusion ratio**

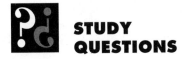 **STUDY QUESTIONS**

SURFACE AREA AND GAS EXCHANGE

Name six major parts of the ventilatory system. (*Hint: Refer to Figure 12.1 in your textbook.*)

1.   4.

2.   5.

3.   6.

ANATOMY OF VENTILATION

Place the following terms in the order that the air reaches them during the inspiratory cycle: bronchioles, trachea, alveoli, and bronchi.

1.

2.

3.

4.

Name the process whereby ambient air is brought into and exchanged with the air in the lungs.

The Lungs

How large is the surface area of the lungs?

The Alveoli

What is the primary function of the alveoli?

MECHANICS OF VENTILATION

List two causes of the changes in lung volume during inspiration and expiration.

1.

2.

Inspiration

List three muscles involved in inspiration.

1.

2.

3.

Expiration

List three factors that bring about the expiration of air from the lungs.

1.

2.

3.

Valsalva Maneuver

What position does the glottis assume during the Valsalva maneuver?

Physiologic Consequences of the Valsalva Maneuver

What are the potential physiologic consequences of the Valsalva maneuver?

Give one reason why individuals with heart and vascular disease should refrain from all-out straining exercises.

LUNG VOLUMES AND CAPACITIES

Static Lung Volumes

Draw and label a spirometer tracing to illustrate the typical values for the various static lung volume measures. (*Hint: Refer to Figure 12.7 in your textbook.*)

Residual Lung Volume

The RLV serves what important physiologic function?

Effects of Previous Exercise

Is the residual lung volume increased or decreased following an acute bout of exercise? Give a possible reason.

Lung Volume Averages for Men and Women

List three factors related to individual differences in lung volumes.

1.

2.

3.

Dynamic Lung Volumes

What two factors determine dynamic lung volumes?

1.

2.

Identify and describe two measures of dynamic lung volume.

Measure   Description

1.

2.

FEV-to-FVC Ratio

Forced expiratory volume provides an indication of what two components of lung function?

1.

2.

Maximum Voluntary Ventilation

Is the MVV usually higher or lower than the ventilation volume observed during maximal exercise? Discuss.

Lung Function, Training, and Exercise Performance

Larger than average breathing capacities in some athletes can be attributed to differences in what two factors?

1.

2.

Training May Benefit Ventilatory Endurance

By about how much can training improve the endurance of the ventilatory muscles?

Exercise and Asthma

Describe exercise-induced bronchospasm.

What is a common test of dynamic lung function to diagnose exercise-induced bronchospasm?

List two environmental factors that increase an individual's susceptibility to exercise-induced bronchospasm.

1.

2.

Sensitivity to Thermal Gradients

How are the rate and magnitude of alterations in pulmonary heat and water exchange related to exercise-induced bronchospasm?

The Environment Makes a Difference

Describe the "best" exercise environment for asthmatics.

Postexercise Coughing

Coughing after exercise is related to what two factors?

1.

2.

PULMONARY VENTILATION

Minute Ventilation

Minute ventilation = _____ × _____

To what extent (as a percent of vital capacity) does the tidal volume generally increase during exercise?

Alveolar Ventilation

Calculate the alveolar ventilation for a tidal volume of 600 mL.

What is the best way to increase alveolar ventilation: increasing the depth or the rate of breathing?

Dead Space versus Tidal Volume

Is there any change in anatomic dead space with an increase in tidal volume?

Physiologic Dead Space

List two conditions that increase the physiologic dead space.

1.

2.

Depth versus Rate

How is total alveolar ventilation increased during moderate and heavy exercise?

- Moderate exercise

- Heavy exercise

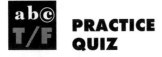 **PRACTICE QUIZ**

MULTIPLE CHOICE

1. **The volume of air that remains in the lungs after a maximal expiration is:**
   a. the expiratory reserve volume
   b. the tidal volume
   c. the residual volume
   d. the inspiratory reserve volume
   e. none of the above

2. **During exercise, tidal volume _____ compared to rest:**
   a. remains the same
   b. increases
   c. decreases
   d. fluctuates randomly
   e. none of the above

3. **A Valsalva maneuver may cause:**
   a. a reduced venous return
   b. a decrease in blood pressure
   c. dizziness
   d. a and b
   e. all of the above

4. **Pulmonary airflow depends on:**
   a. small pressure differences between alveolar and abdominal air
   b. small pressure differences between ambient air and air within the lungs
   c. the vapor pressure of expired air
   d. action of the rhomboid muscle
   e. b and d

5. **Static lung volumes:**
   a. can predict exercise performance
   b. cannot predict exercise performance
   c. are larger for the untrained
   d. are correlated to lactate threshold
   e. none of the above

6. **Measurement of these two lung volumes can detect possible lung disease:**
   a. TV and FRC
   b. RLV and IRV
   c. FEV and MVV
   d. TLC and FVC
   e. none of the above

7. **Lung volume measurements should be:**
   a. expressed relative to body density
   b. based on age and body mass
   c. based on age, sex, and body size
   d. expressed relative to percent body fat
   e. none of the above

8. **Exercise-induced bronchospasm depends on the:**
   a. rate and magnitude of airway cooling and subsequent rewarming
   b. rate and depth of breathing
   c. pressure difference between ambient air and alveolar air
   d. size of lungs and temperature of inspired air
   e. a and d

9. **The ratio of alveolar ventilation to pulmonary blood flow is termed the _____ and is maintained at about ____ during rest and light exercise.**
   a. ventilatory threshold, 1.0
   b. ventilatory pressure gradient, 0.75
   c. Valsalva-perfusion ratio, 0.8
   d. ventilation-perfusion ratio, 0.8
   e. none of the above

10. **Alveolar ventilation is:**
    a. the portion of air that remains in the alveoli after a maximum breath
    b. the total amount of air breathed per minute
    c. the total amount of gas that is exchanged between arterial and venous blood
    d. the portion of the minute ventilation that enters the alveoli and is involved in gaseous exchange with the blood
    e. none of the above

TRUE/FALSE

1. _____ Expiration is the process of air movement into the lungs.

2. _____ Lung volumes should only be evaluated in relation to norms based on age, sex, and body size.

3. _____ The anatomic dead space is the portion of air involved in gaseous exchange with the blood.

4. _____ Expiration at rest is usually a passive process.

5. _____ Alveolar ventilation during heavy exercise increases proportionately depending on one's FVC

6. _____ Exercise-induced bronchospasm is often eliminated when breathing humidified air.

7. _____ Exercise training in the asthmatic can increase air flow reserve and reduce respiratory work.

8. _____ Postexercise coughing is related to the rate of oxygen uptake in relation to the temperature of the gas inhaled.

9. _____ Minute ventilation = breathing rate × tidal volume.

10. _____ The anatomic dead space is the portion of alveolar volume with a poor ventilation-perfusion ratio.

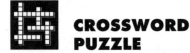

CROSSWORD PUZZLE

ACROSS

2 Major inspiratory muscle

8 Another name for windpipe

9 Residual lung volume + vital capacity (abbr.)

10 Muscle of inspiration

11 Device to measure lung volumes

12 Volume of air moved during normal breathing

15 Air remaining in lungs at end of normal expiration (abbr.)

16 Portion of alveolar volume with poor ventilation-perfusion ration

20 Nondiffusible portion of respiratory tract

25 Air movement into lungs

28 Chemicals that reduce airway resistance

29 Conducting tubes to alveoli

30 Volume remaining in lungs following maximal expiration (abbr.)

31 Primary conduits in lungs

32 Airway obstruction is that point at which less than this percent of vital capacity can be expelled in 1.0 second

DOWN

1 Movement of air into and out of lungs

3 Elongated, narrow opening between vocal cords and larynx

4 Postexercise coughing is related to losses of this compound from respiratory tract

5 Respiratory disorder with recurrent attacks of difficult breathing, particularly on exhalation

6 Forced exhalation against a closed glottis

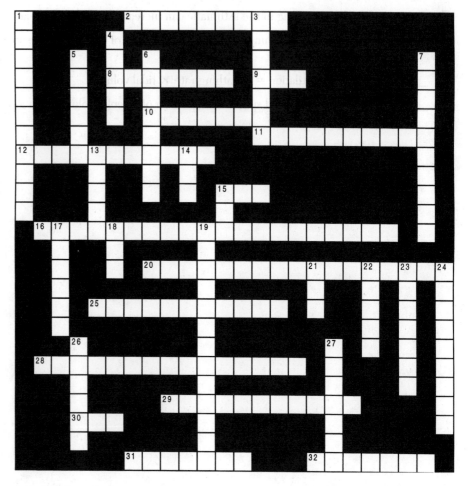

7 Air movement from lungs

13 Organ of ventilation

14 Rapid and deep breathing for 15 seconds extrapolated to 1-minute volume (abbr.)

15 Maximal volume of air moved in one breath (abbr.)

17 Rebreathed gas used to measure residual lung volume

18 Maximum inspiration following normal inspiration (abbr.)

19 Term for air pressure within lungs

21 Maximal exhalation following normal exhalation (abbr.)

22 Exercise tidal volume rarely exceeds this percent of vital capacity

23 Terminal branches of respiratory tract

24 Severe COPD

26 Ultimately, a prolonged Valsalva maneuver _____ blood pressure

27 Inspiratory _____ volume

See page 369 for Crossword Puzzle Solution.

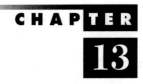

13

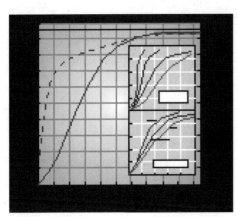

Gas Exchange and Transport

DEFINE KEY TERMS AND CONCEPTS

1. Torr

2. Partial pressure

3. Ambient air

4. Tracheal air

5. P_{O_2}

6. Alveolar air composition

7. Henry's law

8. Pressure differential

9. Solubility

10. Equilibrium

11. **Vol%**

12. **Physical solution**

13. **Venous admixture**

14. **Hemoglobin**

15. **Oxyhemoglobin**

16. **Iron-deficiency anemia**

17. **Oxyhemoglobin dissociation curve**

18. **Percent saturation**

19. **Hematocrit**

20. **Arteriovenous oxygen difference**

21. **Bohr effect**

22. **2,3-Diphosphoglycerate**

23. **Myoglobin**

24. **Bicarbonate**

25. **Carbonic acid**

26. **Carbonic anhydrase**

27. **Chloride shift**

28. **Carbamino compounds**

29. **Haldane effect**

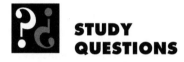

STUDY QUESTIONS

GASEOUS EXCHANGE IN THE LUNGS AND TISSUES

Oxygen supply to the body depends on what two factors related to ambient air?

1.

2.

Concentrations and Partial Pressures of Respired Gases

Give the formula to calculate partial pressure of a gas:

Partial pressure = _____ × _____

Ambient Air

Compute the partial pressures of O_2, CO_2, and N_2 of ambient air at sea level (barometric pressure = 760 mm Hg).

P_{O_2} = _____ × _____

P_{CO_2} = _____ × _____

P_{N_2} = _____ × _____

Tracheal Air

What is the pressure exerted by water vapor and the inspired dry air molecules in tracheal air?

- Water vapor

- Dry air molecules

Alveolar Air

Give the average percentages of O_2, CO_2, and N_2 in alveolar air at sea level.

- O_2

- CO_2

- N_2

Movement of Gas in Air and Fluids

According to Henry's law, the amount of gas that dissolves in fluid is a function of what two factors?

1.

2.

Pressure

The pressure of a specific gas on both sides of a permeable membrane is said to be in equilibrium when:

Solubility

Why is less pressure differential required to move a given amount of CO_2 into or out of a fluid than to move the same quantity of oxygen?

Gas Exchange in the Lungs

What is the average partial pressure of O_2 and CO_2 in the alveoli at rest? How does heavy exercise affect these values?

	P_{O_2}	P_{CO_2}
• Rest		
• Heavy exercise		

Gas Transfer in the Tissues

Give the average partial pressures of O_2 and CO_2 in the tissues at rest. How does heavy exercise affect these values?

	P_{O_2}	P_{CO_2}
• Rest		
• Heavy exercise		

TRANSPORT OF OXYGEN

Transport of Oxygen in the Blood

List the two ways oxygen is transported in the blood.

1.

2.

Oxygen in Solution

Give the amount of oxygen carried in physical solution in:

• 100 mL plasma

• 5000 mL plasma

Oxygen Combined with Hemoglobin

Write the formula for the oxygenation of hemoglobin to oxyhemoglobin.

The oxygenation of hemoglobin to oxyhemoglobin depends on what main factor?

Oxygen-Carrying Capacity of Hemoglobin

List the average hemoglobin values (grams per 100 mL blood) for men and women.

• Men

• Women

Each gram of hemoglobin can combine with _____ mL of oxygen.

P_{O_2} and Hemoglobin Saturation

Draw and label the oxyhemoglobin dissociation curve. (*Hint: Refer to Figure 13.4 in your textbook.*)

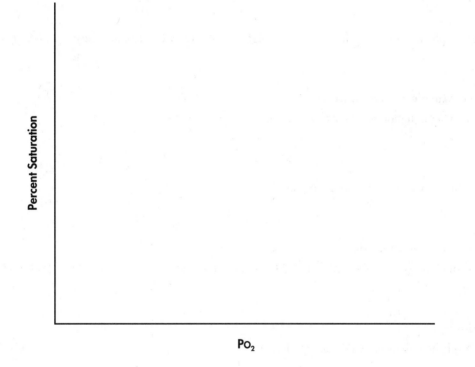

P_{O_2} in the Lungs

Hemoglobin is almost completely saturated at approximately what P_{O_2} value?

Approximately how much oxygen (in mL) is carried in each 100 mL of blood leaving the lungs at sea level?

P_{O_2} in the Tissues

In the tissues during rest, the blood P_{O_2} falls to about _____ mm Hg, and the hemoglobin is about _____ % saturated with oxygen.

The Bohr Effect

List three factors that cause the oxyhemoglobin curve to shift downward and to the right to facilitate the release of oxygen.

1.

2.

3.

Red Blood Cell 2,3-DPG

What effect does the compound 2,3-DPG have on the dissociation of oxygen from hemoglobin?

Where is 2,3-DPG produced and with what does it bind?

• Where produced

• Binds with

What is a possible explanation for why females have a higher level of 2,3-DPG than males?

Myoglobin: The Muscle's Oxygen Store

Complete the following equation for the oxygenation of myoglobin:

$$Mb + O_2 \rightarrow$$

What is the main function of myoglobin in the body?

Oxygen Released at Low Pressures

The greatest quantity of oxygen is released from MbO_2 when the tissue Po_2 drops below _____ mm Hg.

Effects of Training

Can myoglobin levels be enhanced with training? Discuss.

What muscle fiber type has the highest quantity of myoglobin?

Transport of Carbon Dioxide in the Blood

List the three ways in which CO_2 is carried in the blood.

1.

2.

3.

Carbon Dioxide Transport in Solution

How much CO_2 is carried as free CO_2 dissolved in plasma?

Carbon Dioxide Transport as Bicarbonate

In the Tissues

Complete the following equation to show the formation of bicarbonate in the tissues.

$$CO_2 + H_2O \rightarrow$$

What percentage of the total CO_2 in the body is carried as plasma bicarbonate?

In the Lungs

Complete the following equation to show the formation of CO_2 from bicarbonate in the lungs:

$$H^+ + HCO_3^- \rightarrow$$

Carbon Dioxide Transport as Carbamino Compounds

CO_2 reacts with the amino acid molecules of blood proteins to form _____. This is particularly true for the globin portion of hemoglobin, which carries about _____ % of the body's CO_2.

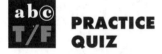 **PRACTICE QUIZ**

MULTIPLE CHOICE

1. **The small amount of free carbon dioxide in solution in plasma:**
    a. establishes the P_{CO_2} of the alveoli
    b. determines the CO_2 gradient between alveoli and ambient air
    c. establishes the P_{CO_2} of the blood
    d. does not take part in metabolism, as it is part of the physiologic dead space
    e. none of the above

2. **The major quantity of carbon dioxide is transported:**
    a. as free CO_2 in the blood
    b. in chemical combination with water and carried as bicarbonate
    c. in combination with myoglobin
    d. in combination with hemoglobin
    e. none of the above

3. **Hemoglobin increases the oxygen-carrying capacity of whole blood about:**
    a. 2 times
    b. 5 times
    c. 10 times
    d. 15 times
    e. none of the above

4. **The interaction between oxygen loading and carbon dioxide release is termed the:**
   a. Bohr effect
   b. Haldane effect
   c. oxyhemoglobin dissociation
   d. ventilatory equivalent
   e. none of the above

5. **Hemoglobin saturation changes very little until the P_{O_2} falls below:**
   a. 80 mm Hg
   b. 60 mm Hg
   c. 40 mm Hg
   d. 20 mm Hg
   e. hemoglobin saturation never changes

6. **_____ augments the blood's oxygen-carrying capacity more than 60 times:**
   a. carbon dioxide
   b. plasma
   c. hemoglobin
   d. bicarbonate
   e. none of the above

7. **What percentage of the total carbon dioxide is carried as plasma bicarbonate?**
   a. 20–40
   b. 40–60
   c. 60–80
   d. above 80
   e. below 20

8. **The small amount of oxygen dissolved in plasma:**
   a. establishes the partial pressure of oxygen in the blood, and thus determines the oxygenation and deoxygenation of hemoglobin
   b. increases the acidity of the blood
   c. determines the P_{O_2} of alveolar air
   d. ultimately combines with serum ferritin
   e. is a good measure of nitrogen elimination

9. **Increases in acidity, temperature, carbon dioxide concentration, and red blood cell 2,3-DPG:**
   a. cause increased $Hb\text{-}O_2$ formation
   b. have no effect on the effectiveness of Hb to hold oxygen
   c. increase hemoglobin's effectiveness to hold oxygen
   d. reduce hemoglobin's effectiveness to hold oxygen
   e. none of the above

10. **Myoglobin:**
    a. has the same oxygen dissociation curve as hemoglobin
    b. holds such small amounts of oxygen that it cannot be considered an "extra" oxygen carrier
    c. only releases oxygen to the mitochondria during rest and light exercise
    d. probably facilitates oxygen transfer to the mitochondria during strenuous exercise because it releases its oxygen at a low P_{O_2}
    e. none of the above

TRUE/FALSE

1. _____ The oxyhemoglobin curve is U shaped.

2. _____ Hemoglobin saturation changes very little until the P_{O_2} falls below 60 mm Hg.

3. _____ Percent saturation = (O_2 combined with Hb ÷ O_2 capacity of Hb) × 100.

4. _____ Oxygen movement into the blood depends on solubility and pressure differential.

5. _____ Exchange of gases between the lungs and blood occurs by active transport.

6. _____ Carbon dioxide is 25 times more soluble in plasma than oxygen.

7. _____ Myoglobin acts as an extra oxygen store in skeletal and cardiac muscle.

8. _____ The major quantity of carbon dioxide in the body is transported as carbamino compounds.

9. _____ Hemoglobin is about 98% saturated with oxygen at the normal alveolar Po_2 of 100 mm Hg.

10. _____ The Bohr effect describes the Hb-O_2 association under normal conditions.

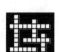

CROSSWORD PUZZLE

ACROSS

1 Ion that moves into blood cell to maintain ionic equilibrium

5 _____ effect refers to interaction between oxygen loading and carbon dioxide release

6 Last word of term describing effects of CO_2, temperature, and acidity on oxyhemoglobin dissociation curve

8 Plot of saturation of hemoglobin with oxygen at various P_{O_2} values is the oxyhemoglobin _____ ___

10 Percent concentration times total pressure of gas mixture = _____ _____

11 Breakdown product of carbonic acid

12 Person who described factors affecting oxygen dissociation curve

15 Clinical condition related to low hemoglobin concentration

18 CO_2 is _____-____ times more soluble in fluid than O_2

19 Law that gas dissolved in fluid depends on pressure and solubility (person's name)

20 Ease of gas movement into solution

22 Iron-containing pigment in muscle

23 When concentration of dissolved substance cannot be exceeded, solution is said to be _____

DOWN

2 Term for percentage volume of blood occupied by erythrocytes

3 Combination of O_2 and Hb forms this compound

4 Refers to environmental conditions

7 Pigmented respiratory protein in erythrocytes

9 Enzyme that accelerates union of CO_2 and H_2O

13 Difference between O_2 content of arterial and mixed venous blood

14 H_2CO_3

16 Organic compound formed from plasma proteins or hemoglobin with CO_2

17 Point where gas movement into fluid equals movement out

21 Unit of atmospheric pressure (abbr.)

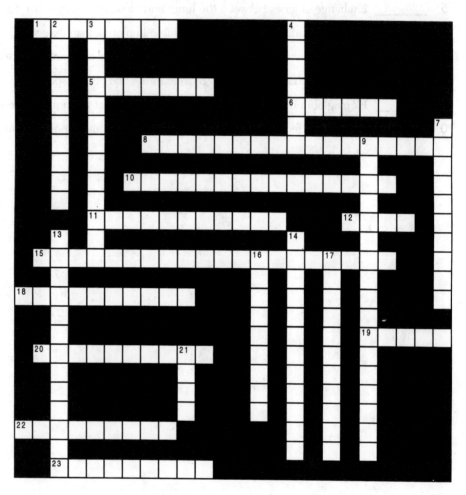

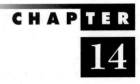

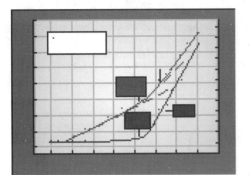

Dynamics of Pulmonary Ventilation

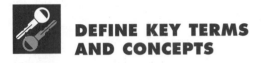

DEFINE KEY TERMS AND CONCEPTS

1. Medulla

2. Chemoreceptors

3. Most important respiratory stimulus

4. "Breakpoint" for breath-hold

5. Hyperventilation

6. Hyperpnea

7. Carotid bodies

8. Mechanoreceptors

9. Phase I ventilatory response

10. Phase II ventilatory response

11. **Phase III ventilatory response**

12. **Ventilatory equivalent**

13. **$\dot{V}_E / \dot{V}_{O_2}$**

14. **OBLA**

15. **Specificity of OBLA**

16. **OBLA and endurance performance**

17. **Energy cost of breathing: rest**

18. **Energy cost of breathing: heavy exercise**

19. **Acid**

20. **Base**

21. **Buffers**

22. **Alkalosis**

23. **Acidosis**

24. **Carbonic acid**

25. **Sodium bicarbonate**

26. **Sodium lactate**

27. **Hemoglobin as a buffer**

28. **Alkaline reserve**

29. **Cortical influence**

30. **Peripheral influence**

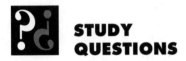

STUDY QUESTIONS

REGULATION OF PULMONARY VENTILATION

Control of Ventilation

List two factors that regulate pulmonary ventilation.

1.

2.

Neural Factors

In addition to the inherent activity of the respiratory center in the medulla, list three other mechanisms for ventilatory control.

1.

2.

3.

Humoral Factors

Pulmonary ventilation at rest is regulated by the _____.

Plasma Po_2 and Peripheral Chemoreceptors

Peripheral chemoreceptors sensitive to the Po_2 of arterial blood are located in the _____ and _____ .

Plasma Po_2 and H^+ Concentration

Describe what happens to the resting $\dot{V}E$ with an increase in inspired Pco_2.

Hyperventilation and Breath-Holding

What primary factor causes the urge to breathe during breath-holding?

Regulation of Ventilation in Exercise

Chemical Control

Why can't chemical stimuli alone entirely explain hyperpnea during exercise?

Nonchemical Control

List three nonchemical factors to explain the rapid increase in ventilation at the onset of exercise.

1.

2.

3.

Neurogenic Factors

List the two neurogenic factors that control pulmonary ventilation.

1.

2.

Influence of Temperature

What role does body temperature have in regulating pulmonary ventilation?

Integrated Regulation

During Exercise

List two factors believed to regulate pulmonary ventilation during exercise.

1.

2.

In Recovery

Why does ventilation abruptly decrease when exercise ceases?

PULMONARY VENTILATION DURING EXERCISE

Ventilation and Energy Demands

Ventilation in Steady-Rate Exercise

Draw and label the relationship between $\dot{V}O_2$ and $\dot{V}E$ during graded exercise up to maximum levels. (*Hint: Refer to Figure 14.5 in your textbook.*)

What is the term for the ratio of minute ventilation to oxygen uptake? Give the average value for this measure for healthy young adults and children during submaximal exercise.

    Term   Average values

• Adults

• Children

Ventilation in Non-Steady-Rate Exercise

Give a typical value for the ventilatory equivalent during light and intense exercise in healthy people.

• Light exercise

• Intense exercise

Onset of Blood Lactate Accumulation (OBLA)

At what average percentage of $\dot{V}O_2$max does blood lactate begin to accumulate in a healthy, untrained person during graded exercise?

Write the chemical reaction for the buffering of lactic acid by sodium bicarbonate.

List two chemical factors associated with the OBLA.

1.

2.

Specificity of the Point of OBLA

Is OBLA specific to the type of exercise? Explain.

Some Independence Between OBLA and $\dot{V}O_2$max

Give possible reasons why the level of OBLA may be improved with aerobic training, independent of any improvement in $\dot{V}O_2$max.

OBLA and Endurance Performance

In addition to $\dot{V}O_2$max, what other variable is a consistent and powerful predictor of aerobic endurance performance?

Energy Cost of Breathing

What percentage of the total oxygen uptake is attributable to the cost of breathing at rest and during heavy exercise?

- Rest

- Heavy exercise

Respiratory Disease

What percentage of the total oxygen uptake during exercise is due to the cost of breathing in patients with severe COPD?

Cigarette Smoking

Describe the acute effects of cigarette smoking on airway resistance to breathing. How might this adversely affect exercise capacity?

- Acute effects

- Exercise capacity

Acute Effects

What is the single most important deleterious effect of cigarette smoking on the acute exercise response?

A Blunted Heart Rate Response

Why is it important to consider a person's smoking status when evaluating fitness data? Explain.

Adaptations in Breathing with Training

List two changes in pulmonary ventilation resulting from aerobic training.

1.

2.

Is the ventilatory response specific or general to the form of exercise used in training? Discuss.

Does Ventilation Limit Aerobic Power and Endurance?

If ventilation limits aerobic power, would there be an increase or decrease in the $\dot{V}E/\dot{V}O_2$ ratio during graded exercise? Discuss.

An Important Exception

What reason is proposed to explain why an elite endurance athlete may be unable to achieve complete arterial oxygen saturation during maximum exercise?

ACID-BASE REGULATION

Buffering

Substances that dissociate in solution and release H^+ are called _____.

A compound that picks up or accepts H^+ to form hydroxide ions is a _____.

The pH of various body fluids ranges from a low of _____ for _____ to a slightly basic pH between _____ and ____ for arterial and venous blood.

Chemical Buffers

Bicarbonate Buffer

What two chemicals provide the body's first line of defense in acid-base regulation?

1.

2.

Phosphate Buffer

List the two chemicals that make up the phosphate buffering system.

1.

2.

Protein Buffer

What is the most important buffer for the H^+ released from the dissociation of carbonic acid?

Relative Power of the Chemical Buffers

List the three most powerful chemical buffers.

1.

2.

3.

Physiologic Buffers

When the chemical buffers are stressed, which physiologic systems contribute to acid-base regulation?

Ventilatory Buffer

Discuss the effect of an increase in the H^+ concentration of extracellular fluid on pulmonary ventilation.

Renal Buffer

Acidity can be regulated by the kidneys via the secretion of _____ and _____ into urine.

Effects of Exercise and Training

What are the extreme low values for pH recorded during maximal exercise?

Does Training Improve Buffering Capacity?

What most likely accounts for the improved tolerance to the acidic condition following anaerobic training?

PRACTICE QUIZ

MULTIPLE CHOICE

1. **In light to moderate exercise, minute ventilation increases:**
   a. linearly with $\dot{V}O_2$
   b. curvilinearly with $\dot{V}O_2$
   c. linearly with arterial PCO_2
   d. directly with inspired PH_2O
   e. none of the above

2. **In non–steady-rate exercise, minute ventilation increases:**
   a. linearly with $\dot{V}O_2$
   b. curvilinearly with plasma protein
   c. linearly with arterial $\dot{V}CO_2$
   d. directly with inspired PH_2O
   e. a, c, and d

3. **OBLA is related to:**
   a. a decrease in H_2CO_3 production
   b. a decrease in $Hb\text{-}O_2$ saturation
   c. the onset of anaerobiosis and subsequent accumulation of plasma lactate
   d. a decrease in non-metabolic carbon dioxide release
   e. a decrease in plasma H^+ concentration

4. **Increases in airway resistance caused by cigarette smoking:**
   a. are not detrimental during heavy aerobic exercise
   b. contribute to increased alkalosis during exercise
   c. are caused by the nicotine in cigarette smoke
   d. are reversible with smoking abstinence
   e. c and d

5. **Aerobic exercise training:**
    a. increases the ventilatory equivalent in submaximal exercise
    b. does not affect the ventilatory equivalent in submaximal exercise
    c. reduces the minute ventilation at $\dot{V}O_2$max
    d. decreases the ventilatory equivalent in submaximal exercise
    e. none of the above

6. **The first line of defense in acid-base regulation is:**
    a. bicarbonate, phosphate, and protein chemical buffers
    b. decrease in the ventilatory equivalent
    c. decrease in the ventilation-perfusion ratio
    d. increase in the ventilation-perfusion ratio
    e. decrease in bicarbonate reserve

7. **Aerobic exercise training:**
    a. decreases an individual's buffering capacity
    b. has essentially no effect on an individual's buffering capacity
    c. increases an individual's buffering capacity
    d. decreases buffering capacity and increases one's tolerance for elevated H^+ concentration
    e. a, b, and c

8. **$H_2O + CO_2 \rightarrow H_2CO_3 \rightarrow H^+ + HCO_3^-$:**
    a. is an expression of alkalosis
    b. usually occurs during light exercise
    c. is an expression of acidosis
    d. usually occurs during rest
    e. a and c

9. **Nonchemical regulatory factors for ventilatory adjustments to exercise include:**
    a. cortical activation
    b. elevation in body temperature
    c. peripheral sensory input from mechanoreceptors
    d. a and c
    e. all of the above

10. **What does <u>not</u> reduce the effectiveness of Hb to hold oxygen?**
    a. increase in acidity
    b. increase in temperature
    c. increase in carbon dioxide concentration
    d. increase in thyroxine
    e. none of the above

TRUE/FALSE

1. _____ A buffering system consists of a weak acid and the salt of that acid.

2. _____ In general, training increases the tidal volume in submaximal exercise.

3. _____ An increase in pH above the normal average of 7.4 is termed alkalosis.

4. _____ A decrease in pH above the normal average of 7.4 is termed alkalosis.

5. _____ The kidneys stand as the final buffering system by excreting H^+.

6. _____ The lowest pH tolerated by humans is 5.5.

7. _____ For men and women, the point of OBLA is a consistent and powerful predictor of aerobic exercise performance.

8. _____ Pulmonary function probably is not the "weak link" in the oxygen transport system of healthy individuals with an average to moderately high aerobic capacity.

9. _____ There is substantial reversal in the increased oxygen cost of breathing with only one day of abstinence from smoking.

10. _____ Decreased minute ventilation is often called hyperpnea.

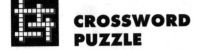

CROSSWORD PUZZLE

ACROSS

1 Sensitive to decreased arterial P_{O_2} and P_{CO_2}
4 Arterial P_{CO_2} of about 50 mm Hg is the _____ for breath-hold
7 Danish chemist who devised pH scale
8 Respiratory center
9 Phase of ventilatory control involving "fine tuning" through peripheral feedback mechanisms
11 Compounds formed when CO_2 combines with protein
12 Peripheral arterial chemoreceptors
13 Overbreathing
15 Brain area responsible for immediate, rapid rise in exercise ventilation
16 _____ buffers provide the rapid first line of defense
18 Condition of abnormally high $[H^+]$
20 Chemicals that minimize changes in $[H^+]$
21 Peripheral receptors sensitive to muscle action
23 Minute ventilation $\div \dot{V}_{O_2}$ is termed ventilatory _____

DOWN

1 Most important respiratory stimulus
2 This many days of smoking abstinence reverses increased cost of breathing
3 Condition of abnormally low $[H^+]$
5 Term relating to chemical base

6 With COPD, resistance is greatest in this phase of the ventilatory cycle
10 Another word for increased exercise ventilation
13 The point for OBLA is somewhat _____ than for the lactate threshold
14 Specificity of ventilatory response to training is related to a lower blood level of blood _____

17 In light to moderate exercise, ventilation increases in this manner with $\dot{V}_{O_2}$ and $\dot{V}_{CO_2}$
19 Onset of blood lactic acid buildup (abbr.)
20 Binds with H^+
22 Liberates H^+ in solution

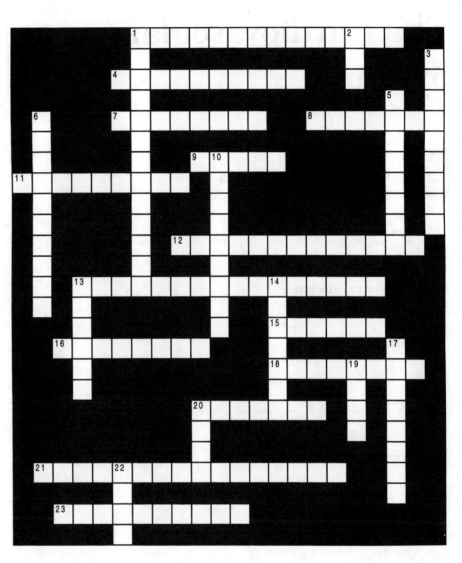

See page 370 for Crossword Puzzle Solution.

The Cardiovascular System

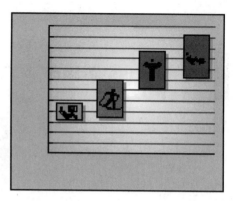

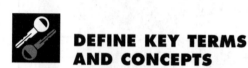

DEFINE KEY TERMS AND CONCEPTS

1. **Myocardium**

2. **Pulmonary circulation**

3. **Systemic circulation**

4. **Septum**

5. **Atrioventricular valves**

6. **Tricuspid valve**

7. **Bicuspid valve**

8. **Semilunar valves**

9. **Isovolumetric contraction period**

10. **Arteries**

11. **Aorta**

12. **Arterioles**

13. **Systolic blood pressure**

14. **Systole**

15. **Diastole**

16. **Diastolic blood pressure**

17. **Peripheral resistance**

18. **Mean arterial pressure**

19. **Metarterioles**

20. **Capillaries**

21. **Precapillary sphincter**

22. **Venules**

23. **Inferior vena cava**

24. **Superior vena cava**

25. **Mixed venous blood**

26. **Blood reservoirs**

27. **Varicose veins**

28. **Venous pooling**

29. **Edema**

30. **Active cool-down**

31. **Hypertension**

32. **Borderline hypertension**

33. **Hypotensive response to previous exercise**

34. **Coronary circulation**

35. **Coronary sinus**

36. **Anterior cardiac veins**

37. **Angina pectoris**

38. **Thrombus**

39. **Myocardial infarction**

40. **RPP**

41. **Ischemia** _____

_____

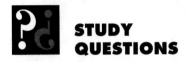

STUDY QUESTIONS

COMPONENTS OF THE CARDIOVASCULAR SYSTEM

List the four major components of the cardiovascular system.

1.   3.

2.   4.

The Heart

What type of muscle makes up the myocardium?

List two functions of the left and right sides of the heart.

       Left heart   Right heart

1.   1.

2.   2.

Name two different heart valves.

1.

2.

The Arterial System

The Arteries

What is the main function of the arteries and arterioles?

Explain why the arterioles are referred to as "resistance vessels."

Blood Pressure

Systolic Blood Pressure

Where are the three most accessible places on the body to feel the pulse?

1.

2.

3.

What is a "normal" systolic blood pressure during rest?

Systolic blood pressure provides an estimate of what two physiologic factors?

1.

2.

Systolic blood pressure can be measured by changes in sounds with the _____ method.

Diastolic Blood Pressure

What is a "normal" diastolic blood pressure during rest?

Diastolic blood pressure provides an indication of what physiologic factor?

Mean Arterial Pressure

What does the mean arterial pressure represent?

Cardiac Output and Total Peripheral Resistance

Write the formulas for cardiac output and total peripheral resistance.

- CO =

- TPR =

The Capillaries

The capillaries contain approximately what percentage of the total blood volume?

How much time is needed for one blood cell to pass through the typical capillary at rest?

Blood Flow in Capillaries

What capillary structure regulates blood flow within specific tissues?

Capillary blood flow is _____ _____ to the vasculature's cross-sectional area.

The Veins

What is the name of the largest vein in the body?

Venous Return

What do veins have that arteries do not? What is the function of these structures?

What is the advantage of having the blood in the venous system under low pressure?

An Active Vasculature
Discuss the role of veins as blood reservoirs.

Varicose Veins
Where do varicose veins usually appear? Why?

Venous Pooling
What is the main cause for fainting in the tilt table experiment?

The Active Cooldown
Why is it always beneficial to actively cool down after exercise in comparison to more passive procedures?

HYPERTENSION
Give the general statistics for hypertension in the United States.

Effects of Regular Exercise
Does regular aerobic exercise lower blood pressure? By how much?

Give one contributing factor for the exercise-induced lowering of resting blood pressure.

BLOOD PRESSURE AND EXERCISE
Static and Dynamic Resistance Exercise
Does straining-type exercise increase or decrease total peripheral resistance?

Is the active muscle mass or the exercise intensity more important in causing increases in blood pressure during straining-type exercise?

Chronic Effects of Resistance Training
Describe the effect of long-term resistance exercise training on resting blood pressure.

Do body builders show increased or decreased blood pressure response during resistance exercise compared to the untrained?

Steady-Rate Exercise

Describe the normal systolic and diastolic blood pressure response during the first few minutes of rhythmic submaximal exercise.

Graded Exercise

Describe the general response pattern for systolic and diastolic blood pressure during continuous, graded treadmill exercise. (*Hint: Refer to Figure 15.9 in your textbook.*)

Blood Pressure in Upper-Body Exercise

Describe the difference in the blood pressure response during upper-body exercise compared to walking at a similar level of oxygen uptake.

In Recovery

Is blood pressure reduced following sustained submaximum exercise? By how much?

Body Inversion

Is the inversion technique prudent for hypertensive individuals? Explain.

THE HEART'S BLOOD SUPPLY

At rest, normal blood flow to the myocardium is approximately what percentage of total cardiac output?

Myocardial Oxygen Utilization

How much oxygen is extracted from the coronary blood flow at rest?

List the two factors that increase coronary blood flow during vigorous exercise.

1.

2.

The Rate-Pressure Product: An Estimate of Myocardial Work

Write the equation for the rate-pressure product.

The RPP is highly related to _____.

Myocardial Metabolism

Approximately what percentage of circulating lactate is used for energy by the myocardium?

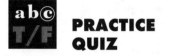

PRACTICE QUIZ

MULTIPLE CHOICE

1. **At rest, approximately what percentage of the oxygen flowing through the coronary arteries is extracted by the myocardium?**
   a. 30%
   b. 60%
   c. 80%
   d. 100%
   e. none of the above

2. **Following exercise, blood pressure:**
   a. remains elevated for 1 to 2 hours
   b. immediately returns to the pre-exercise level
   c. remains elevated only for 10 to 15 minutes
   d. falls below pre-exercise levels for several hours or longer
   e. none of the above

3. **The main substrates used by the heart for energy include all of the following except:**
   a. amino acids
   b. fatty acids
   c. glucose
   d. lactic acid
   e. pyruvic acid

4. **The brief interval in the cardiac cycle when ventricular tension rises but the heart volume and muscle fiber length remain unchanged is termed the _____ period:**
   a. Frank-Starling
   b. isometric contraction
   c. isovolumetric contraction
   d. stretch-recoil
   e. refractory

5. **Snow shoveling is a potentially dangerous physical activity for the cardiac patient because it:**
   a. causes a significant reduction in cardiac output
   b. augments the release of the oxygen-wasting hormone acetylcholine
   c. greatly reduces the contractile capacity of the myocardium
   d. results in a significant increase in the RPP
   e. eliminates the Frank-Starling mechanism

6. **Large quantities of blood can move from peripheral veins into the central circulation by means of:**
   a. venous dilation
   b. venous constriction
   c. arterial stability
   d. arterial constriction
   e. none of the above

7. **Gradually cooling down after exercise is recommended because:**
   a. a sudden drop in core temperature results if exercise is stopped abruptly
   b. abrupt cessation of upright exercise may lead to a drop in venous return
   c. abrupt cessation of upright exercise causes an increase in lactic acid production
   d. abrupt cessation of upright exercise may lead to a drop in cardiac output
   e. b and d

8. **Which is the <u>false</u> statement concerning the myocardium?**
   a. myocardial tissue is almost totally dependent on the energy from aerobic metabolism
   b. whereas skeletal muscle can increase its oxygen supply by increasing its a-v O_2 difference and blood supply, the myocardium is almost totally dependent on increased blood flow to increase its oxygen supply.
   c. the work of the myocardium in exercise is nicely estimated from the product of heart rate and systolic blood pressure
   d. the hormones epinephrine and norepinephrine generally reduce myocardial contractility
   e. none of the above

9. **Which is the <u>false</u> statement concerning the blood pressure response of healthy people during moderate steady-rate exercise?**
   a. diastolic blood pressure remains relatively unchanged and may even decrease slightly
   b. systolic blood pressure increases rapidly and levels off between 140 and 160 mm Hg
   c. compared to steady-rate leg exercise, arm exercise at the same oxygen uptake is generally performed with a lower systolic blood pressure
   d. the magnitude of one's blood pressure is intimately linked to the cardiac output and the total peripheral resistance
   e. none of the above

10. **This term refers to systolic ejection against the resistance encountered to arterial blood flow:**
    a. preload
    b. Starling effect
    c. afterstretch
    d. afterload
    e. prestretch

TRUE/FALSE

1. _____ Afterload is a more complete emptying during systole despite an increasing systolic pressure.
2. _____ Heart rate times diastolic blood pressure provides a good estimate of the heart's workload.
3. _____ Systolic pressure is higher at similar power outputs performed with the arms than with the legs.
4. _____ The inferior vena cava empties blood into the lower half of the body.
5. _____ The volume of flow in a blood vessel is directly proportional to the pressure gradient between the two ends of the vessel, and not the absolute pressure within the vessel.
6. _____ Diastolic plus systolic pressures × one-third of HR provides a good estimate of the heart's workload.
7. _____ When performing heavy resistance exercise training, the systolic and diastolic blood pressures mirror the hypertensive state of an individual.
8. _____ Static-type exercises tend to increase the myocardial oxygen uptake disproportionately compared to rhythmic or dynamic exercise at the same oxygen uptake.
9. _____ In terms of energy metabolism, the heart uses whatever substrate is available to it on a physiologic level.
10. _____ The RPP is an estimate of the relative stress of exercise based on perception of strain or effort.

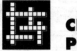

CROSSWORD PUZZLE

ACROSS

2   Heart valve between right atrium and right ventricle

6   Atypical accumulation of fluid in the interstitial space

9   Valves between atria and ventricles

11 Heart attack (abbr.)

13 Diseased vein

14 Contraction phase of cardiac cycle

15 Blood clot that forms in the vascular circuit

19 Blood pressure = cardiac output × total _____ _____

25 Index of relative cardiac work (abbr.)

27 Accumulation of blood in veins of lower extremities

29 High blood pressure

31 Method for measuring blood pressure that involves sound

32 Small artery that supplies blood to capillaries

DOWN

1   Instrument to measure blood pressure

3   Component of circulatory system that delivers (and returns) blood to all tissues except lungs

4   Vein leading into right atrium

5   Relaxation phase of cardiac cycle

7   Carries blood away from the heart

8   Crown-like grouping of arteries

10 Deficiency of tissues' oxygen supply

12 Ventricular contraction period where heart volume and muscle fiber length remain unchanged

16 Valve that prevents backflow from left ventricle to left atrium

17 Small vein

18 Blood vessels that contain valves

20 Sensory organ that could be adversely affected by inversion exercise

21 Neurohormone released by vagus nerve

22 Muscular partition between the right and left sides of the heart

23 Chest pain with ischemic myocardium

24 Blood vessel where diffusion occurs

26 Another word for heart muscle

28 Major artery from the heart

30 Component of coronary circulation that receives blood from tissues of left ventricle

31 Exercise with this musculature causes a larger increase in blood pressure

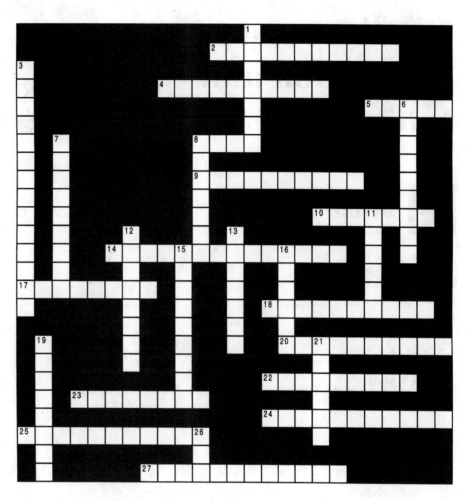

See page 370 for Crossword Puzzle Solution.

Cardiovascular Regulation and Integration

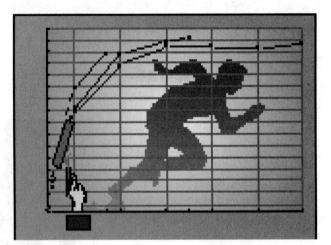

 DEFINE KEY TERMS AND CONCEPTS

1. Intrinsic regulation

2. S-A node

3. A-V node

4. Bundle of His

5. A-V bundle

6. Purkinje system

7. ECG

8. P wave

9. QRS complex

10. **T wave**

11. **Refractory period**

12. **Extrinsic regulation**

13. **Ventrolateral medulla**

14. **Catecholamines**

15. **Tachycardia**

16. **Adrenergic fibers**

17. **Cholinergic fibers**

18. **Vasomotor tone**

19. **Acetylcholine**

20. **Bradycardia**

21. **Vagus nerve**

22. **Baroreceptors**

23. **Exercise pressor reflex**

24. **Carotid artery palpation**

25. **Venoconstriction**

26. **Poiseuille's law**

27. **Autoregulatory mechanisms**

28. **Orthotopic transplantation**

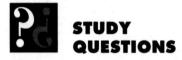

STUDY QUESTIONS

INTRINSIC REGULATION OF HEART RATE

Name the heart's "pacemaker" and indicate its role.

- Name

- Role

List the route for the electrical impulse of the heart from the S-A node into the ventricles. (*Hint: Refer to Figure 16.1 in your textbook.*)

The Heart's Electrical Activity

Where does the electrical impulse for the heart originate?

The Electrocardiogram (ECG)

Draw and label a typical ECG tracing.

List two uses for the ECG.

1.

2.

EXTRINSIC REGULATION OF THE HEART AND CIRCULATION

Name the cardiovascular control center that regulates the output of blood from the heart and its distribution.

Sympathetic and Parasympathetic Neural Input

What autonomic neural fibers stimulate the atria and ventricles?

- Atria

- Ventricles

Sympathetic Influence

What effects do the catecholamines have on heart rate?

Name the two catecholamines.

1.

2.

The sympathetic constrictor fibers are called _____ fibers.

Cholinergic nerve fibers release _____, and their action is _____.

Parasympathetic Influence

Parasympathetic fibers are carried by the _____ nerve.

What influence does acetylcholine exert on heart rate?

Training Effects

Explain why exercise training results in significant bradycardia.

Input From Higher Centers: A Central Command

Discuss the role of "central command" in cardiovascular regulation.

The heart is "turned on" in exercise by a decrease in _____ neural activity and an increase in _____ neural activity.

Peripheral Input

Indicate the effect of increased blood pressure on heart rate. Why is this beneficial?

Why isn't the carotid artery the best location to record heart rate in all conditions?

DISTRIBUTION OF BLOOD

Discuss how vasodilation and constriction contribute to maintenance of adequate exercise blood flow and blood pressure during exercise.

Physical Factors That Affect Blood Flow

List the two factors that determine the amount of blood flow through a vessel.

1.

2.

Name the "law" that governs the relationship between pressure, resistance, and fluid flow.

Effect of Exercise

List two characteristics of blood vessels that determine their volume of flow.

1.

2.

Local Factors

List two important functions served by the opening of dormant capillaries.

1.

2.

Hormonal Factors

List the two hormones from the adrenal medulla that act as chemical messengers to bring about a generalized constrictor response.

1.

2.

INTEGRATED RESPONSE IN EXERCISE

Describe the effects of neural, chemical, and hormonal factors on the cardiovascular adjustment to exercise.

• Neural

• Chemical

• Hormonal

EXERCISING AFTER CARDIAC TRANSPLANTATION: A "SLUGGISH" CIRCULATORY RESPONSE

Describe the sluggishness of the transplanted heart's response to exercise. (*Hint: Refer to Figure 16.7 in your textbook.*)

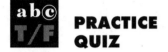 **PRACTICE QUIZ**

MULTIPLE CHOICE

1. Cholinergic fibers release _____, which causes _____.
   a. norepinephrine, vasodilation
   b. acetylcholine, vasoconstriction
   c. acetylcholine, vasodilation
   d. norepinephrine, vasoconstriction
   e. none of the above

2. Other than the active muscle, this organ receives the greatest redistribution of the blood flow during moderate exercise:
   a. kidney
   b. brain
   c. liver
   d. skin
   e. gallbladder

3. If left to its inherent rhythmicity (without any neural input), the human heart would beat steadily at about ____ beats per minute.
   a. 20
   b. 40
   c. 80
   d. 100
   e. 120

4. The heart's "pacemaker" is the:
   a. A-V node
   b. Purkinje system
   c. A-V bundle
   d. ECG
   e. none of the above

5. Cardiac muscle, unlike skeletal muscle, cannot be tetanized with repeated stimulation because of its relatively long:
   a. isovolumetric period
   b. refractory period
   c. latency period
   d. residual period
   e. prestretch-overload period

6. This part of the electrocardiogram represents repolarization of the left ventricle:
   a. S-T segment
   b. P wave
   c. QRS complex
   d. T wave
   e. b and d

7. **Which of the following are <u>true</u> statements?**
   a. the slowing of the heart rate is termed bradycardia
   b. stimulation of the vagus nerve tends to increase the left ventricle's contractility
   c. exercise training creates an imbalance between the tonic activity of the sympathetic accelerator and parasympathetic depressor neurons in favor of greater sympathetic dominance.
   d. The central command in the central nervous system provides the greatest control over the heart rate during exercise.
   e. a and d

8. **Which of the following is <u>not</u> a component of Poiseuille's law?**
   a. blood vessel length
   b. state of training
   c. blood vessel diameter
   d. blood viscosity
   e. a, b, and c

9. **Autoregulatory mechanisms to increase local blood flow include:**
   a. temperature effects
   b. carbon dioxide effects
   c. pH effects
   d. all of the above
   e. none of the above

10. **If fully dilated, the blood vessels of an adult could hold about this many liters of blood:**
    a. 5
    b. 10
    c. 20
    d. 30
    e. 40

TRUE/FALSE

1. _____ The A-V node initiates the cardiac rhythm.

2. _____ The heart's refractory period provides sufficient time for ventricular filling between heart beats.

3. _____ Adrenergic fibers are responsible for vasoconstriction.

4. _____ Catecholamines are the hormones of the parasympathetic nervous system.

5. _____ During near-maximal exercise, blood flow to the kidneys can be reduced by as much as four-fifths the resting value.

6. _____ The neural center that controls the cardiovascular system is located in the hypothalamus.

7. _____ In exercising muscles, the diameter of the arterioles increases as the intensity of exercise increases.

8. _____ Vasoconstriction permits large quantities of blood to move from peripheral veins into the central circulation.

9. _____ At rest, in a healthy, active person the myocardium receives approximately 250 mL of blood per minute, and this increases approximately 4 to 5 times during maximal exercise.

10. _____ The sinoatrial system is a specialized group of fibers that rapidly transmit the heart's electrical impulse throughout the left and right ventricles.

CROSSWORD PUZZLE

ACROSS

3 Period when ventricles cannot be stimulated

4 Blood flow is related to blood vessel's _____ raised to fourth power

6 Chemicals that act as neurotransmitters (epinephrine and norepinephrine)

9 Slow heart rate

11 State of stiffening of venous circulation

14 Nerve that slows heart rate

15 ECG component indicating atrial depolarization

18 Aspect of exercise cardiac response blunted in heart transplant patients

20 Excessive external pressure on this artery could slow heart rate

21 Pacemaker

22 Neurotransmitter that stimulates skeletal muscle

23 Opposite of cholinergic

DOWN

1 Neural tone relating to control of blood vessel diameter

2 Organ with greatly reduced blood supply during exercise

5 Graphic record of electrical changes during cardiac cycle (abbr.)

7 Described laminar fluid flow through a tube

8 Receptors sensitive to changes in blood pressure

10 Location of cardiovascular center

12 ECG component indicating ventricular repolarization

13 Rapid heart rate

16 Nerve fibers that secrete acetylcholine

17 ECG component indicating ventricular depolarization

18 Bundle of ____

19 Specialized fibers that speed impulse over ventricles

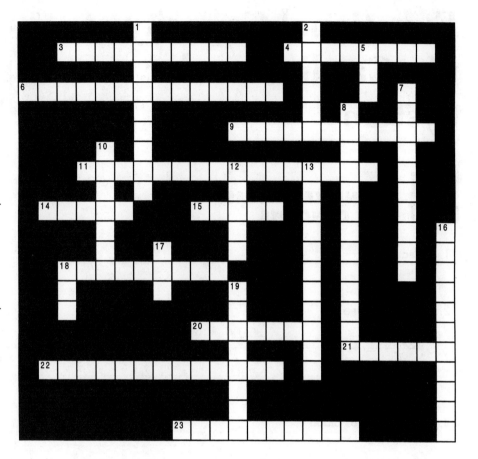

See page 370 for Crossword Puzzle Solution.

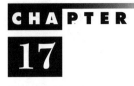

Functional Capacity of the Cardiovascular System

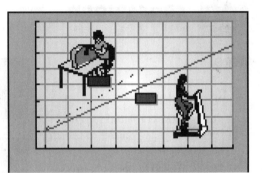

 DEFINE KEY TERMS AND CONCEPTS

1. Heart rate

2. Stroke volume

3. Cardiac output

4. Mixed venous blood

5. Fick equation

6. Invasive technique

7. Indicator dilution method

8. Noninvasive technique

9. CO_2 rebreathing

10. **End-diastolic volume**

11. **Systolic emptying**

12. **Starling's law of the heart**

13. **Preload**

14. **Afterload**

15. **Heart's functional residual volume**

16. **Eccentric hypertrophy**

17. **Shunting of blood**

18. **Visceral organs**

19. **a-$\bar{v}$ O$_2$ difference**

20. **Microcirculation**

21. **Cardiac hypertrophy**

22. **Athlete's heart**

23. **Echocardiography**

24. **Concentric hypertrophy**

25. **Pathologic hypertrophy**

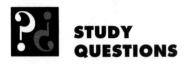

STUDY QUESTIONS

CARDIAC OUTPUT

Cardiac output = _____ × _____ .

Measurement of Cardiac Output

List three methods for measuring cardiac output.

1.

2.

3.

Direct Fick Method

Write the equation for cardiac output using the Fick procedure.

Calculate cardiac output for a person who has a $\dot{V}O_2$ of 400 mL·min^{-1} and an a-$\bar{v}O_2$ difference of 7 mL O_2·100 mL^{-1}.

Indicator Dilution Method

Describe the rationale for the indicator dilution method for cardiac output measurement.

CO_2 Rebreathing Method

List two advantages to using the CO_2 rebreathing method.

1.

2.

CARDIAC OUTPUT AT REST

Untrained

Give a typical resting cardiac output for an untrained male and female.

• Male

• Female

Endurance Athletes

What is the difference in the resting cardiac output between the trained and the untrained?

CARDIAC OUTPUT DURING EXERCISE

Draw and label the relationship between cardiac output during progressively increasing exercise oxygen uptake.

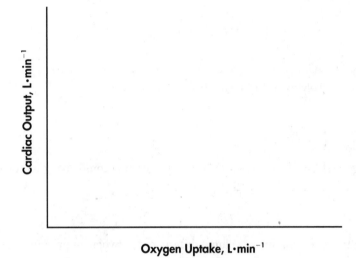

How can aerobically trained athletes achieve a higher maximum cardiac output than the untrained, even though they may have a slightly reduced maximum heart rate?

Stroke Volume in Exercise: Training Effects

Give three different statements concerning stroke volume differences between a sedentary and an aerobically trained person in response to exercise.

1.

2.

3.

Stroke Volume and $\dot{V}O_2$max

Draw and label the relationship between $\dot{V}O_2$max and maximum stroke volume for individuals who vary widely in $\dot{V}O_2$max.

Stroke Volume: Systolic Emptying versus Diastolic Filling

List two physiologic mechanisms that regulate stroke volume.

1.

2.

Enhanced Diastolic Filling

Enhanced diastolic filling is most likely to occur in what body position?

Greater Systolic Emptying

Complete the sentence: "A greater systolic ejection, with or without an accompanying increase in end-diastolic volume, is possible because _____."

Training Effects

Give three different statements concerning stroke volume differences between an untrained and an aerobically trained person in response to exercise.

1.

2.

3.

Heart Rate During Exercise: Training Effects

Draw and label the relationship between heart rate and $\dot{V}O_2$ during graded exercise for an untrained and an aerobically trained person.

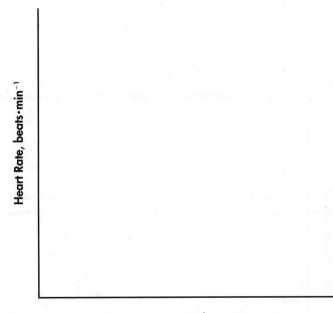

DISTRIBUTION OF CARDIAC OUTPUT

Blood Flow at Rest
Blood Flow during Exercise

Blood Flow to the Heart and Brain

Indicate the relative distribution (percent of cardiac output) of total blood flow at rest and during heavy exercise to the following organs:

	Rest	Exercise
• Muscles		
• Digestive tract		
• Liver		
• Kidneys		

Redistribution of Blood

Which two body tissues cannot tolerate a reduction in blood flow?

1.

2.

Blood Flow to the Heart and Brain

Does blood flow to the myocardium increase with increasing exercise? Discuss.

CARDIAC OUTPUT AND OXYGEN TRANSPORT

At Rest

How much oxygen is carried in each liter of a healthy person's blood?

During Exercise

At a cardiac output of 5 L·min^{-1}, how much total oxygen moves through the body each minute?

Close Association Between Maximum Cardiac Output and $\dot{V}O_2$max

Draw and label the relationship between $\dot{V}O_2$max and maximum cardiac output.

Differences in Cardiac Output Between Men and Women

Give one reason why females have a larger cardiac output than males at the same absolute submaximum $\dot{V}O_2$.

EXTRACTION OF OXYGEN: THE a-v̄ O_2 DIFFERENCE

Write the equation for calculating the a-v̄ O_2 difference.

Give an average a-v̄ O_2 difference during rest and maximum exercise.

• Rest

• Maximum exercise

a-v̄ O_2 Difference at Rest

At rest, how much of the oxygen returns "unused" to the heart in the mixed venous blood?

a-v̄ O_2 Difference in Exercise

Discuss how aerobic training can increase the a-v̄ O_2 difference.

In Heart Disease

How can a heart disease patient improve aerobic capacity if there is little training improvement in maximum cardiac output?

Factors That Affect a-$\bar{v}$ O_2 Difference in Exercise

List two factors that determine the capacity for oxygen extraction (i.e., a-$\bar{v}$ O_2 difference).

1.

2.

CARDIOVASCULAR ADJUSTMENTS TO UPPER-BODY EXERCISE

Maximal Oxygen Uptake

$\dot{V}o_2$max attained during arm exercise is about what percent different than that attained during leg exercise?

Submaximal Oxygen Uptake

What is the general trend for the difference between submaximal $\dot{V}o_2$ during arm exercise and that during leg exercise at a similar exercise power output?

Physiologic Response

List three physiologic variables that are larger during submaximal upper-body exercise compared to lower-body exercise at the same oxygen uptake.

1.

2.

3.

Implications

In terms of physiologic response, what is the main point the exercise specialist should know when designing an exercise program using upper-body and lower-body exercise?

CARDIAC HYPERTROPHY AND THE "ATHLETE'S HEART"

Discuss two of the characteristics of cardiac hypertrophy in an exercise-trained healthy heart.

1.

2.

Specific Nature of Training Hypertrophy

Give an example of how specific training can affect structural and dimensional characteristics of the hearts of different types of athletes. (*Hint: Refer to Table 17.6.*)

Functional versus Pathologic Hypertrophy

Describe one major difference between the "athlete's heart" and the enlarged heart of the individual with chronic hypertension.

Other Training Adaptations

List three adaptations of the heart that can result from regular exercise training:

1.

2.

3.

**abc
T/F PRACTICE
QUIZ**

MULTIPLE CHOICE

1. **Each 100 mL of normal blood carries about how much oxygen?**
   a. 10 mL
   b. 20 mL
   c. 50 mL
   d. 65 mL
   e. more than 65 mL

2. **Cardiac hypertrophy is a response to:**
   a. heart attack
   b. sedentary lifestyle
   c. increased protein intake
   d. increased work load placed on the myocardium
   e. all of the above

3. **Which statement is <u>true</u> about resting cardiac output?**
   a. it is about equal for the trained and the nontrained
   b. it is greater for the trained than for the nontrained
   c. it is greater for the nontrained than for the trained
   d. it is estimated by $HR \times a\text{-}\bar{v} \ O_2$
   e. a and d

4. **The average $a\text{-}\bar{v} \ O_2$ difference between arterial blood and mixed venous blood at rest is about:**
   a. 5 mL of O_2/10 mL of blood
   b. 5 mL of O_2/100 mL of blood
   c. 10 mL of O_2/50 mL of blood
   d. 30 mL of O_2/100 mL of blood
   e. none of the above

5. **The oxygen uptake is 3200 mL per minute, the $a\text{-}\bar{v} \ O_2$ difference is 160 mL O_2 per liter of blood, and the weather is cloudy. The cardiac output is _____ L per minute.**
   a. 5
   b. 10
   c. 15
   d. 20
   e. 25

6. **Cardiac output can increase about _____ times the resting level during maximal exercise in a highly trained endurance athlete.**
   a. 2 to 4
   b. 6 to 8
   c. 10 to 12
   d. 16 to 18
   e. 20 to 22

7. An anatomical "mixing chamber" that reflects the oxygen content of mixed venous blood is the:
   a. inferior vena cava
   b. hepatic vein
   c. coronary sinus
   d. right ventricle
   e. c or d

8. Which of the following is a realistic value for the maximum stroke volume of an elite male endurance athlete?
   a. 180 mL
   b. 130 mL
   c. 90 mL
   d. 60 mL
   e. none of these values are realistic

9. With an exercise cardiac output of 30 L per minute, approximately ____ L of oxygen is circulated through the arterial system each minute (assume normal levels of blood hemoglobin and arterial saturation).
   a. 3
   b. 4
   c. 5
   d. 6
   e. 8

10. Which of the following is generally **not** a physiologic characteristic of a 30-year-old elite male endurance athlete?
    a. a maximum heart rate usually between 180 and 200 beats per minute
    b. a maximum cardiac output usually between 30 and 40 L·min^{-1}
    c. eccentric ventricular hypertrophy
    d. sinus tachycardia at rest
    e. c and d

TRUE/FALSE

1. _____ At rest, approximately 4 to 7 mL of blood is delivered each minute to every 100 grams of muscle.

2. _____ Sex differences in cardiac output occur because men have lower heart rates than women.

3. _____ The larger maximum cardiac output of the aerobically trained athlete compared to the nonathlete is mainly due to the trained athlete's lower maximum heart rate.

4. _____ During rest, the total blood volume circulates around the body about 5 times per minute.

5. _____ During maximal running in an aerobically trained runner, the maximal a-v̄ O_2 difference is as large as 4 vol%.

6. _____ Fick is the last name of the person who described the method for measuring cardiac output from measures of oxygen uptake and a-v̄ O_2 difference.

7. _____ The enlarged left ventricular volume of aerobically trained athletes is termed eccentric hypertrophy.

8. _____ A person with a maximum heart rate of 196 beats per minute and a maximum stroke volume of 154 mL per beat generates a maximum cardiac output of 24.2 L per minute.

9. _____ For any level of oxygen uptake or percent of maximum, the physiologic strain is greater in upper-body than in lower-body exercise.

10. _____ The myocardium of resistance-trained athletes tends to demonstrate what is termed concentric hypertrophy.

CROSSWORD PUZZLE

ACROSS

1 This cardiac volume is extremely large in endurance athletes

3 Term for lying down

5 Endurance training increases the influence of this nerve on the heart

8 $\dot{V}O_2 = 2.4$ L·min^{-1} and a-$\bar{v}$ O_2 difference = 12 vol%; the cardiac output is _____ L·min^{-1}

9 Method not requiring entering a body cavity

11 Physiologist who described force-length characteristics of cardiac muscle

13 Ultrasound technique to study heart structure

16 Hypertrophy that reflects enlarged ventricular chamber

20 Related to arterial pressure that a ventricle must overcome during systolic ejection

21 Cardiac output measurement technique involving CO_2

22 One of the small vessels that increase in number with aerobic training

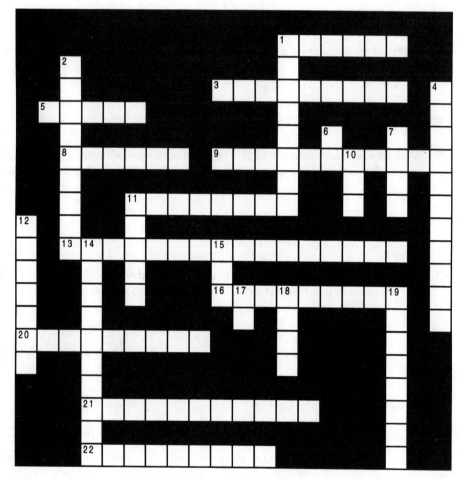

DOWN

1 Diversion of blood from one body region to another

2 Number of ventricular contractions per minute

4 Increase in muscle fiber size

6 Amount of blood pumped by the left ventricle each beat (abbr.)

7 Man who developed invasive method for measuring cardiac output

10 Physiologic strain is great during this form of exercise

11 The _____ of HR-$\dot{V}O_2$ line differs between trained and untrained

12 Increased filling during diastole

14 Hypertrophy that reflects enlarged ventricular mass

15 Dilution technique to measure cardiac output

17 Volume of blood pumped by left ventricle in 1 minute (abbr.)

18 Ultrasound waves map the heart's structure (abbr.)

19 Flexible tube inserted into blood vessel

See page 371 for Crossword Puzzle Solution.

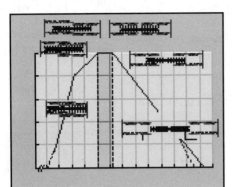

Skeletal Muscle: Structure and Function

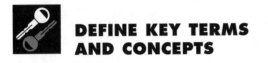

DEFINE KEY TERMS AND CONCEPTS

1. **Endomysium**

2. **Perimysium**

3. **Fasciculus**

4. **Epimysium**

5. **Fusiform**

6. **Pennate**

7. **Physiological cross-sectional area (PCSA)**

8. **Tendons**

9. **Periosteum**

10. **Origin**

11. **Insertion**

12. **Sarcolemma**

13. **Sarcoplasm**

14. **Sarcoplasmic reticulum**

15. **Myoglobin**

16. **Fibrils/myofibrils**

17. **Filaments/myofilaments**

18. **Actin**

19. **Myosin**

20. **Troponin**

21. **Tropomyosin**

22. **Sarcomere**

23. **Striated**

24. **T-tubule system**

25. **Crossbridges**

26. **Triad**

27. **Sliding-filament theory**

28. **Actomyosin**

29. **Myosin ATPase**

30. **Excitation-contraction coupling**

31. **Rigor mortis**

32. **Fast-twitch muscle fiber**

33. **Slow-twitch muscle fiber**

34. **Type I fiber**

35. **Type II fiber**

36. **FOG fiber**

37. **FG fiber**

38. **Type IIc fiber**

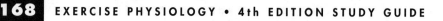

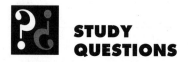

STUDY QUESTIONS

GROSS STRUCTURE OF SKELETAL MUSCLE

Draw and label a muscle's cross section. (*Hint: Refer to Figure 18.1 in your textbook.*)

Levels of Organization

Give one difference between the endomysium and epimysium.

The stable skeletal part to which the muscle attaches is the _____; the distal attachment of the muscle to the moving bone is the _____.

Chemical Composition

Indicate the percentage composition of skeletal muscle for the following:

- Water

- Protein

- Other

List the three most abundant muscle proteins.

1.

2.

3.

Blood Supply

Describe the effect of straining-type muscular activities on blood flow in the active muscle.

Capillarization of Muscle

The capillarization of skeletal muscle is about ____% greater in endurance athletes than in untrained counterparts.

There are approximately ____ capillaries per square millimeter of skeletal muscle.

Ultrastructure of Skeletal Muscle

Draw a diagram showing the microscopic anatomy of a muscle sarcomere. Identify the actin and myosin filaments, the I and A bands, the Z line, and the H zone. (*Hint: Refer to Figure 18.2 in your textbook.*)

The Sarcomere

Which cellular component gives the muscle fiber its striated appearance?

Name the functional unit of the muscle fiber.

Name the two contractile proteins found in the sarcomere.

1.

2.

Alignment of Sarcomeres in a Muscle Fiber

Which muscle arrangement type, fusiform or pennate, allows for packing a larger number of fibers into a relatively small cross-sectional area?

Fiber Length to Muscle Length Ratio

What is the normal ratio of individual fiber length to a muscle's total length?

Describe the difference in the muscle force-muscle length and the muscle force-muscle velocity relationships for fusiform and pennate muscle. (*Hint: Refer to Figure 18.5 in your textbook.*)

• Fusiform

• Pennate

Actin-Myosin Orientation

What is the structural link between thin and thick myofilaments?

List the two proteins of the myofibrillar complex and their function.

Protein   Function

1.

2.

Intracellular Tubule Systems

Describe the function of the triad and T-tubule system.

CHEMICAL AND MECHANICAL EVENTS DURING CONTRACTION AND RELAXATION
Sliding-Filament Theory

List five important facts in the sequencing of muscle action according to the sliding-filament theory.

1.

2.

3.

4.

5.

Mechanical Action of the Crossbridges

Discuss the role of the globular head of the myosin crossbridge in muscle action.

Sarcomere Length-Isometric Tension Curve in an Isolated Fiber

Draw and label a typical "length-tension" curve for skeletal muscle. (*Hint: Refer to Figure 18.11 in your textbook.*)
Link Between Actin, Myosin, and ATP

Write the formula for the dissociation of actomyosin.

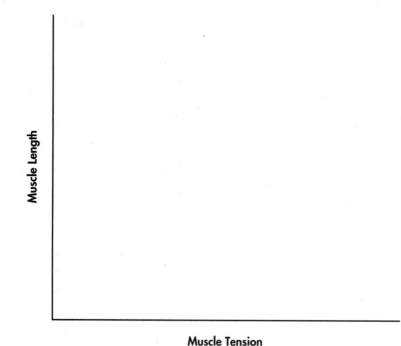

Excitation-Contraction Coupling

Describe the role of calcium in the process of excitation-contraction coupling.

Relaxation

List two purposes of "deactivation" during the relaxation period.

1.

2.

Describe the dynamics of intracellular calcium when a muscle is no longer stimulated.

Sequence of Events in Muscle Action

With several key words, describe nine main events in muscle action.

1.   6.

2.   7.

3.   8.

4.   9.

5.

MUSCLE FIBER TYPE

List the two muscle fiber types and classify each by its contractile and metabolic characteristics.

Type	Contractile Characteristics	Metabolic Characteristics
1.		
2.		

Fast-Twitch Fibers

Fast-twitch fibers are activated in what types of physical activity?

Slow-Twitch Fibers

Slow-twitch muscle fibers are activated in what types of physical activity?

Fast-Twitch Subdivisions

Name the three subdivisions of the fast-twitch fiber group.

1.

2.

3.

Species Differences: A Brief Comparative Look

Describe one difference in muscle fiber type between humans and other nonhuman species.

Differences Between Athletic Groups

Which athletic group has the highest percentage of slow-twitch muscle fibers?

True or False: There is a clear-cut distinction between exercise performance and muscle fiber composition for elite athletes.

Can Muscle Fibers Type Be Changed?

Is it possible to change muscle fiber type with training? Discuss.

Metabolic Adaptations Are Real and Significant

List three changes that occur in skeletal muscle with specific exercise training. (*Hint: Refer to Table 18.3 in your textbook.*)

1.

2.

3.

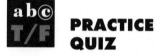 **PRACTICE QUIZ**

MULTIPLE CHOICE

1. **The percentage distribution of muscle fiber type among humans:**
   a. is predominantly slow twitch
   b. does not differ significantly
   c. can differ significantly
   d. is predominantly fast twitch
   e. b and c

2. **The metabolic capacity of:**
   a. slow-twitch fibers does not improve with specific endurance and power training
   b. fast-twitch fibers does not improve with specific endurance and power training
   c. both slow-twitch and fast-twitch fibers improves markedly with specific endurance and power training
   d. muscle fibers is fixed by genetic code and cannot improve with specific endurance and power training
   e. muscle fibers depends solely on hypertrophic neurotransmitters

3. **Muscle fibers are generally classified by their:**
   a. size and color
   b. size and neuronal innervation
   c. contractile and metabolic characteristics
   d. nutrient use and fatigue characteristics
   e. none of the above

4. **The major function of tropomyosin is to:**
   a. stimulate crossbridge shortening
   b. inhibit calcium uptake by the mitochondria
   c. inhibit actin and myosin interaction
   d. enable motor neuron excitation
   e. all of the above

5. **There is some research evidence that:**
   a. specific training (and perhaps inactivity) may induce an actual conversion of type I to type II fibers (or vice versa)
   b. FOG fibers can be converted to SO fibers with anaerobic training
   c. general aerobic training induces the transformation of type I to type IIa fiber
   d. SO fibers are converted into FG fibers with aerobic training
   e. a and b

6. **When a muscle is no longer stimulated, the flow of calcium:**
    a. increases and troponin is free to inhibit actin-myosin interaction
    b. increases and troponin levels decrease
    c. increases to cause an uncoupling of actin and myosin
    d. increases and actin is inhibited
    e. none of the above

7. **The sliding-filament theory proposes that muscle fibers shorten or lengthen because:**
    a. thick and thin myofilaments slide past each other and change length
    b. thick and thin myofilaments slide into each other
    c. thick and thin myofilaments slide past each other and retain length
    d. the sliding-filament theory does not propose that muscles shorten or lengthen
    e. thick and thin filaments require magnesium during depolarization

8. **Which of the following statements is true:**
    a. type I fibers are fast-twitch
    b. type IIa fibers are fast-twitch
    c. type IIb fibers are slow-twitch
    d. type IIc fibers are the most common
    e. b and c

9. **The fiber type with high capacity for both aerobic and anaerobic energy transfer is:**
    a. FG
    b. SO
    c. FOG
    d. FO
    e. none of the above

10. **Aerobic exercise training:**
    a. probably does not alter muscle fiber type to any large degree
    b. makes type I muscle fibers act like type II fibers
    c. results in dramatic changes in muscle function and fiber type
    d. increases the actual number of motor units
    e. a and b

TRUE/FALSE

1. _____ The sarcomere is the functional unit of the muscle cell.

2. _____ The crossbridges provide the structural link between tropomyosin and the sarcoplasmic reticulum.

3. _____ The microtransportation network for spreading the action potential from the fiber's outer membrane inward to the deep regions of the cell is the sarcoplasmic reticulum.

4. _____ The percentage distribution of muscle fiber type is largely determined by genetic code.

5. _____ Muscle action occurs when calcium activates actin, causing the myosin crossbridges to attach to active sites on the actin filaments.

6. _____ Seventy-five percent of skeletal muscle is composed of protein.

7. _____ Improved exercise capacity with training may occur by decreases in capillary density of the trained muscles.

8. _____ Tropomyosin has a high affinity for calcium ions.

9. _____ Fast-twitch fibers are predominantly activated during endurance activities.

10. _____ The metabolic capacity of muscle fiber types can be improved by specific training.

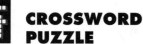

CROSSWORD PUZZLE

ACROSS

1 Blood flow is occluded when muscle generates about ____ percent of its force-generating capacity

2 Globular "lollipop-like" heads on myosin filaments

5 Repeating pattern of two vesicles and T tubules in region of each Z line

6 Muscle form resembling a feather

9 Layer of connective tissue surrounding entire muscle

13 One of two major myofibril proteins

17 Muscle protein of actin filaments

18 Skeletal muscle is this classification

20 Theory that explains muscle contraction

27 _____ reticulum is the extensive network of tubular channels in muscle fiber

29 Region where the tendon joins a relatively stable skeletal part

30 Rare subdivision of fast-twitch fibers

31 Spindle-shaped type of muscle with long fibers

33 Physiological cross-sectional area (abbr.)

34 Muscle-bone attachment distal to body

DOWN

2 Crucial mineral in muscle

3 Functional unit of muscle fiber

4 When muscle becomes stiff and rigid soon after death

5 Slow-twitch muscle fibers

7 Outermost covering of skeleton

8 Layer of connective tissue surrounding a fasciculus

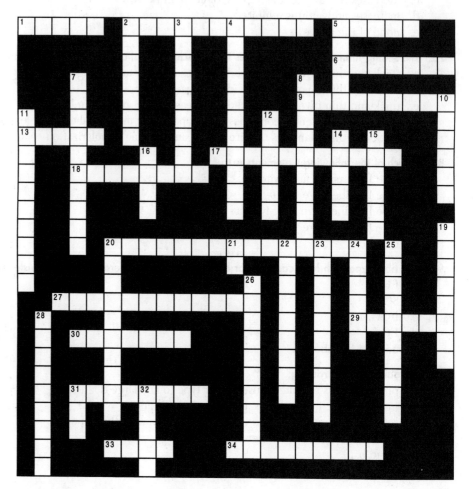

10 Protein found in thick filaments

11 Fiber type with high capability for power activities

12 Fast-twitch muscle fibers

14 Type of athlete favored by type II fibers

15 Series of sarcomeres

16 ____-twitch fibers have a high level of myosin ATPase

19 Muscle protein in the actin fibers

20 Cytoplasm of muscle fiber

21 Muscle fiber type with fast contraction speed and high anaerobic power (abbr.)

22 Efferent system that activates viscera

23 Connective tissue layer around each muscle fiber

24 Connects both ends of the muscle to outermost covering of skeleton

25 Bundle of up to 150 muscle fibers

26 Interaction of these protein filaments causes movement

28 Functional unit of muscle

31 Intermediate type of fast-twitch fiber with high oxidative capacity (abbr.)

32 High _____ is produced in FF motor units

See page 371 for Crossword Puzzle Solution.

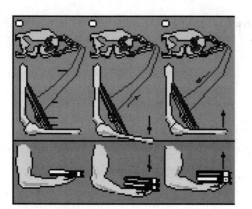

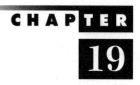

Neural Control of Human Movement

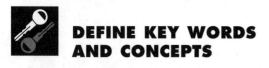

DEFINE KEY WORDS AND CONCEPTS

1. Central nervous system

2. Peripheral nervous system

3. Brain stem

4. Reticular formation

5. Cerebellum

6. Hypothalamus

7. Telencephalon

8. Limbic system

9. Spinal cord

10. Efferent neurons

11. **Afferent neurons**

12. **Ascending nerve tracts**

13. **Chemoreceptors**

14. **Baroreceptors**

15. **Descending nerve tracts**

16. **Pyramidal tract**

17. **Alpha motoneurons**

18. **Extrapyramidal tract**

19. **Reticular formation**

20. **Peripheral nervous system**

21. **Somatic nerves**

22. **Autonomic nervous system**

23. **Sympathetic nervous system**

24. **Parasympathetic nervous system**

25. **Reflex arc**

26. **Motor unit**

27. **Anterior motoneuron**

28. **Axon**

29. **Dendrites**

30. **Myelin sheath**

31. **Nodes of Ranvier**

32. **Neuromuscular junction**

33. **Action potential**

34. **Cholinesterase**

35. **EPSP**

36. **Temporal summation**

37. **Neuronal facilitation**

38. **IPSP**

39. **All-or-none principle**

40. **Motor unit recruitment**

41. **Size principle**

42. **Asynchronous motor unit firing**

43. **EMG**

44. **Proprioceptors**

45. **Muscle spindles**

46. **Extrafusal fibers**

47. **Intrafusal fibers**

48. **Gamma-efferent fibers**

49. **Stretch reflex**

50. **Golgi tendon organs**

51. **Reflex inhibition**

52. **Pacinian corpuscles**

53. **Generator potential**

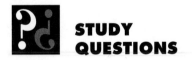 **STUDY QUESTIONS**

ORGANIZATION OF THE NEUROMOTOR SYSTEM

List the two major parts of the human nervous system.

1.

2.

Central Nervous System—The Brain

List the six main areas of the brain and give one fact about each.

Main Area   Fact

1.

2.

3.

4.

5.

6.

Central Nervous System—The Spinal Cord

There are _____ [number] vertebrae in the human spinal column.

What are the functional roles of the ventral and dorsal horns of the spinal cord?

- Ventral horn

- Dorsal horn

Ascending Nerve Tracts

The ascending nerve tracts send _____ information from _____ receptors to the _____.

Sensory Receptors

List four factors monitored by the body's peripheral sensory receptors.

1.   3.

2.   4.

Descending Nerve Tracts

Name and give the function of the two major pathways that constitute the descending nerve tracts.

Pathway   Function

1.

2.

List the four structures that interconnect with the reticular formation.

1.   3.

2.   4.

Peripheral Nervous System

List the two types of peripheral efferent nerves.

1.

2.

What is always the result of somatic efferent nerve firing?

List the number of pairs of spinal nerves for the following regions of the spinal cord.

- Cervical

- Thoracic

- Lumbar

- Sacral

- Coccygeal

Autonomic Nerves

What is the major function of the autonomic nervous system?

Sympathetic and Parasympathetic Nervous System

Indicate the areas of the body innervated by the sympathetic and parasympathetic nervous systems.

- Sympathetic

- Parasympathetic

The Reflex Arc

Draw and label a typical autonomic reflex arc in the spinal cord. (*Hint: Refer to Figure 19.5 in your textbook.*)

Motor Unit Anatomy

List the two components of a motor unit

1.

2.

Anterior Motoneuron

List and give the function for three parts of an anterior motoneuron.

    Part   Function

1.

2.

3.

Explain how the structure and location of motor units result in a more effective application of force and a diminished mechanical stress.

Neuromuscular Junction (Motor Endplate)

What is the primary function of the neuromuscular junction?

Excitation

What is the role of acetylcholine in neuromuscular excitation?

Facilitation

Describe two situations in which temporal summation could enhance exercise performance.

1.

2.

Inhibition

What happens if a motoneuron is subjected to both excitatory and inhibitory influences, and the IPSP is large?

Motor Unit Physiology

Fill in the following table concerning the physiologic and mechanical properties of muscle fiber types and motor units.

Motor Unit Type	Force Production	Contraction		Muscle Fiber Type
		Speed	Fatigue	
Fast Fatigable (FF)				
Fast-Fatigue Resistance (FR)				
Slow (S)				

Twitch Characteristics

List the three categories of motor units with respect to speed, force, and fatigue characteristics.

1.

2.

3.

All-or-None Principle

State the all-or-none principle in 20 words or less.

Graduation of Force

List the two factors contributing to one's ability to vary the force of muscular action.

1.

2.

Motor Unit Recruitment

Why don't all of the motor units in a muscle fire at the same time during a submaximal muscle action?

Neuromuscular Fatigue

List four factors that could explain muscular fatigue during exercise.

1.   3.

2.   4.

RECEPTORS IN MUSCLES, JOINTS, AND TENDONS: THE PROPRIOCEPTORS

List the three variables that are monitored by the body's proprioceptors:

1.

2.

3.

Muscle Spindles

Describe the major function of muscle spindles.

List the three main components of the stretch reflex.

1.

2.

3.

Golgi Tendon Organs

What is the major function of the Golgi tendon organs?

Pacinian Corpuscles

List the two sensory variables monitored by the pacinian corpuscles.

1.

2.

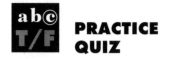

PRACTICE QUIZ

MULTIPLE CHOICE

1. **The function of the pyramidal tract is to regulate:**
   a. postural movements
   b. background level of neuromuscular tone
   c. discrete muscle movements
   d. facial movements only
   e. none of the above

2. **The basic neural component for controlling so-called automatic muscular movements is the:**
   a. cerebellum
   b. basal ganglia
   c. reflex arc
   d. motor unit
   e. none of the above

3. **The number of muscle fibers in a motor unit depends upon:**
   a. size of the muscle
   b. strength of the muscle
   c. movement function of the muscle
   d. the resting level of cholinesterase at the neuromuscular junction
   e. all of the above

4. **Fast-twitch muscle fibers are commonly associated with all of the following except:**
   a. large motoneurons with fast conduction velocities
   b. high peak tension
   c. resistance to fatigue
   d. great force capacity
   e. none of the above

5. **The function of the pacinian corpuscles is to detect:**
   a. quick movement and deep pressure
   b. changes in muscle tension
   c. changes in length of the muscle fiber
   d. motor unit firing pattern
   e. none of the above

6. **The functional unit of the muscle cell is the:**
   a. motor unit
   b. sarcomere
   c. endomysium
   d. neuron
   e. none of the above

7. **The _____ is the major comparing, evaluating, and integrating center that provides the "fine tuning" for muscular movement:**
   a. spinal cord
   b. sensorimotor cortex
   c. cerebellum
   d. brain stem
   e. cerebrum

8. **The anterior motoneuron:**
   a. transmits electrochemical nerve impulses to the spinal cord from the muscles
   b. transmits electrochemical nerve impulses from the spinal cord to the muscle
   c. is the major interface between the spinal cord and the muscle fiber
   d. is the major integrating center for movement
   e. transmits sensory root information to the presynaptic clefts

9. **Strength improvements with training, especially during the early stages of training, can be largely explained by:**
   a. increases in the actual number of motor units
   b. increases in the size of the trained muscles
   c. alterations in motor unit recruitment and firing patterns
   d. decreases in the size of the neuromuscular junction
   e. alterations in the sensitivity to epinephrine

10. **Golgi tendon organs function to:**
   a. increase the size of muscle fibers during training
   b. change electrical potential of the nerve endings
   c. decrease motor unit firing during light exercise
   d. protect the muscle and its connective tissue harness from injury due to an excessive load
   e. c and d

TRUE/FALSE

1. _____ The anterior motoneuron transmits the nerve impulse from the spinal cord to the muscle.

2. _____ The IPSP excites the neuron, increasing the likelihood of its firing.

3. _____ Changes in fiber type explain a large portion of strength improvements with resistance training.

4. _____ The interneurons receive information from the sensory root of the reflex arc.

5. _____ The reticular formation transmits impulses that inhibit neurons to the antigravity muscles.

6. _____ The functional significance of the muscle spindle is that it senses deep pressure under stress.

7. _____ The differential control of the motor unit firing pattern is the same in skilled and unskilled performers.

8. _____ It is not possible to "fatigue" the neuromuscular junction.

9. _____ Excitation occurs everywhere in the muscle except the neuromuscular junction.

10. _____ The "all-or-none law" only relates to the functioning of cardiac muscle.

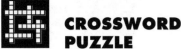

CROSSWORD PUZZLE

ACROSS

2 Nervous system that includes brain and spinal cord (abbr.)

4 Sensory nerve fibers enter the spinal cord through the _____ horn

6 Neuron that carries impulses toward the brain

7 Law stating that a motor unit either responds completely or not at all to a stimulus

8 Nerve tract that transmits impulses from brain to spinal cord

12 Part of the brain responsible for posture, locomotion, and equilibrium

15 This nervous system includes the cranial and spinal nerves

18 Component of nervous system associated with forebrain and concerned with emotional behavior and learning

22 Large efferent neurons that innervate striated muscle

28 Tracing of brain's electrical activity (abbr.)

29 These nodes speed transmission of nerve impulses

30 This effect on neurons makes them harder to fire (abbr.)

31 Nerve fibers that carry impulses away from the CNS

32 Pertaining to the body

33 Adding more motor units to increase force production is called motor unit _____

DOWN

1 Regulates autonomic nervous system and endocrine glands

2 Another term for pyramidal tract

3 First word of sensory receptors in ligaments

5 Transmits nerve impulses toward cell body of neuron

6 Transmits nerve impulses away from cell body of neuron

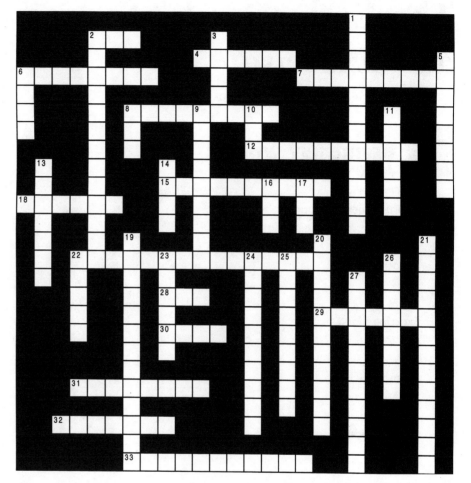

8 Nervous system that includes spinal nerves (abbr.)

9 Anterior motoneuron and specific muscle fibers it innervates

10 Reflex _____ composed of a sensory neuron, spinal interneurons, and anterior motoneuron

11 Nerve cell

13 Monitors changes in muscle length and tension

14 This effect on neurons makes them easier to fire (abbr.)

16 Tracing of muscle's electrical activity

17 Autonomic nervous system (abbr.)

19 Receptor stimulated by chemical state of fluid bathing it

20 Neuron that relays information to various levels of cord

21 Sensory organ in muscles, tendons, and joints

22 These motoneurons control skeletal muscle activity

23 Lipid-protein sheath around axon

24 Specialized fibers attached in parallel to regular muscle fibers

25 Basic unit of involuntary neural control

26 Specialized sensory receptor corpuscles in the skin that respond to firm pressure and quick movement

27 A _____ pattern of motor unit firing occurs in weightlifting

See page 371 for Crossword Puzzle Solution.

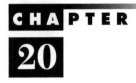

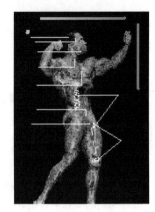

The Endocrine System and Exercise

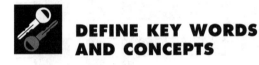

DEFINE KEY WORDS AND CONCEPTS

1. **Neuroendocrine organ**

2. **Endocrine gland**

3. **Exocrine gland**

4. **Hormone**

5. **Prostaglandins**

6. **Hormone-receptor binding**

7. **Host gland**

8. **Receptor organ**

9. **Target cells**

10. **Up-regulation**

11. **Downregulation**

12. **Cyclic AMP**

13. **Allosteric modulation**

14. **Hormonal stimulation**

15. **Humoral stimulation**

16. **Neural stimulation**

17. **Hypophysis**

18. **POMC**

19. **Somatomedin**

20. **Somatotropin**

21. **Somatostatin**

22. **TSH**

23. **ACTH**

24. **PRL**

25. **FSH**

26. **LH**

27. **Neurohypophysis**

28. **ADH**

29. **Oxytocin**

30. **Thyroxine**

31. **Triiodothyronine**

32. **Adrenal medulla**

33. **Adrenal cortex**

34. **Catecholamines**

35. **Adrenocortical hormones**

36. **Mineralocorticoids**

37. **Aldosterone**

38. **Angiotensin**

39. **Glucocorticoids**

40. **Cortisol**

41. **Androgens**

42. **Acini**

43. **Islets of Langerhans**

44. **Alpha cell secretion**

45. **Beta cell secretion**

46. **Insulin**

47. **Glucose-insulin feedback interaction**

48. **Catecholamine suppression of insulin**

49. **Type I diabetes**

50. **Type II diabetes**

51. **The "insulin antagonist"**

52. **Improved insulin sensitivity**

53. **Opioid peptides**

54. **URTI**

55. **NK cells**

56. **T cells** _____

_____

57. **Natural immune function** _____

_____

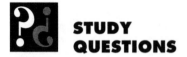 **STUDY QUESTIONS**

ENDOCRINE SYSTEM OVERVIEW
ENDOCRINE SYSTEM ORGANIZATION

List the three components of the endocrine system.

1.

2.

3.

What determines whether a gland is classified as endocrine or exocrine?

Nature of Hormones

List three chemical categories of hormones.

1.

2.

3.

Hormone-Target Cell Specificity

What is the major function of hormones? Indicate three ways this function is accomplished.

- Function
- Accomplished by

1.

2.

3.

Hormone-Receptor Binding

List the three factors that determine a target cell's activation.

1.

2.

3.

Cyclic AMP: The Intracellular Messenger
What is the "first messenger in hormone function"?

What is the role of cyclic AMP as an intracellular messenger?

List three factors that initiate the action of cyclic AMP.

1.

2.

3.

Effects on Enzymes
List the three ways in which hormones increase enzyme activity.

1.

2.

3.

Factors That Determine Hormone Levels
List three ways that endocrine glands are stimulated and give one example of each.

	Stimulation	Example
1.		
2.		
3.		

List two factors that determine blood hormone concentration.

1.

2.

RESTING AND EXERCISE-INDUCED ENDOCRINE SECRETIONS
ANTERIOR PITUITARY HORMONES
What is another name for the pituitary gland?

List six different hormones secreted from the pituitary gland.

1.   4.

2.   5.

3.   6.

Growth Hormone

What is the major function of GH?

In what way can GH contribute to one's ability to perform endurance exercise and respond to training?

- Endurance exercise

- Training response

GH, Exercise, and Tissue Synthesis

What is the GH response during a bout of exercise?

Give one possible way GH secreted during exercise enhances protein synthesis.

What is IGF?

Thyrotropin

What is the major function of TSH?

Corticotropin

What is the major function of ACTH?

Prolactin

What is the major function of PRL?

Gonadotropic Hormones

List two gonadotropic hormones and their major function.

Hormone	Function
1.	
2.	

POSTERIOR PITUITARY HORMONES

List two posterior pituitary hormones and their major function.

Hormone	Function
1.	
2.	

THYROID HORMONES

List two thyroid hormones and their major function.

	Hormone	Function
1.		
2.		

ADRENAL HORMONES

List two parts of the adrenal gland.

1.

2.

Adrenal Medulla Hormones

List two hormones of the adrenal medulla and their major function.

	Hormone	Function
1.		
2.		

Discuss the term "sympathoadrenal response."

Adrenocortical Hormones

List three groups of adrenocortical hormones and their major function.

	Hormone	Function
1.		
2.		
3.		

Cortisol

List three major effects of cortisol release on metabolism.

1.

2.

3.

PANCREATIC HORMONES

Name two types of pancreatic tissue and the function of each.

	Tissue	Function
1.		
2.		

Insulin

Describe the major function of insulin in carbohydrate regulation and lipid metabolism.

• Carbohydrate

• Lipid

Glucose-Insulin Interaction

What substance controls insulin secretion?

Describe the effects of the catecholamines on insulin release.

Do simple carbohydrates cause the same potential for insulin over-release when consumed during exercise as when consumed prior to exercise? Explain.

Diabetes Mellitus

List and describe the two major classifications of diabetes mellitus.

1.

2.

Indicate four beneficial aspects of exercise for patients with NIDDM.

1.

2.

3.

4.

Give four recommendations to a well-controlled type I diabetic who wishes to engage in a strenuous exercise program with minimal risk.

1.

2.

3.

4.

Diabetes and Exercise

What is the most common disturbance in glucose homeostasis during exercise for diabetics receiving exogenous insulin?

Physical Activity and Risk for NIDDM

Discuss the effect of regular exercise on the risk for developing NIDDM.

Which ethnic group has the highest incidence of NIDDM in the United States?

Exercise Benefits for NIDDM

List four benefits of exercise for those with NIDDM.

1.

2.

3.

4.

Exercise Risks for NIDDM

List three adverse effects of exercise for the patient with NIDDM. (*Hint: Refer to Figure 20.17 in your textbook.*)

1.

2.

3.

Exercise Guidelines for Type I Diabetics

List four exercise guidelines for the patient with type I diabetes.

1.

2.

3.

4.

Glucagon

Give the major function of glucagon.

EXERCISE TRAINING AND ENDOCRINE FUNCTION

During standard-load exercise, is the hormonal response higher or lower in the trained compared to the untrained? Discuss.

List six different hormones and the response of each to exercise training. (*Hint: Refer to Table 20.3 in your textbook.*)

          Hormone   Training Response

1.

2.

3.

4.

5.

6.

FSH, LH, and Testosterone
Women
In addition to alterations in FSH and LH, list two factors that may contribute to menstrual dysfunction.

1.

2.

Men
Is an impaired gonadotropin release with training responsible for reduced testosterone levels in the trained state?

Adrenal Hormones
Aldosterone
Cortisol
Describe changes in aldosterone and cortisol secretion with exercise training.

• Aldosterone

• Cortisol

Epinephrine and Norepinephrine
Describe the most familiar aspect of the sympathoadrenal training response.

Pancreatic Hormones
Insulin and Glucagon
List the two ways that regular exercise blunts the insulin response (i.e., improves insulin sensitivity) during rest and moderate exercise.

1.

2.

Exercise Training in Diabetes

Type I Diabetes

Describe the situation in which type I diabetics must be cautious regarding regular exercise.

Type II Diabetes

List four beneficial aspects of exercise for patients with NIDDM.

1.

2.

3.

4.

RESISTANCE TRAINING AND ENDOCRINE FUNCTION

List the two hormones involved in resistance training adaptations and indicate possible sex differences in the release of these hormones.

Hormone	Sex Differences

1.

2.

OPIOID PEPTIDES AND EXERCISE

List three opioid peptides.

1.

2.

3.

Explain the so-called "exercise euphoria" that results from moderate to intense exercise.

EXERCISE, INFECTIOUS ILLNESS, CANCER, AND IMMUNE RESPONSE

What level of exercise is related to increased risk of upper respiratory tract infection?

What two factors in addition to exercise have a direct effect on immune status?

1.

2.

Upper Respiratory Tract Infections

Describe the relationship between exercise intensity and the risk of upper respiratory tract infections. (*Hint: Refer to Figure 20.22 in your textbook.*)

Acute Exercise Effects

Describe the immune function responses to a bout of moderate exercise and a bout of exhaustive exercise.

• Moderate exercise

• Exhaustive exercise

Effects of Chronic Exercise

What effects does chronic exercise have on immune function?

Describe the "open-window" phenomena for exercise and infection.

THE EXERCISE-CANCER CONNECTION

Give one hypothesis for why exercise may decrease cancer risk.

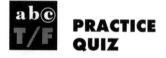 **PRACTICE QUIZ**

MULTIPLE CHOICE

1. **Exocrine glands:**
    a. have no ducts
    b. secrete their substances directly into the extracellular spaces around a gland
    c. include the pancreas
    d. are under nervous system control
    e. are located within the sac-like structure of the endocrine glands

2. **Which is a method for altering the rates of specific cellular reactions of specific "target cells"?**
    a. altering the rate of synthesis of intracellular proteins
    b. changing the rate of enzyme activity
    c. modifying cell membrane transport
    d. inducing secretory activity
    e. all of the above

3. **Which is not a method for stimulating endocrine glands?**
   a. changing levels of P_{N_2} in inspired air
   b. hormones influencing the secretion of other hormones
   c. changing levels of ions and nutrients in the blood
   d. nerve fibers stimulating hormone release
   e. a and c

4. **Which statement is false about growth hormone?**
   a. it promotes cell division and cellular proliferation throughout the body
   b. it facilitates protein synthesis
   c. its secretion decreases with increasing exercise intensity
   d. it decreases carbohydrate utilization
   e. none of the above

5. **The major function of ADH is to:**
   a. stimulate the ovaries to secrete estrogen
   b. control the excretion of water by the kidneys
   c. stimulate the contraction of muscle in the uterus
   d. stimulate carbohydrate and lipid metabolism
   e. none of the above

6. **Which is not a function of cortisol?**
   a. stimulating protein breakdown to amino acids in all cells of the body except the liver
   b. controlling reabsorption of sodium in the kidneys
   c. supporting the action of other hormones in the gluconeogenic process
   d. inhibiting glucose uptake and oxidation
   e. a, b, and c

7. **Which statement is false about insulin?**
   a. it regulates glucose metabolism in all tissues except the brain
   b. it directly controls blood glucose level
   c. it causes protein deposition in cells
   d. when it is present fatty acids are mobilized and used in place of sugar
   e. a and d

8. **Which is an exercise benefit for non-insulin-dependent diabetes mellitus:**
   a. improved glycemic control
   b. improved cardiovascular effects
   c. weight loss
   d. decreased disease risk
   e. all of the above

9. **Which statement is true about the pancreatic hormones and exercise:**
   a. physical training decreases a person's sensitivity to insulin
   b. physical training lowers the insulin requirement
   c. exercise requires a larger insulin output to clear excess glucose
   d. physical training causes insulin and glucagon levels in the blood to be higher than resting values
   e. none of the above

10. **Exercise-induced elevation of which of the following opioids produces euphoria and increased pain tolerance?**
    a. beta-endorphins
    b. beta-lipotropins
    c. dynorphin
    d. a and c
    e. b and c

TRUE/FALSE

1. _____ A target cell's ability to respond to a hormone depends largely on the presence of specific protein receptors.

2. _____ The adrenal gland secretes at least six different hormones and influences the secretion of several others.

3. _____ ACTH concentrations in the blood increase with exercise duration if intensity is higher than 25% of $\dot{V}O_2$max.

4. _____ During exercise, blood levels of "free" T_4 increase.

5. _____ Aldosterone acts by regulating calcium reabsorption in the distal tubules of the kidneys.

6. _____ The pancreas gland is composed of alpha cells that secrete insulin and beta cells that secrete glucagon.

7. _____ Type I diabetes usually occurs in younger individuals.

8. _____ The magnitude of hormonal response to a standard exercise load declines with endurance training.

9. _____ Plasma concentrations of epinephrine and norepinephrine decrease during the first weeks of training.

10. _____ Testosterone and growth hormone are the two hormones primarily involved in resistance training adaptations.

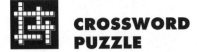

CROSSWORD PUZZLE

ACROSS

2 Another name for growth hormone

4 Inhibits testosterone (abbr.)

7 Second messenger to facilitate hormone function

9 Testosterone is a ____oid-type hormone

10 _____ cells are cells on which hormones act

13 Renin stimulates release of this kidney hormone

15 Underproduction of this hormone causes Addison's disease

18 Adrenocortical hormones that regulate electrolytes

23 Stimulates production and release of cortisol (abbr.)

25 ____cagon is "insulin antagonist"

26 Male sex hormones

28 Hormone in birthing and lactation

29 Islets composed of alpha and beta cells

30 Promotes retention of sodium by kidneys

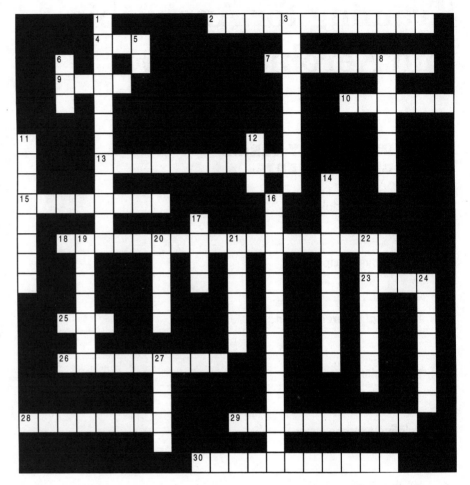

DOWN

1 Target cells form more receptors in response to increasing hormone levels

3 T_4

5 Hormone that stimulates estrogen production (abbr.)

6 Stimulates thyroxine release (abbr.)

8 Cap-like gland above each kidney

11 Type of gland (e.g., sweat gland)

12 A gonadotropic hormone

14 Another word for pituitary gland

16 Epinephrine and norepinephrine

17 ____erior portion of pituitary gland resembles true neural tissue

19 Produced by beta cells of pancreas

20 Pancreas exocrine cells that secrete digestive enzymes

21 Type of peptide that exerts morphine-like effects

22 Disease caused by inadequate insulin

24 Chemical messenger

27 Tissue classified as endocrine or exocrine

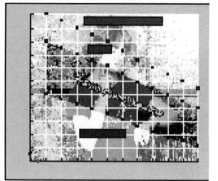

CHAPTER 21

Training for Anaerobic and Aerobic Power

 DEFINE KEY TERMS AND CONCEPTS

1. Overload principle

2. Specificity principle

3. Individual differences principle

4. Reversibility principle

5. Relative exercise stress

6. HR threshold

7. Conversational exercise

8. Training-sensitive zone

9. HR threshold = HR_{rest} + 0.60 (HR_{max} − HR_{rest})

10. Age-predicted maximum heart rate

11. **RPE training**

12. **Lactate threshold training**

13. **Recommended training duration**

14. **Recommended training frequency**

15. **Lactate stacking**

16. **Interval training**

17. **Relief interval**

18. **Repetitions**

19. **Sets**

20. **Continuous training**

21. **LSD training**

22. **Fartlek training**

23. **Overtraining**

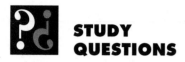

STUDY QUESTIONS

PRINCIPLES OF TRAINING

List the four principles of training.

1.

2.

3.

4.

Overload Principle

List four variables that can be manipulated to achieve exercise overload.

1.

2.

3.

4.

Specificity Principle

Give an example to support the statement: "Specific exercise elicits specific adaptations creating specific training effects."

Specificity of $\dot{V}O_2max$

Give one example of exercise training specificity.

Specificity of Local Changes

How does the overload of specific muscle groups in endurance training contribute to enhanced exercise performance and aerobic power?

Individual Differences Principle

Give one example why the principle of individual differences is important in formulating an exercise program.

Reversibility Principle

What are the effects of detraining on $\dot{V}O_2max$ and related functions? (*Hint: Refer to Table 21.2 of your textbook.*)

PHYSIOLOGIC CONSEQUENCES OF TRAINING

Anaerobic System Changes

List three physiologic changes that occur with sprint- and power-type training.

1.

2.

3.

Aerobic System Changes

Metabolic Adaptations

List five metabolic adaptations that occur with aerobic training.

1.

2.

3.

4.

5.

Cardiovascular and Pulmonary Adaptations

List five cardiovascular and pulmonary adaptations that occur with aerobic training.

1.

2.

3.

4.

5.

Other Adaptations

In addition to metabolic, cardiovascular, and pulmonary function changes, list three other important changes that occur with aerobic training.

1.

2.

3.

Practical Implications

What cellular adjustments account for a trained person's ability for prolonged steady-rate exercise at a large percentage of $\dot{V}O_2$max? (*Hint: Refer to Figure 21.5 in your textbook.*)

FACTORS THAT AFFECT THE AEROBIC TRAINING RESPONSE

List four factors that have a significant effect on the aerobic training response.

1.

2.

3.

4.

Initial Level of Aerobic Fitness

What is the generally expected range for percent improvement in $\dot{V}O_2$max with aerobic training?

Exercise Intensity

List five ways to express intensity of exercise.

1.

2.

3.

4.

5.

In terms of upper-body and lower-body exercise, give an important point to remember when using heart rate to establish training intensity.

Train at a Percentage of HRmax

Write the formula for calculating the heart rate training threshold as a percentage of HRmax.

Is Strenuous Training More Effective?

What is the "ceiling" for training intensity for exercise heart rate and percent $\dot{V}O_2$max?

- Heart rate

- % $\dot{V}O_2$max

The "Training-sensitive Zone"

Calculate your exercise training-sensitive zone.

Running versus Swimming and Other Forms of Upper-Body Exercise

What is the difference in maximum heart rate between running and swimming, and other forms of upper-body exercise?

Is Less Intense Training Effective?

How can exercise duration be altered to effect a training response with a lower intensity of exercise?

Train at a Perception of Effort

How is it possible to determine training intensity based on "how you feel" during exercise?

Train at the Lactate Threshold

Discuss the influence of exercising at the lactate threshold on the aerobic training response.

Training Duration

Give the generally recommended minimum threshold of exercise duration necessary to induce an aerobic training effect.

Training Frequency

What is generally believed to be the minimum frequency of training sessions per week to induce an aerobic training effect?

Give a general recommendation of exercise for weight loss.

Exercise Mode

Discuss the influence of exercise mode on the training response.

How Long Does It Take Before Improvements Are Noted?

Discuss the general time course for improvement in aerobic capacity with training. (*Hint: Refer to Figure 21.10 in your textbook.*)

Maintenance of Aerobic Fitness

Discuss the roles of exercise frequency, duration, and intensity in the maintenance of aerobic fitness.

- Frequency

- Duration

- Intensity

METHODS OF TRAINING

List three main training methods to improve metabolic capacity.

1.

2.

3.

Anaerobic Training

The Intramuscular High-Energy Phosphates

Discuss how interval training can overload the immediate energy system.

Lactic Acid-Generating Capacity

Why should anaerobic power training occur at the end of a conditioning session?

Aerobic Training

List two important factors in formulating an aerobic training program. (*Hint: Refer to Figure 21.12 in your textbook.*)

1.

2.

Interval Training

What four factors formulate the exercise prescription in interval training?

1.

2.

3.

4.

Rationale for Interval Training

Describe a practical method for determining the appropriate exercise and relief intervals for interval training. (*Hint: Refer to Table 21.7.*)

Continuous Training

List one important advantage of continuous exercise training.

Fartlek Training

How does fartlek training differ from interval training?

OVERTRAINING: TOO MUCH OF A GOOD THING

List three symptoms of overtraining. (*Hint: Refer to Table 21.7 in your textbook.*)

1.

2.

3.

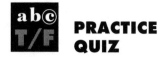

PRACTICE QUIZ

MULTIPLE CHOICE

1. **The major objective of exercise training is to:**
    a. maintain an ideal body weight
    b. protect against cardiovascular diseases
    c. cause biologic adaptations to physiologic systems to improve functioning
    d. increase one's endurance capacity
    e. none of the above

2. **Maximum heart rate during arm exercise compared to leg exercise is:**
    a. lower in arm exercise by 10 to 15 beats·min^{-1}
    b. higher in arm exercise by 10 to 15 beats·min^{-1}
    c. equal for arm and leg exercise
    d. higher in arm exercise by 5 to 10 beats·min^{-1}
    e. none of the above

3. **Maximum heart rate during swimming averages _____ beats per minute lower than during running:**
    a. 2 to 5
    b. 6 to 9
    c. 20 to 25
    d. 25 to 30
    e. none of the above

4. **Which statement is <u>true</u> of the effects of regular aerobic training on resting blood pressure?**
    a. training reduces systolic and increases diastolic blood pressure
    b. training reduces diastolic and increases systolic blood pressure
    c. training reduces systolic and diastolic blood pressure
    d. training increases systolic and diastolic blood pressure
    e. none of the above

5. **Which is <u>not</u> a method for improving aerobic fitness?**
    a. fartlek training
    b. interval training
    c. plyometric training
    d. continuous training
    e. all of the above

6. **Which is <u>not</u> a metabolic change that occurs with short-duration, power-type training?**
    a. increase in $\dot{V}O_2$max
    b. increase in resting levels of anaerobic substrates
    c. increase in the quantity and activity of anaerobic enzymes
    d. increase in the capacity to generate high levels of blood lactate
    e. increase in ATP and CP

7. **Conditioning of the aerobic system occurs as long as the exercise heart rate is within:**
    a. 10–30% of maximum
    b. 30–50% of maximum
    c. 50–70% of maximum
    d. 70–90% of maximum
    e. all of the above

8. Which is <u>not</u> an adaptation that usually occurs with aerobic training?
   a. mitochondria increase their capacity to generate ATP
   b. increased reliance on lipid oxidation
   c. increased level of succinic dehydrogenase
   d. increased capacity to oxidize carbohydrate
   e. decrease in lean body mass

9. Which statement is <u>true</u> about cardiovascular adaptations to aerobic exercise training?
   a. cardiac hypertrophy occurs in the right ventricle
   b. plasma volume increases within several training sessions
   c. heart's stroke volume decreases at rest
   d. heart's maximum cardiac output decreases
   e. a and b

10. Which statement is <u>false</u> about pulmonary adaptations to a standard exercise load with aerobic exercise training?
    a. training increases the submaximal exercise tidal volume
    b. training decreases the submaximal exercise breathing rate
    c. training increases the submaximal exercise breathing rate
    d. training decreases the submaximal exercise minute ventilation
    e. a and d

TRUE/FALSE

1. _____ The four principles of training are overload, specificity, individual differences, and reversibility.

2. _____ Anaerobic training decreases the capacity for blood lactate accumulation during all-out exercise.

3. _____ Aerobic training causes large increases in total muscle blood flow during maximal exercise.

4. _____ Exercise frequency, intensity, duration, and body composition are all important factors in determining appropriate exercise overload.

5. _____ Trained muscle exhibits a greater capability to oxidize lipids than untrained muscle.

6. _____ Specific exercise elicits general adaptations that create general training effects.

7. _____ The beneficial effects of exercise training are transient and reversible.

8. _____ The step test is an effective method of using heart rate to evaluate the efficiency of the cardiovascular response to aerobic exercise.

9. _____ Moderate aerobic exercise compromises fetal oxygen supply for the physically active, healthy woman.

10. _____ A minimum of 60 minutes per exercise session is desirable for training the aerobic system.

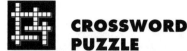

CROSSWORD PUZZLE

ACROSS

1. Continuous activity of 3 minutes and longer mainly engages this system of energy transfer
6. Type of training used by endurance athletes
8. Recommended minimum number of days per week for aerobic training
9. People respond differently to training. This is the _____ difference principle
10. Step test is named for this Michigan city
15. Method for estimating training heart rate that uses "heart rate reserve"
18. This principle operative when training stops
22. This fist-sized muscle thickens with pressure overload
24. All-out exercise for 60 seconds mainly engages this energy transfer system
25. Blood will do this in peripheral tissue if exercise stops abruptly
26. Max HR decreases with this variable
27. Lower recovery HR on this weight-bearing exercise test indicates higher aerobic fitness

DOWN

2. The lower the _____ fitness level, the greater the potential for improvement
3. 70% HRmax is minimum threshold for training sensitive-_____
4. Step test is named for this New York college
5. Endurance swimmers are not necessarily good endurance runners (training principle)

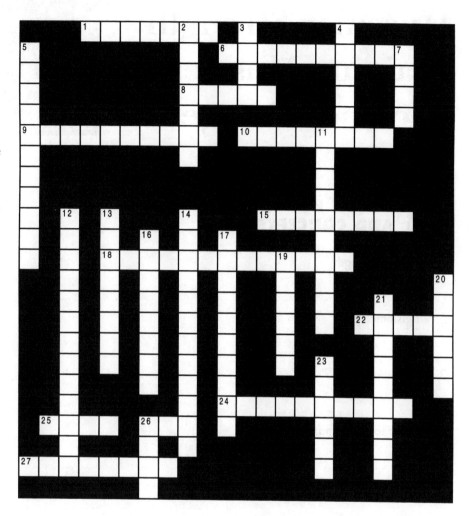

7. Principle related to specificity of training (abbr.)
11. Anaerobic training requires high levels of this psychological factor
12. About 70 to 90% of HRmax is called the training-_____ _____
13. Lower exercise intensity is offset by longer exercise _____
14. Another term for $\dot{V}O_2$max
16. A fundamental training principle
17. Repetitive stair sprinting will train the _____ _____ phosphates

19. Acid produced during repetitive bouts of near-maximum exercise
20. First word in abbreviation RPE
21. Second word in abbreviation RPE
23. A rest-_____ interval is period of passive recovery in interval training
26. Initials for professional sports medicine organization

See page 372 for Crossword Puzzle Solution.

Muscular Strength: Training Muscles to Become Stronger

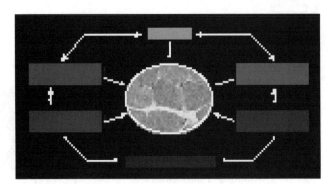

 DEFINE KEY TERMS AND CONCEPTS

1. Muscle strength

2. Tensiometry

3. Dynamometry

4. One-repetition maximum

5. Isokinetic dynamometer

6. Absolute strength

7. Relative strength

8. Muscle plus bone cross-sectional area

9. Allometric scaling

10. **Muscular overload**

11. **Concentric muscle action**

12. **Eccentric muscle action**

13. **Isometric muscle action**

14. **Isotonic**

15. **PRE**

16. **Periodization**

17. **Macrocycle**

18. **Low back pain syndrome**

19. **Isometric strength training**

20. **Specificity of training response**

21. **Accommodating resistance exercise**

22. **Variable-resistance exercise**

23. **Peak torque**

24. **Plyometrics**

25. **Drop-jumping**

26. **EMG**

27. **Bidirectional muscle exercise**

28. **Double concentric muscle actions**

29. **QNF**

30. **Neural facilitation**

31. **"Psyching"**

32. **Muscular hypertrophy**

33. **Hyperplasia**

34. **Longitudinal splitting**

35. **Motor unit recruitment**

36. **Patellar tendon reflex response**

37. **CRT**

38. **Nautilus**

39. **Cybex**

40. **Hydra-fitness**

41. **DOMS**

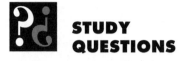

STUDY QUESTIONS

STRENGTH MEASUREMENT AND RESISTANCE TRAINING
Measurement of Muscle Strength
List four methods for measuring muscular strength.

1.

2.

3.

4.

Cable Tensiometry
List two advantages of cable tensiometry testing.

1.

2.

Dynamometry
Describe the principle for the operation of hand-grip and back-lift steel dynamometers.

One-Repetition Maximum
Write the equations for estimating the 1-RM for untrained and trained individuals.

• Untrained

• Trained

Computer-Assisted, Electromechanical, and Isokinetic Methods
What is a major advantage of strength testing with isokinetic methods?

Categories of Resistance Training Equipment

List the three categories of resistance training equipment.

1. Category I

2. Category II

    a.

    b.

3. Category III

Strength Testing Considerations

List four important considerations when performing strength testing.

1.

2.

3.

4.

Sex Differences in Muscle Strength

Give two approaches to evaluate strength differences between males and females.

1.

2.

Strength in Relation to Muscle Cross-Section

How much force can be generated per square centimeter of muscle area?

Absolute Muscle Strength

What are the sex differences in absolute muscle strength of the upper and lower body?

• Upper body

• Lower body

Sex Differences in Weightlifting Championships
Relative Muscle Strength

What evidence shows that the upper-body and lower-body strength of males is greater than that of females?

Allometric Scaling

Discuss the nature of the relationship between body mass and muscle strength.

Write the general allometric scaling equation.

Training Muscles to Become Stronger

List three common exercise systems for training muscles to become stronger.

1.

2.

3.

Different Forms of Muscle Action

List the three types of muscle action and give one fact about each.

1.

2.

3.

Resistance Training for Children

Outline a prudent recommendation for a resistance training program for children.

Progressive-Resistance Weight Training

Progressive-Resistance Exercise (PRE)

Describe the original method for PRE.

Variations of PRE

List five general observations regarding the optimal number of sets and repetitions, and the frequency and relative intensity required to improve muscle strength.

1.

2.

3.

4.

5.

Periodization

In periodization, what is the purpose of fractionating the resistance-training cycle?

Describe a typical mesocycle in periodization. (*Hint: Refer to Figure 22.9 in your textbook.*)

Is periodization sport specific? Explain.

Practical Recommendations for Initiating a Weight-Training Program
List three recommendations to consider when starting resistance training.

1.

2.

3.

The Lower Back
What role can resistance training play in reducing the risk of low back pain syndrome?

Resistance Training plus Aerobic Training Often Equals Less Strength Improvement
Discuss whether it is possible to concurrently maintain both resistance and aerobic training programs at equally high levels.

Isometric Strength Training
What is the average duration of a typical isometric muscle action during isometric training?

Limitations of Isometric Exercise
List two limitations of isometric training.

1.

2.

Benefits of Isometric Exercise
In what setting is isometric exercise best suited?

Which Are Better, Static or Dynamic Methods?
Is one method of resistance training "better" than another? Discuss.

Specificity of the Training Response
Practical Implications
How does the interaction between the nervous and muscular systems help to explain the large specificity of the strength training response?

Supplemental Resistance Training with Modified Sports Equipment
Describe two sport-specific resistance training examples.

1.

2.

Isokinetic Resistance Training

Isokinetics versus Standard Weightlifting

Discuss the distinction between a muscle loaded during weightlifting exercise and one loaded with an isokinetic dynamometer. (*Hint: Refer to Figure 22.6 in your textbook.*)

Experiments with Isokinetic Exercise and Training

Plot the relationship between peak torque output and angular velocity for power and endurance athletes.

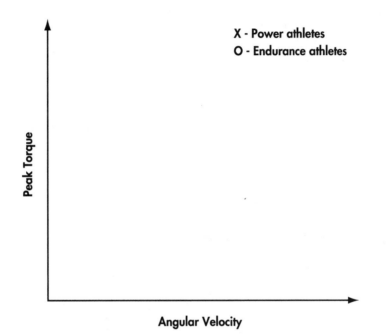

Fast versus Slow Isokinetic Training

Which type of isokinetic training, fast or slow, appears to give a more "general" strength improvement? Why?

Plyometric Training

Give the general rationale for plyometric training.

Practical Application of Plyometrics

Describe an example of plyometric training for a track athlete.

Physical Testing in the Occupational Setting: The Role of Specificity

Discuss the use of a 12-minute run to estimate the aerobic capacity of firefighters for their specific job.

Electromyography (EMG) during Maximal Ballistic Muscle Action

Describe the EMG pattern during rapid, ballistic movements.

EMG During Concentric Bidirectional Muscle Work

Describe the EMG pattern during bidirectional, concentric muscle actions.

ADAPTATIONS WITH RESISTANCE TRAINING

List six factors that influence the development and maintenance of muscle mass.

1.

2.

3.

4.

5.

6.

Factors That Modify the Expression of Human Strength

Psychological/Neural Factors

List four possible neural adaptations with resistance training.

1.

2.

3.

4.

Muscular Factors

List two physiologic and two anatomic factors within the muscle itself that significantly affect muscle strength.

- Anatomic
  1.
  2.

- Physiologic
  1.
  2.

Muscle Hypertrophy

What is the primary requirement for initiating muscle hypertrophy?

Even the Very Elderly Respond

List two benefits of resistance training for the elderly.

1.

2.

Muscle Hyperplasia: Are New Muscle Fibers Made?

Describe the evidence for longitudinal muscle fiber splitting with resistance training.

Which factor, hyperplasia or hypertrophy, accounts for most of the increase in muscle size with resistance training?

Changes in Muscle Fiber-Type Composition

List three changes in fiber composition resulting from resistance training.

1.

2.

3.

Comparative Training Responses of Men and Women

Muscle Strength and Hypertrophy

What is the current thinking concerning muscle hypertrophy with resistance training for women?

What is the basic sex difference in response to resistance training?

Is Muscle Strength Related to Bone Density?

Discuss the relationship between muscle strength and bone density.

Detraining

What is known about the detraining response for muscle strength?

Metabolic Stress of Resistance Training

Give an explanation of why a typical resistance training program does not provide an adequate stimulus for cardiovascular training.

Circuit Resistance Training (CRT)

Describe the circuit resistance method of training.

Muscle Soreness and Stiffness

List four possible causative factors for muscle soreness.

1.

2.

3.

4.

Soreness Occurs Predominantly with Eccentric Actions

What is it about eccentric actions that contribute to muscle damage and resulting soreness?

Actual Cell Damage

List three specific cellular changes that occur with DOMS

1.

2.

3.

Current Model For Doms

Describe the major events in the development of DOMS. (*Hint: Refer to Figure 22.26 in your textbook.*)

abc T/F PRACTICE QUIZ

MULTIPLE CHOICE

1. **Which of the following is <u>not</u> used to measure the maximum force or tension generated by a muscle:**
    a. tensiometry
    b. dynamometry
    c. plyometry
    d. one-repetition maximum
    e. all of the above are used

2. **To determine true "sex differences" in muscle strength, strength is most appropriately evaluated:**
    a. in relation to muscle cross-sectional area
    b. on an absolute basis as total force exerted
    c. as relative strength per unit body mass
    d. as strength per unit percent body fat
    e. in relation to the lean-to-fat ratio

3. **Which is <u>not</u> an appropriate explanation for the muscle soreness and stiffness that often accompany resistance training?**
    a. high levels of lactic acid build up
    b. minute tears in the muscle tissue
    c. overstretching of muscle and connective tissue tears
    d. repetitive eccentric muscle actions
    e. b and d

4. What type of training utilizes the inherent stretch-recoil characteristics of the neuromuscular system?
   a. isometric
   b. isokinetic
   c. plyometric
   d. periodization
   e. none of the above

5. As movement velocity increases, greater torque is achieved by individuals with a higher percentage of which type of muscle fibers?
   a. fast-twitch
   b. slow-twitch
   c. equal percentages of fast-twitch and slow-twitch
   d. type I
   e. SO

6. Which is <u>false</u> about a concentric muscle action?
   a. it occurs in dynamic activity
   b. the muscle lengthens while generating force
   c. joint movement occurs as tension is developed
   d. an example is raising a dumbbell from the extended to the flexed-elbow position
   e. all of the above

7. Which statement is <u>false</u> about progressive resistance training?
   a. the most effective number of repetitions for increasing muscle strength is 3 to 9-RM
   b. performing one set of an exercise is more effective for strength improvement than two or three sets
   c. training four or five days a week may be less effective for increasing strength than two or three times a week
   d. a fast rate of movement may generate greater strength improvement than lifting at a slower rate
   e. none of the above

8. At what minimum percentage of a muscle's force-generating capacity should resistance be set to ensure that strength increases?
   a. 10–20%
   b. 20–40%
   c. 60–80%
   d. 80–90%
   e. greater than 90% is generally recommended

9. This type of exercise causes the greatest DOMS:
   a. eccentric
   b. concentric
   c. isometric
   d. isokinetic
   e. plyometric

10. This is <u>not</u> a factor believed to have an impact on the development and maintenance of muscle mass:
    a. genetics
    b. race
    c. nutritional status
    d. endocrine influence
    e. pattern of nervous system activation

TRUE/FALSE

1. _____ On an absolute basis, men are usually stronger than women.

2. _____ Overload is created by increasing the load and decreasing the speed of muscle contraction.

3. _____ Heavy resistance training does not bring about adaptations that enhance aerobic energy transfer.

4. _____ Increased muscle size with overload training occurs mainly by enlargement of individual muscle fibers.

5. _____ Isokinetic resistance training offers an effective alternative for combining the muscle-training benefits of resistance exercise with the cardiovascular benefits of continuous dynamic exercise.

6. _____ It is imprecise to term eccentric or concentric muscle actions as isotonic movements.

7. _____ Humans generate between 2 and 5 kg of force per square centimeter of muscle cross section, regardless of sex.

8. _____ The lower back is not susceptible to significant injury with resistance training.

9. _____ Absolute increases in muscle girth with resistance training are less for women than for men.

10. _____ Resistance training programs using moderate levels of concentric exercise can improve the strength of preadolescent children without adverse effects.

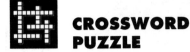

CROSSWORD PUZZLE

ACROSS

1 DOMS prevalent after this type of muscle action
5 Cable _____
9 First word in PRE
10 First four letters of factor that accounts for rapid increase in strength early in training
11 ____metric training is static resistance
12 Area of body susceptible to injury with improper resistance training
14 Strength measurement device using steel spring
18 First four letters of hormone that exerts anabolic effect
20 Weight _____
21 Force- _____ curve
22 The weakest point in joint range of motion is termed "sticking _____"
23 Rotational force on an isokinetic dynamometer
24 Form of training that uses pre-stretch prior to force application
25 Greatest sex difference when strength expressed in this manner

DOWN

2 Weight training is considered dynamic form of progressive resistance _____
3 This demand relatively low with standard resistance training
4 Abbr. describing muscle pain day after unaccustomed exercise

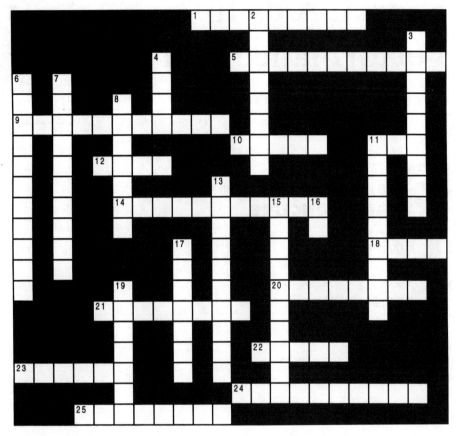

6 Enlargement of individual muscle fibers
7 Maximum force generated throughout movement at pre-set, constant speed
8 CRT significantly increases metabolic ____ of resistance training
11 Static resistance training popularized by German researchers in mid-1950s
13 Muscle shortens while developing tension

15 A theory to explain muscle soreness
16 1-____ is a measure of strength
17 First word in CRT
19 Differences in body size and composition mainly account for strength differences between _____

See page 372 for Crossword Puzzle Solution.

Special Aids to Performance and Conditioning

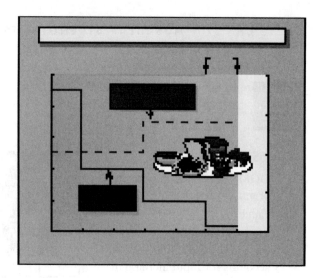

DEFINE KEY WORDS AND CONCEPTS

1. Ergogenic aid

2. Anabolic steroid

3. Steroid stacking

4. Gynecomastia

5. Human growth hormone

6. Recombinant human GH

7. Acromegalic syndrome

8. Amphetamine

9. Benzedrine

10. **Sympathomimetic**

11. **Caffeine**

12. **Caffeine content of coffee**

13. **Pangamic acid**

14. **Bicarbonate loading**

15. **TMJ repositioning**

16. **MORA**

17. **Blood doping**

18. **Autologous transfusion**

19. **Homologous transfusion**

20. **Vitamin B$_{15}$**

21. **Hormonal blood boosting**

22. **Erythropoietin**

23. **General warm-up**

24. **Specific warm-up**

25. **Hyperoxic gas mixtures**

26. **Glycogen supercompensation**

27. **Glycogen synthetase**

28. **Carbohydrate loading**

29. **L-Carnitine**

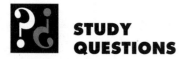

STUDY QUESTIONS

PHARMACOLOGIC AGENTS
Anabolic Steroids

Structure and Action

What is an anabolic steroid and what is its mode of action?

• Anabolic steroid

• Mode of action

Are They Effective?

What are some sources of confusion concerning the effectiveness of anabolic steroids as an ergogenic aid?

Are There Risks?

List five potential harmful side effects or health risks from using anabolic steroids

1.

2.

3.

4.

5.

Steroid Use and Life-Threatening Disease

What is considered a therapeutic dose of anabolic steroids?

Steroid Use and Plasma Lipoproteins

Describe the effects of anabolic steroids on blood lipids.

ACSM Position Statement on Anabolic Steroids

Summarize the ACSM position on the use and abuse of anabolic-androgenic steroids in sports.

Steroid Use by Females

List two possible negative effects unique to females using anabolic steroids.

1.

2.

Growth Hormone: The Next Magic Pill?

What is the normal medical use for human growth hormone, and what are the risks of its unsupervised use?

• Medical use

• Risks

Nutritional Supplements for an Anabolic Effect

Discuss the scientific evidence on the use of specific amino acids for anabolic purposes.

Amphetamines

List three effects of amphetamines on normal physiologic function.

1.

2.

3.

Dangers of Amphetamines

List four potentially dangerous side effects of amphetamine use in athletics.

1.

2.

3.

4.

Amphetamine Use and Athletic Performance

Describe the general research findings concerning the ergogenic effects of amphetamines.

Caffeine

How does caffeine exert its ergogenic effect on endurance performance?

Proposed Mechanism for Ergogenic Action

Explain the main facilitating effect of caffeine as an ergogenic aid.

Endurance Effects Are Often Inconsistent

List two factors that may blunt the ergogenic benefit of caffeine for endurance exercise.

1.

2.

Effects on Muscle

What is the proposed ergogenic effect of caffeine on neuromuscular function?

Warning

List three negative side effects of caffeine.

1.

2.

3.

Pangamic Acid

What is another name for pangamic acid?

Explain the proposed ergogenic benefit of pangamic acid and describe the research findings concerning this benefit.

- Proposed benefit
- Research findings

Buffering Solutions

How does ingestion of a pre-exercise buffering solution enhance short-term exhaustive exercise performance?

Effect Related to Dosage and Degree of Anaerobiosis

What dose of bicarbonate facilitates H^+ efflux from the cell?

TEMPOROMANDIBULAR JOINT (TMJ) REPOSITIONING

Briefly explain the rationale for TMJ repositioning as a possible exercise enhancer.

RED BLOOD CELL REINFUSION—BLOOD DOPING

How It Works

Outline the general procedure of red blood cell reinfusion for ergogenic purposes.

Give a quantitative example of how the addition of red blood cells can increase the oxygen-carrying capacity of blood.

Describe a potential danger of blood doping.

What are the physiologic and performance benefits of red blood cell reinfusion?

A NEW TWIST—HORMONAL BLOOD BOOSTING

Describe the physiologic function of erythropoietin and discuss its danger as an ergogenic aid.

- Physiologic function
- Potential danger

WARM-UP (PRELIMINARY EXERCISE)

Psychological Considerations

What is the psychological basis for warming up?

Physiologic Considerations

List four physiologic mechanisms by which warm-up could potentially improve subsequent exercise performance.

1.

2.

3.

4.

Effects on Performance

Describe the ergogenic benefits of warming up and give a recommendation concerning its use.

- Ergogenic benefits
- Recommendation

Sudden Strenuous Exercise

What research evidence justifies the potential cardiovascular benefits of warming up prior to sudden, strenuous exercise?

OXYGEN INHALATION (HYPEROXIA)

Give the physiologic rationale for breathing oxygen-enriched gas mixtures prior to, during, or in recovery from strenuous exercise.

PRE-EXERCISE OXYGEN BREATHING

Explain why pre-exercise breathing of a hyperoxic gas mixture has no ergogenic benefit.

Oxygen Breathing during Exercise

Outline the research findings on the ergogenic benefits of breathing hyperoxic gas during submaximal and maximal aerobic exercise.

• Submaximal exercise

• Maximal exercise

Why does breathing hyperoxic gas during exercise provide an ergogenic effect in aerobic exercise?

Oxygen Breathing during Recovery

What is the effect of breathing hyperoxic gas in recovery from strenuous exercise?

MODIFICATION OF CARBOHYDRATE INTAKE

Nutrient-Related Fatigue during Prolonged Exercise

Is it possible to avoid "hitting the wall"? Explain.

Glycogen Supercompensation

How much glycogen can be packed into skeletal muscle with carbohydrate loading?

Classic Carbohydrate Loading Procedure

List five steps in the classic carbohydrate loading procedure.

1.

2.

3.

4.

5.

Carbohydrate Loading Not Necessary for All Competition

Outline a prudent approach to carbohydrate loading for the athlete who wants to try it for the first time.

Negative Aspects

List two potential negative aspects of the "classic" carbohydrate loading procedure.

1.

2.

Modified Loading Procedure

List four steps of the modified carbohydrate loading procedure.

1.

2.

3.

4.

L-CARNITINE

What physiologic function is served by L-carnitine?

Discuss the ergogenic effect of L-carnitine supplementation.

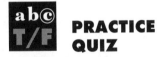 **PRACTICE QUIZ**

MULTIPLE CHOICE

1. **Hyperoxic gas breathed during exercise:**
   a. enhances endurance activities at high altitude
   b. increases running economy at high altitude
   c. enhances anaerobic activities at high altitude
   d. facilitates high-altitude acclimatization
   e. none of the above

2. **Which statement is _false_ about anabolic steroids?**
   a. they are drugs that function similarly to the male hormone estrogen
   b. they bind with specific receptor sites on the muscle
   c. they contribute to the male secondary sex characteristics
   d. they contribute to the sex differences in muscle mass and strength
   e. none of the above

3. **Which is _not_ a consequence of taking anabolic steroids?**
   a. impaired normal testosterone endocrine function
   b. increased concentration of circulating estradiol, a major female hormone
   c. gynecomastia
   d. decreased response of stress-related hormones
   e. acne

4. **Which is true of steroid use and plasma lipoproteins?**
   a. steroid use lowers high-density lipoprotein cholesterol
   b. steroid use lowers low-density lipoprotein cholesterol
   c. steroid use lowers triglycerides
   d. b and c
   e. none of the above

5. **Which is not a function of growth hormone?**
   a. stimulation of amino acid uptake and protein synthesis by muscle
   b. increased lipid breakdown
   c. prevention of lactic acid buildup in muscle
   d. decreased quantity of carbohydrate used by the body
   e. a and c

6. **The following exerts a powerful stimulating effect on central nervous system function:**
   a. TMJ adjustment
   b. pangamic acid
   c. amphetamines
   d. buffering solutions
   e. none of the above

7. **Which statement is true concerning pangamic acid?**
   a. it is commonly known as vitamin B_{10}
   b. it increases the cell's efficiency to use protein for fuel
   c. it reduces lactic acid buildup and enhances endurance performance
   d. it serves no particular nutritive role for the body
   e. none of the above

8. **The following physiologic adjustments occur in response to red blood cell reinfusion (blood doping):**
   a. red blood cell count and hemoglobin levels increase
   b. the added blood volume contributes to a larger maximal cardiac output
   c. the blood's oxygen-carrying capacity increases
   d. a and c
   e. all of the above

9. **Which is a purported benefit attributed to "warming up"?**
   a. increased speed of muscle contraction and relaxation
   b. facilitated oxygen utilization by the muscles
   c. facilitated nerve transmission
   d. increased blood flow through active tissues
   e. all of the above

10. **Which of the following is not a benefit to breathing hyperoxic gas during exercise?**
    a. reduced maximal oxygen uptake
    b. reduced blood lactate levels
    c. reduced submaximal heart rate
    d. reduced submaximal minute ventilation
    e. a and c

TRUE/FALSE

1. _____ "Stacking" is a term that refers to using anabolic steroids every other week.

2. _____ Anabolic steroids can increase aerobic power.

3. _____ Human growth hormone can cause gigantism in children and acromegaly symptoms in adults.

4. _____ The ergogenic effect of caffeine occurs by the facilitated use of lipid as fuel for exercise.

5. _____ Bicarbonate loading is completely safe and causes no adverse effects to the body.

6. _____ A large infusion of packed red blood cells could increase blood viscosity and cause a decrease in cardiac output.

7. _____ Erythropoietin is a hormone that stimulates the muscle to produce red blood cells.

8. _____ Adaptation of coronary blood flow to sudden and vigorous exercise occurs instantaneously as exercise begins.

9. _____ Breathing high concentrations of oxygen after strenuous exercise greatly increases oxygen transport by hemoglobin.

10. _____ The side effects of amphetamines include drug dependency, headache, and confusion.

CROSSWORD PUZZLE

ACROSS

1 Anabolic _____ is a drug that functions similarly to testosterone

3 _____ hormone may replace anabolic steroids as abused ergogenic aid

4 Methylxanthine

5 "Pep pill"

6 Erythrocyte (abbr.)

8 Oxygen-enriched gas

13 Ergogenic technique that enhances anaerobic capacity

16 _____ acid is another name for vitamin B_{15}

17 Person's own blood

DOWN

1 Term for compound that mimics action of catecholamine

2 Last seven letters of kidney hormone that stimulates bone marrow to produce RBCs

3 Type of warm-up involving calisthenics and stretching

7 Red blood cell reinfusion

9 Something that enhances exercise capacity

10 ____cythemia is increased concentration of red blood cells

11 Progressively increasing steroid dose in oral and injectable form

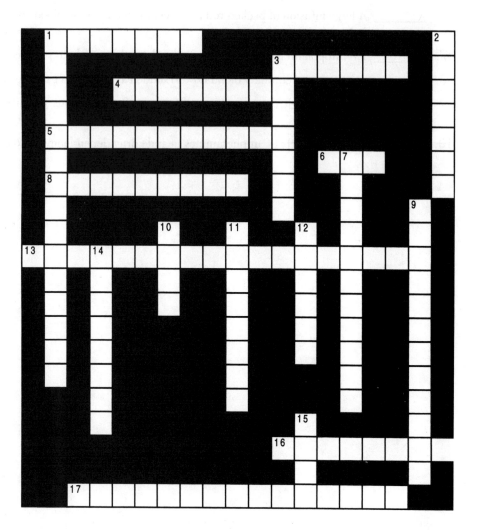

12 _____trophic hormone is another term for human growth hormone

14 Tissue building

15 First four letters of chemicals known as "downers"

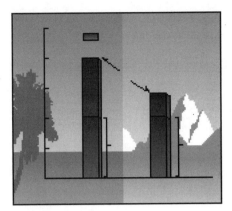

Environmental Factors and Exercise

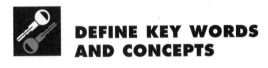

DEFINE KEY WORDS AND CONCEPTS

1. High altitude

2. Oxygen transport cascade

3. Ambient P_{O_2} at sea level

4. Ambient P_{O_2} at 3048 m

5. Acclimation

6. Alveolar P_{O_2} on Mt. Everest

7. Density of air

8. $\dot{V}_{O_2}$max on Mt. Everest

9. Acclimatization

10. Hyperventilation and alveolar P_{O_2}

11. **Arterial chemoreceptors**

12. **AMS**

13. **HAPE**

14. **HACE**

15. **Respiratory alkalosis**

16. **Lactate paradox**

17. **Polycythemia**

18. **Erythropoietin**

19. **Hyperbaric chamber**

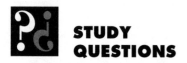

STUDY QUESTIONS

EXERCISE AT MEDIUM AND HIGH ALTITUDE

What is the major physiologic challenge of altitude?

THE STRESS OF ALTITUDE

Indicate the partial pressure of oxygen (PO_2) in ambient air at each of the following terrestrial elevations. (*Hint: Refer to Figure 24.1 in your textbook.*)

- Sea level

- 5,000 ft

- 10,000 ft

- 15,000 ft

- 20,000 ft

Oxygen Loading at Altitude

Give two quantitative examples of the effect of various altitudes on $\dot{V}O_2$max in comparison to values at sea level.

1.

2.

ACCLIMATIZATION

Present three broad guidelines concerning the length of time required to acclimatize to various altitudes. (*Hint: Refer to Table 24.1 in your textbook.*)

1.

2.

3.

Immediate Responses to Altitude

List two rapid physiologic responses that occur to compensate for the decrease in alveolar oxygen pressure at terrestrial elevations above 2300 m.

1.

2.

Hyperventilation

Discuss why hyperventilation is a desirable immediate first line of defense against exposure to high altitude.

Increased Cardiovascular Response

Why is an increased cardiac output during submaximal exercise at altitude compared to sea level a beneficial physiologic adjustment?

The increase in systemic arterial blood pressure during high altitude exposure is related to what factor?

Submaximum ventilation during moderate exercise increases approximately how much for each 1000-m increase in altitude? (*Hint: Refer to Figure 24.5 in your textbook.*)

Altitude-Related Medical Problems

Name the three medical conditions that can pose serious problems to one's overall health and safety at high altitude.

1.

2.

3.

Acute Mountain Sickness

List three major symptoms of acute mountain sickness.

1.

2.

3.

How soon do acute mountain sickness symptoms appear?

High-Altitude Pulmonary Edema (HAPE)

How soon do HAPE symptoms appear following rapid ascent to high altitude?

List three significant symptoms of HAPE.

1.

2.

3.

High-Altitude Cerebral Edema (HACE)

List two significant symptoms of HACE.

1.

2.

Why is it necessary to diagnose and treat HACE?

Other High-Altitude Conditions

List several high-altitude medical conditions other than AMS, HAPE, and HACE.

Fluid Loss

Why are people who exercise and train at altitude at an increased risk of becoming dehydrated?

Longer-Term Adjustments to Altitude

List four important longer-term adjustments to a prolonged stay at altitude.

1.

2.

3.

4.

Acid-Base Readjustment

Describe the effects of the "blowing-off" of the body's content of carbon dioxide in a hypoxic environment.

Reduced Buffering Capacity and the "Lactate Paradox"

Give a possible explanation for the blunted lactate production during anaerobic exercise at altitude.

Hematologic Changes

Give the most important longer-term adaptation to altitude exposure.

Decrease in Plasma Volume

Discuss the diagnosis of the body's fluid balance during a prolonged stay at high altitude.

Increase in Red Blood Cell Mass

Contrast hematocrit values of high-altitude natives with those of lowlanders.

Cellular Adaptations

List three important cellular adaptations during a prolonged altitude exposure.

1.

2.

3.

Changes in Body Mass and Composition

Describe the effects of long-term altitude exposure on body composition.

TIME REQUIRED FOR ACCLIMATIZATION

About how long is required to adapt to altitudes up to 2300 m?

How rapidly are the benefits of acclimatization lost on return to sea level?

METABOLIC, PHYSIOLOGIC, AND EXERCISE CAPACITIES AT ALTITUDE

Maximal Oxygen Uptake

Describe the relationship between $\dot{V}O_2$max and increases in altitude.

Does the degree of physical conditioning prior to altitude exposure offer protection to the altitude-related decrease in $\dot{V}O_2$max? Discuss.

Circulatory Factors

Submaximal Exercise

What causes the eventual reduction in exercise cardiac output in submaximal exercise during a prolonged stay at altitude?

Maximal Exercise

What is a possible cause for the reduced stroke volume observed at high altitude?

Performance Measures

By about how much is running performance decreased for 1- to 3-mile distances during exposure to medium altitudes?

ALTITUDE TRAINING AND SEA-LEVEL PERFORMANCE
AEROBIC CAPACITY ON RETURN TO SEA LEVEL

Give two effects of altitude training on subsequent performance on return to sea level.

1.

2.

Possible Negative Effects

List two physiologic changes that occur during prolonged altitude exposure that may negate the potential positive effects of acclimatization on exercise performance upon return to sea level.

1.

2.

Can Training Be Maintained at Altitude?

Why is it desirable for athletes to periodically return from altitude to sea level for intensive training?

Is Altitude Training More Effective Than Sea-Level Training?

Describe an experiment that evaluated the effect of aerobic training at altitude compared to equivalent training at sea level.

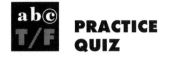

PRACTICE QUIZ

MULTIPLE CHOICE

1. This condition in ambient air causes the immediate physiologic adjustments to high altitude:
   a. reduced P_{CO_2}
   b. increased P_{CO_2}
   c. reduced P_{O_2}
   d. increased P_{O_2}
   e. decreased P_{N_2}

2. Which is a long-term adjustment to altitude exposure?
   a. increased red blood cell 2,3-DPG
   b. acid-base readjustment
   c. increased oxygen-carrying capacity of blood
   d. increased concentration of capillaries in skeletal muscle
   e. all of the above

3. The percent concentration of oxygen in ambient air at an altitude of 5000 m is:
   a. 20.93
   b. 19.93
   c. 18.93
   d. 17.93
   e. 16.93

4. Concerning the physiologic stress and exercise performance effects of altitude:
   a. there is only a small decrease in the percentage of arterial saturation of hemoglobin up to an altitude of about 2000 m.
   b. performance in short-term anaerobic power activities is not negatively affected at altitude
   c. the $\dot{V}_{O_2}max$ is reduced by about 50% at the summit of Mt. Everest
   d. $\dot{V}_{O_2}max$ decreases between 1.5 and 3.5% for every 1000 feet above an altitude of 5000 feet
   e. a, b, and d

5. Which of the following is <u>not</u> considered an immediate response of a native lowlander to acute altitude exposure?
   a. hyperventilation
   b. increase in submaximal heart rate
   c. increase in submaximal cardiac output
   d. increase in hemoglobin and hematocrit
   e. a and d

6. The reduced arterial P_{O_2} at altitude stimulates an increase in the total number of red blood cells through the action of the hormone:
   a. thyroxine
   b. erythropoietin
   c. erythrocytin
   d. testosterone
   e. estrogen

7. Which of the following is <u>false</u> concerning the longer-term adjustments to altitude hypoxia?
   a. decrease in maximum heart rate
   b. decrease in maximum cardiac output
   c. decrease in total number of red blood cells
   d. increase in red blood cell 2,3-DPG
   e. c and d

8. **Hyperventilation in response to acute altitude exposure:**
   a. increases alveolar P_{O_2}
   b. increases alveolar P_{CO_2}
   c. decreases blood pH
   d. stimulates production of urine
   e. all of the above

9. **As a broad guideline, how many weeks are required to adapt to altitudes up to 2300 m?**
   a. 1
   b. 2
   c. 3
   d. 4
   e. 7

10. **Which of the following physiologic changes that occur during prolonged altitude exposure may actually negate adaptations that might improve aerobic performance on return to sea level?**
    a. decrease in heart's stroke volume
    b. increase in production of erythropoietin
    c. increase in red blood cell 2,3-DPG
    d. renal excretion of base
    e. all of the above

TRUE/FALSE

1. _____ A reduced loading of hemoglobin with oxygen occurs at high altitudes.

2. _____ Aerobic capacity decreases linearly with increases in altitude.

3. _____ The adaptive physiologic responses that improve one's tolerance to altitude hypoxia are broadly described by the letters HACE.

4. _____ The term "lactate paradox" refers to an increase in blood lactate concentration during all-out exercise with large muscle groups following altitude acclimatization.

5. _____ Altitude acclimatization significantly improves aerobic capacity and endurance performance immediately on return to sea level.

6. _____ The most important and clear-cut immediate response of the native lowlander to altitude exposure is hyperventilation brought on by reduced arterial P_{O_2}.

7. _____ Appetite suppression can be severe during the early stages of a high-altitude stay and may reduce energy intake by about 40%.

8. _____ The life-threatening altitude complication called HAPE causes a significant amount of fluid to accumulate in the peripheral tissues of the lower body.

9. _____ For well-acclimatized mountaineers, the blood's oxygen-carrying capacity is between 35 and 40 mL of oxygen per 100 mL of blood.

10. _____ There is significant loss in lean body mass and body fat during long-term exposure to high altitude.

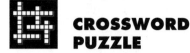

CROSSWORD PUZZLE

ACROSS

1 This chamber simulates altitude
4 Pulmonary disorder at altitude (abbr.)
5 This macronutrient is well tolerated and potentially beneficial at high altitude
7 A condition of abnormally high pH
9 Concentration of this iron-containing protein compound in muscle increases with long-term altitude acclimatization
15 The body's immediate first line of defense to altitude exposure
19 Upper limit of beneficial percentage increase in hemoglobin concentration at altitude is about _____ percent
20 This quality of the ambient gaseous environment decreases progressively with increasing altitude
21 Loss of this body composition component at altitude negatively affects strength and power performance
22 This category of activities is negatively affected at high altitude
23 Abnormally high concentration of red blood cells

DOWN

2 Neural bodies sensitive to decrease in arterial P_{O_2}
3 Maladaptation to high altitude that affects central nervous system (abbr.)
6 Percentage of _____ in air on Mt. Everest is 20.9

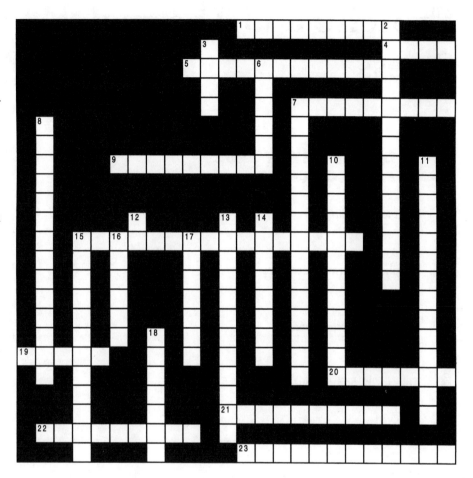

7 Adaptive response that improves tolerance to altitude hypoxia
8 Describes the reduced maximal lactate concentration during all-out exercise at altitude
10 H_2CO_3
11 This hormone stimulates production of red blood cells
12 A dietary deficiency in this mineral hinders acclimatization (abbr.)

13 This component of cardiac function decreases at altitude
14 The length of altitude acclimatization depends on this factor
15 Altitudes between 3048 and 5486 m and higher
16 _____ fluid volume decreases during the first several days of altitude exposure
17 Highest mountain in the world
18 Pertaining to the surrounding environment

See page 372 for Crossword Puzzle Solution.

Exercise and Thermal Stress

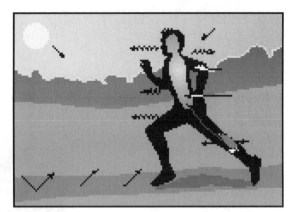

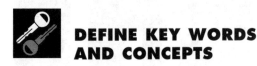

**DEFINE KEY WORDS
AND CONCEPTS**

1. Core temperature

2. Peripheral thermal receptors

3.. Posterior hypothalamus

4. Anterior hypothalamus

5. Radiation

6. Conduction

7. Convection

8. Evaporation

9. Insensible perspiration

10. Relative humidity

11. **ADH**

12. **Aldosterone**

13. **Heat loss through the head**

14. **The ideal winter clothes**

15. **Peak water loss by sweating**

16. **Diuretic-induced dehydration**

17. **Primary aim of fluid replacement**

18. **Hyperhydration**

19. **Heat acclimatization**

20. **Heat illness**

21. **Heat cramps**

22. **Heat exhaustion**

23. **Heat stroke**

24. **Oral versus rectal temperature in exercise**

25. **Thermal conductivity: water versus air**

26. **WB-GT index**

27. **Ama divers**

28. **Wind chill index**

29. **Balaclava**

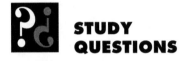

STUDY QUESTIONS

THERMAL BALANCE

How much energy (in calories) can be generated in sustained vigorous exercise?

Explain how the circulatory system provides the "fine tuning" for temperature regulation.

HYPOTHALAMIC REGULATION OF TEMPERATURE

Discuss the role of the hypothalamus in temperature regulation.

THERMOREGULATION IN COLD STRESS: HEAT CONSERVATION AND HEAT PRODUCTION

Vascular Adjustments

What causes the constriction of peripheral blood vessels during cold exposure?

Muscular Activity

In what way do shivering and physical activity contribute to thermoregulation during cold stress?

Hormonal Output

Name three hormones that increase the body's resting heat production.

1.

2.

3.

THERMOREGULATION IN HEAT STRESS: HEAT LOSS

Heat Loss by Radiation

Describe how radiation contributes to the body's heat loss.

Heat Loss by Conduction

Describe how conduction contributes to the body's heat loss.

Heat Loss by Convection

Describe how convection contributes to the body's heat loss.

Heat Loss by Evaporation

Describe how evaporation contributes to the body's heat loss.

Evaporative Heat Loss at High Ambient Temperature

What heat loss mechanisms are blunted when ambient temperature exceeds body temperature?

Heat Loss in High Humidity

List three factors that affect the total sweat vaporized from the skin.

1.

2.

3.

What role does the relative humidity of ambient air play in the effectiveness of evaporative heat loss?

Integration of Heat-Dissipating Mechanisms

Circulation

Discuss how the circulatory system serves as the "workhorse" in temperature regulation.

Evaporation

Discuss how circulation and evaporation work hand-in-hand in thermoregulation.

Hormonal Adjustments

What role does the pituitary gland play in the body's adjustment to heat stress?

EFFECTS OF CLOTHING ON THERMOREGULATION

Cold-Weather Clothing

Identify three characteristics of appropriate clothing for exercise in cold weather.

1.

2.

3.

Warm-Weather Clothing

Identify three characteristics of appropriate clothing for exercise in warm weather.

1.

2.

3.

Football Uniforms

Why do football uniforms pose a unique problem to thermoregulation during exercise in the heat?

CARDIOVASCULAR EXERCISE IN THE HEAT

Circulatory Adjustments

When exercising in the heat, the body is faced with what two competitive demands?

1.

2.

Is cardiac output higher, lower, or the same during submaximum exercise in the heat compared to the cold?

Vascular Constriction and Dilation

Can prolonged reduction in blood flow to certain tissues cause complications? Explain.

Maintenance of Blood Pressure

In addition to redirecting blood to areas in great need, what other hemodynamic role does vasoconstriction serve during exercise in the heat?

Core Temperature during Exercise

Higher Core Temperatures Are Regulated

Plot the general relationship between esophageal temperature (y axis) and oxygen uptake as a percent of a person's $\dot{V}O_2$ max during graded exercise (x axis). (*Hint: Refer to Figure 25.4 in your textbook.*)

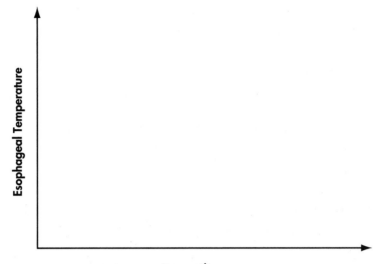

Water Loss In Heat—Dehydration

Magnitude of Fluid Loss

Discuss the following statement: "Excessive output of sweat in high humidity contributes little to the body's cooling."

Significant Consequences

Indicate the effects of dehydration (use + for increase, − for decrease) of the following physiologic functions during exercise compared to conditions of normal hydration.

   Variable   Effect of Dehydration
- Rectal temperature

- Heart rate

- Sweat rate

- $\dot{V}O_2max$

Physiologic and Performance Decrements

The reduction in peripheral blood flow and the increase in core temperature during exercise are proportional to the level of _____.

Approximately how much does exercise heart rate increase for each liter of sweat-loss dehydration?

Quantify the relationship between performance decrements and level of dehydration.

Use of Diuretics

What is a unique negative effect of inducing dehydration with diuretics?

Water Replacement: Rehydration

The primary aim of fluid replacement during exercise is to maintain _____.

The most effective defense against heat stress is _____.

Adequacy of Rehydration

How can a person know if he or she has adequately rehydrated following exercise?

Electrolyte Replacement

A Small Amount of Salt May Be Beneficial

Discuss two reasons why a small amount of electrolytes added to fluid may contribute to a more complete rehydration than water alone.

1.

2.

Factors That Modify Heat Tolerance

Acclimatization

List five important physiologic adjustments that occur during the process of heat acclimatization.

1.

2.

3.

4.

5.

Training

Give two important beneficial effects of exercise training on the body's ability to adjust to environmental heat stress.

1.

2.

Age

What is the general effect of age on thermoregulatory function?

Children

List three differences between children and adults with respect to sweating and core temperature during heat stress.

1.

2.

3.

Sex

Indicate the sex difference in thermoregulatory function for the following variables:

- Sweating

- Evaporative versus circulatory cooling

- Ratio of body surface area to volume

- Effect of menstruation

Level of Body Fat

Discuss why excessive body fat is a liability when exercising in the heat.

Complications from Excessive Heat Stress

List four signs of heat stress.

1.

2.

3.

4.

List the major forms of heat illness in order of increasing severity.

1.

2.

3.

Heat Cramps

What probably causes heat cramps?

Heat Exhaustion

What is a likely cause of heat exhaustion?

List five symptoms of heat exhaustion.

1.

2.

3.

4.

5.

Heat Stroke

What causes heat stroke?

Why is heat stroke considered a "medical emergency"?

Don't Rely on Oral Temperature

Explain why oral temperature is often a poor indicator of core temperature.

How Hot Is "Too Hot"?

Give the formula for calculating the WB-GT index.

List three general guidelines that can be applied to athletic activities to minimize the chances of heat injury.

1.

2.

3.

Compute the Heat Stress Index for an ambient temperature of 90°F and 75% relative humidity.

EXERCISE IN THE COLD

How much greater is heat conduction in water than in air at equivalent temperatures?

Body Fatness, Exercise, and Cold Stress

Give the benefit of body fat during exposure to environmental cold stress.

Explain why the stress of environmental cold is said to be highly relative.

Acclimatization to the Cold

Do humans adapt better to cold or heat stress? Explain.

Give two unique aspects of the Korean Ama divers.

1.

2.

Give three examples of the body's limited adaptation to environmental cold stress.

1.

2.

3.

How Cold Is "Too Cold"?

The Wind Chill Index

List three environmental factors that contribute to the Wind Chill Index.

1.

2.

3.

The Respiratory Tract During Cold-Weather Exercise

Describe the effect on the respiratory tract of breathing extremely cold air.

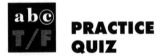 **PRACTICE QUIZ**

MULTIPLE CHOICE

1. **Which statement is <u>true</u> about the hypothalamus?**
   a. it receives input from receptors in the blood that are sensitive to changes in $\dot{V}O_2$
   b. it is the "thermostat" for temperature regulation
   c. it is activated during strenuous exercise only
   d. it receives input from receptors in the blood that are sensitive to changes in acidity
   e. all of the above

2. **Which provides the "fine tuning" for temperature regulation?**
   a. hormonal adjustments
   b. receptor adjustments
   c. circulatory adjustments
   d. ventilatory adjustments
   e. none of the above

3. **What provides the major physiologic defense against overheating?**
   a. heat loss by radiation
   b. heat loss by conduction
   c. heat loss by convection
   d. heat loss by evaporation
   e. none of the above

4. **Which of the following statements is <u>true</u>?**
   a. one should wear one single bulky layer of clothing when exercising in the cold
   b. the thinner the zone of trapped air next to the body, the more effective is the insulation
   c. wool or synthetics such as polypropylene insulate well and dry quickly.
   d. when clothing becomes wet from sweating, the effectiveness of insulation is increased
   e. a and c

5. Which statement is <u>false</u> about exercising in cold weather?
   a. in severe cold, cutaneous blood flow approaches zero
   b. exercise $\dot{V}O_2$ tends to be lower when exercising in the cold
   c. skin temperature falls toward the temperature of the environment
   d. a and b
   e. b and c

6. Which is a consequence of pre-exercise dehydration?
   a. increase in rectal temperature
   b. decrease in sweat rate
   c. decrease in $\dot{V}O_2$max
   d. a and b
   e. all of the above

7. Which of the following is a factor that can modify heat tolerance?
   a. acclimatization
   b. training
   c. fatness
   d. a and c
   e. all of the above

8. Which statement is <u>true</u>?
   a. humans possess less capacity for adaptation to cold than to heat exposure
   b. humans possess greater capacity for adaptation to cold than to heat exposure
   c. humans possess similar capacities for adaptation to cold and to heat exposure
   d. humans possess less capacity for adaptation to cold than to heat exposure only at sea level
   e. humans possess greater capacity for adaptation to cold than to heat exposure only at sea level

9. Which of the following variables is <u>not</u> considered in the Wind Chill Index?
   a. ambient temperature
   b. wind speed
   c. altitude
   d. relative humidity
   e. c and d

10. For each liter of water that evaporates from the skin's surface, this much heat is extracted from the body and transferred to the environment:
    a. 9 kcal
    b. 100 kcal
    c. 275 kcal
    d. 327 kcal
    e. 580 kcal

TRUE/FALSE

1. _____ The amount of body surface exposed to the environment is the most important factor determining the effectiveness of evaporative heat loss.

2. _____ With extreme heat stress, 15 to 25% of the cardiac output passes through the skin.

3. _____ For some athletes, fluid loss from sweating can represent 6 to 10% of body mass.

4. _____ The most effective defense against heat stress is "cold treatments" to the head.

5. _____ Exercise training causes sweating to begin at a lower body temperature.

6. _____ Women possess fewer heat-activated sweat glands per unit skin area than men.

7. _____ Fatal heat stroke occurs 3.5 times more frequently in young adults who are overweight.

8. _____ Cold ambient air can significantly damage the respiratory passages.

9. _____ A reduced loading of hemoglobin with oxygen occurs at high altitudes.

10. _____ Aerobic capacity shows a linear decrease with increases in altitude.

CROSSWORD PUZZLE

ACROSS

2 This temperature is a poor indicator of core temperature after strenuous exercise
3 Index of ambient cold
5 Heat transfer involving air or fluid movement
10 Major physiologic defense against overheating
12 Sweat glands are of this type
15 Hormone released from adrenal cortex to increase sodium reabsorption
18 Regulation of body temperature
22 A calorigenic hormone
26 Deeper body tissues
28 The major portion of sweat is drawn from this body fluid
29 Another term for perspiration
30 Fluid intake related to excess water content of the body
32 _____ perspiration

DOWN

1 Cold-weather clothing that covers nose and mouth
3 Cools body 2 to 4 times faster than air at same temperature
4 Thirty to forty percent of heat is lost from this body area
6 Electrolyte that when added in small amounts to fluid may sustain thirst drive (abbr.)
7 Group at high risk when working in the heat
8 This American sport and its equipment pose a significant challenge to thermoregulation
9 Elite marathoners frequently experience fluid losses in excess of ____ liters during competition
11 Women divers of Korea and southern Japan

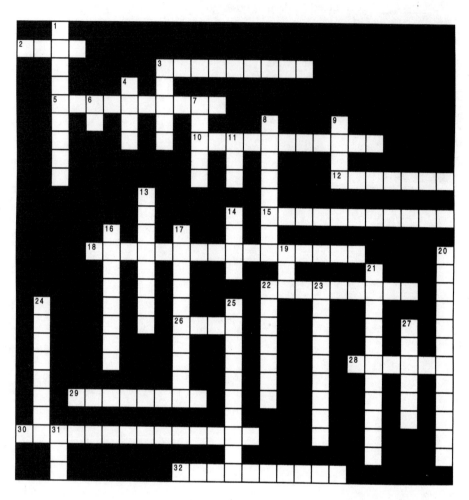

13 Drug or substance that promotes body water loss
14 Heat stress index that uses temperature, humidity, and radiant heat (abbr.)
16 This group demonstrates a lower rate of sweating and a higher core temperature during heat stress
17 Direct molecular transfer of heat through liquid, solid, or gas
19 Acts on kidneys to conserve water during heat stress (abbr.)
20 Coordinating center for temperature regulation

21 This system is the "workhorse" for temperature regulation
22 _____ balance is achieved when heat loss equals heat gain
23 Heat transfer via electromagnetic waves
24 Moisture content of air
25 Most serious and complex of the heat-stress maladies
27 This tissue "wins out" in competition for blood in hot-weather exercise
31 First 3 letters of gland that releases ADH

See page 373 for Crossword Puzzle Solution.

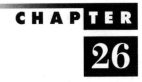

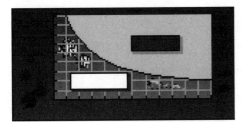

Sport Diving

DEFINE KEY TERMS AND CONCEPTS

1. Boyle's law

2. One atmosphere pressure

3. Snorkel size limit

4. Blackout

5. Breakpoint for breath-hold

6. Lung squeeze

7. Scuba

8. Open-circuit scuba

9. Closed-circuit scuba

10. Lung burst

11. **Air embolism**

12. **Emboli**

13. **Pneumothorax**

14. **Mask squeeze**

15. **Aerotitis**

16. **Eustachian tubes**

17. **Popping the ears**

18. **Aerosinusitis**

19. **Nitrogen narcosis**

20. **Rapture of the deep**

21. **The bends**

22. **Zero decompression limits**

23. **Decompression sickness**

24. **Oxygen poisoning**

25. **Carbon monoxide poisoning**

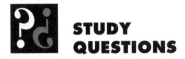

STUDY QUESTIONS

PRESSURE-VOLUME RELATIONSHIPS AND DIVING DEPTH

Diving Depth and Pressure

List two factors that determine the water pressure against a diver's body under water.

1.

2.

What would be the pressure exerted by fresh water at a depth of 33 ft?

Diving Depth and Gas Volume

Quantify the changes in a 6-L lung volume as a breath-hold diver progressively descends below the water's surface.

SNORKELING AND BREATH-HOLD DIVING

Limits to Snorkel Size

List two factors to consider when increasing snorkel size for underwater swimming.

1.

2.

Inspiratory Capacity with Diving Depth

Why is it not possible to breathe through a tube when immersed to a depth of about 3 ft?

Snorkel Size with Pulmonary Dead Space

Give the ideal snorkel size (length and inside diameter) based on average values for anatomic dead space.

Breath-Hold Diving

Give the changes in arterial P_{O_2} and P_{CO_2} during a normal breath-hold.

- P_{O_2}
- P_{CO_2}

Hyperventilation and Breath-Hold Diving: Blackout

List three reasons for loss of consciousness during an extended breath-hold dive.

1.

2.

3.

Discuss the physiological rationale for hyperventilation prior to a breath-hold dive.

Additional Considerations

List two risks of hyperventilation preceding a breath-hold dive.

1.

2.

Depth Limits with Breath-Hold Diving: Thoracic Squeeze

What is the critical depth for breath-hold diving without danger of lung squeeze?

Other Problems

What is the reason for eardrum rupture during an underwater dive?

SCUBA DIVING

List the two basic scuba designs.

1.

2.

Open-Circuit Scuba

What is the basic purpose of a scuba system?

List one major drawback of the open-circuit scuba system.

How long could a diver stay underwater at a depth of 10 m with a tank containing 80 ft^3 of air compressed to 3000 p.s.i.?

Closed-Circuit Scuba

List two main problems encountered with the use of closed-circuit scuba.

1.

2.

SPECIAL PROBLEMS BREATHING GASES AT HIGH PRESSURES
Air Embolism

Discuss the danger in breath-holding during ascent from a dive with scuba.

At what depths do the changes in pressure have the greatest effect on lung volume during ascent from a dive?

Pneumothorax: Lung Collapse

What is a sure way to eliminate the danger of air embolism and pneumothorax during scuba diving?

Mask Squeeze

What is one advantage of using a standard face mask compared to goggles during breath-hold diving?

Aerotitis: Middle-Ear Squeeze

Why is it sometimes necessary to swallow, yawn, or move the jaws from side to side during air travel in nonpressurized aircraft?

Explain why divers with an upper respiratory infection often suffer severe pain in the ears when immersed only a few feet under water.

Never Dive with Earplugs

Explain why it is undesirable to dive with earplugs.

Aerosinusitis

What is the major cause of "sinus squeeze"?

Nitrogen Narcosis: Rapture of the Deep

Give the inspired P_{N_2} during scuba diving at a depth of 60 m.

List two factors that determine nitrogen uptake at the tissue level during scuba diving.

1.

2.

Give an explanation for why divers breathing compressed air will sometimes remove their scuba gear for no apparent reason during a dive of 30 m or deeper.

What is the maximum recommended depth range for recreational scuba divers?

Decompression Sickness: The Bends

Under what conditions does decompression sickness occur?

Why are women generally at greater risk for decompression sickness?

Zero Decompression Limits

Give the upper limit for diving depth and duration before sufficient nitrogen becomes dissolved and poses a danger for the bends.

Give a prudent recommendation for the sport diver in terms of depth and duration for compressed-air diving. (*Hint: Refer to Figure 26.6 in your textbook.*)

Consequences of Inadequate Decompression

When do symptoms of decompression sickness usually appear following a dive?

Give the most common symptom of inadequate decompression from a compressed-air dive.

Describe the common treatment for the bends.

Oxygen Poisoning

What is the maximum diving depth recommended when breathing pure oxygen?

List two ways in which a high P_{O_2} negatively affects bodily functions.

1.

2.

Carbon Monoxide Poisoning

What are some problems that could occur when filling scuba tanks with compressed air?

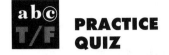 **PRACTICE QUIZ**

MULTIPLE CHOICE

1. **Although it increases breath-hold capacity, hyperventilation is dangerous because:**
    a. it may reduce cerebral blood flow
    b. it results in an increase in plasma carbon dioxide
    c. it results in an acid-base imbalance
    d. a and c
    e. a and b

2. **The maximum depth for breath-hold diving is generally determined by the:**
    a. amount of CO_2 in the lungs at the start of the dive
    b. amount of oxygen in the alveoli at the start of the dive
    c. point where the diver's lung volume is compressed to residual volume
    d. oxygen uptake during the dive
    e. diver's pain tolerance

3. **The maximum recommended depth for breathing compressed air is generally:**
    a. 30 m
    b. 45 m
    c. 60 m
    d. 90 m
    e. > 90 m

4. **If a scuba diver ascends toward the surface too rapidly, the excess nitrogen:**
    a. cannot exit through the lungs and escapes from the dissolved state and forms bubbles in the tissues.
    b. exits the lungs into the atmosphere
    c. remains in the cells until an equilibrium of all gases is reached in the body's tissues
    d. is buffered and exits the body as nitrous dioxide
    e. decreases in volume until the air passages equilibrate

5. **Carbon monoxide:**
    a. is able to combine with hemoglobin 200 times more readily than oxygen
    b. does not readily combine with hemoglobin
    c. has the same affinity for hemoglobin as oxygen
    d. has the same affinity for hemoglobin as carbon dioxide
    e. a, b, and c

6. **Aerosinusitis refers to the condition where:**
    a. air escapes into the sinus cavities from surrounding tissues in an attempt to equalize pressure differentials
    b. blood rushes into the sinus cavities due to high pressures of dissolved nitrogen
    c. sinus cavities become inflamed due to the elevated inspired P_{N_2}
    d. inflamed and congested sinus cavities prevent the air pressure in these cavities from equalizing during diving; this results in bleeding in the sinus membranes as blood moves in to equalize the pressure differential
    e. none of the above

7. **During deep-water diving the total pressure of the respired gas:**
    a. decreases in direct proportion to the total gas availability
    b. increases in direct proportion to the depth of the dive
    c. remains the same throughout the dive
    d. becomes volatile and the total pressure no longer equals the sum of the partial pressures
    e. none of the above

8. **An increase in the pressure and quantity of dissolved nitrogen causes:**
   a. physical and mental reactions characterized by a general state of euphoria called nitrogen narcosis
   b. internal bleeding in the sinuses called nitrogen bends
   c. nitrogen gas to escape into the tissues at a rate that causes oxygen dilution and eventual asphyxia
   d. oxygen and carbon dioxide to reach an equilibrium that results in a general state of euphoria similar to alcohol intoxication
   e. nitrogen to escape into the lung cavity, causing breathing to become compromised

9. **A full inhalation of compressed air in 6 ft of water can cause serious overdistention of lung tissue during ascent if the diver does not:**
   a. continue to inhale
   b. continue to exhale
   c. continue to breath-hold
   d. inhale at a rate equal to the rate of ascent
   e. none of the above

10. **One major problem with closed-circuit scuba is:**
   a. the use of cumbersome equipment that makes movement difficult
   b. the inability to use 100% oxygen instead of compressed air
   c. serious injury can occur if carbon dioxide output exceeds its rate of absorption in the closed system
   d. the inability to go deeper than 30 m due to the escape of oxygen from the system
   e. absorption of nitrogen gas from the inspired air

TRUE/FALSE

1. _____ Hyperventilation increases breath-hold time but also can contribute to underwater blackout.

2. _____ Snorkel size is limited by the underwater depth at which the skin diver can generate sufficient inspiratory force to breathe.

3. _____ Significant hazards of scuba diving are air embolism, pneumothorax, mask and middle-ear squeeze, and aerosinusitis.

4. _____ Excess oxygen in the tissues is often termed the "bends."

5. _____ Oxygen poisoning occurs when the inspired P_{O_2} exceeds 2 atm (1520 mm Hg).

6. _____ Symptoms of decompression sickness can begin immediately after ascent.

7. _____ The most common symptom of decompression sickness is shortness of breath.

8. _____ The deeper the descent, the less time can be spent underwater without danger from decompression sickness.

9. _____ "Rapture of the deep" refers to sounds heard during underwater diving while wearing a face mask in depths greater than 30 m.

10. _____ If you have a cold it is advisable to dive with earplugs to allow the pressure to equalize in various air cavities.

CROSSWORD PUZZLE

ACROSS

2 Condition caused by breathing high pressures of O_2

5 Only effective treatment for air embolism is rapid _____

7 Air breathed at water depth of 10 meters _____ in volume when brought to the surface

9 Inflamed and congested sinuses that prevent air pressure in these cavities from equalizing

11 Potentially dangerous ventilatory maneuver prior to breath-hold diving

16 Condition in which dissolved nitrogen moves out of solution and forms bubbles in body tissues

19 Second word in term describing effects of excess nitrogen dissolved in body fluids

20 Diving women of Korea and Japan

21 Barometric pressure is about 760 mm Hg at this elevation

23 Person who described relation between gas volume and pressure

24 Middle-ear squeeze

DOWN

1 Another term for lung collapse

2 This gas becomes poisonous when breathed in excess of 2 atmospheres pressure

3 Only form of scuba system recommended in sport diving

4 Breakpoint for breath-hold corresponds to arterial P_{CO_2} of about ____ mm Hg

6 Air cavities in skull

8 Scuba system useful for military operations

10 Sudden loss of consciousness in breath-hold diving

12 Force per unit area exerted by gas or liquid

13 "Rapture of the deep" is caused by accumulation of this gas

14 ____ _____ occurs when lung volume is compressed below residual volume

15 Equivalent to depth of about 32 ft

17 J-shaped tube used in skin diving

18 Tube leading from tympanic cavity to nasopharynx

21 Open-circuit diving system (abbr.)

22 Bubbles caused by expansion of air in respiratory tract causing lung tissue to rupture

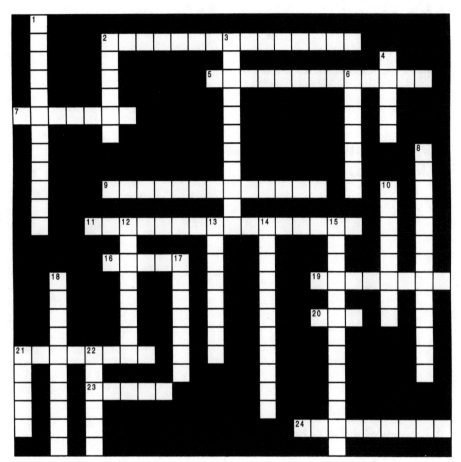

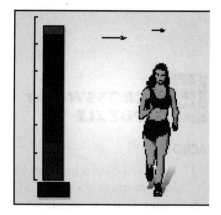

Body Composition Assessment

DEFINE KEY TERMS AND CONCEPTS

1. Height-weight tables

2. Morbidity

3. BMI

4. Overweight

5. Five-level model of body composition

6. Dr. Albert Behnke

7. Reference man and woman

8. Essential fat

9. Sex-specific fat

10. Storage fat

11. **Fat-free body mass**

12. **Lean body mass**

13. **Minimal body mass**

14. **Underweight**

15. **Oligomenorrhea**

16. **Amenorrhea**

17. **"Critical level" of body fat**

18. **Hydrostatic weighing**

19. **Specific gravity**

20. **Density**

21. **Archimedes' principle**

22. **William Siri**

23. **Fat mass**

24. **Body volume**

25. **Buoyancy**

26. **Subcutaneous fatfolds**

27. **Fatfold caliper**

28. **Generalized equations**

29. **Body profile**

30. **BIA**

31. **NIR**

32. **MRI**

33. **Ultrasound**

34. **Arm x-ray**

35. **DEXA**

36. **CT scan**

37. **Desirable body mass**

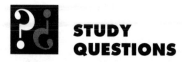

STUDY QUESTIONS

BODY COMPOSITION ASSESSMENT

List the three structural components of the body and their percentages for the reference man and woman.

	Structural Component	Reference Man	Reference Woman
1.			
2.			
3.			

Give one major criticism of the standard height-weight tables.

The Body Mass Index: A Somewhat Better Alternative

Give the desirable BMI range for women and men.

• Women

• Men

Example Computation of BMI

Compute your BMI.

Limitations of BMI

Under what condition is the BMI likely to be misleading as an index of obesity?

COMPOSITION OF THE HUMAN BODY

Describe the anthropologist Matiega's model of body composition.

Give the density values of storage fat mass and the fat-free mass components of the body.

• Storage fat mass

• Fat-free mass

Behnke Reference Man and Woman
Essential and Storage Fat

Give the generalized locations for essential and storage fat in the body.

1. Essential fat

2. Storage fat

Give the whole-body density of Behnke's reference man and woman.

• Man

• Woman

Fat-Free Mass and Lean Body Mass

Describe the difference between fat-free body mass and lean body mass.

Minimal Standards for Leanness

Indicate the components that make up the minimal body mass in females.

Minimal Body Mass

What is the lowest healthy weight for adult males and females?

1. Male

2. Female

Calculation of Minimal Mass

Give the formula for calculating minimal body mass.

Five-Level Model of Body Composition

List the five levels for quantifying body composition and give one fact about each.

	Level	Fact
1.		
2.		
3.		
4.		
5.		

Underweight and Thin

What precisely is meant by the terms "underweight" and "thin"?

- Underweight

- Thin

Leanness, Regular Exercise, and Menstrual Irregularity

Give the lower limit of body fat believed to trigger menstrual irregularity.

Describe the association between menstrual irregularity and body fat.

Leanness Is Not the Only Factor

List four factors associated with menstrual dysfunction.

1.

2.

3.

4.

Delayed Onset of Menstruation and Cancer Risk

Can a delayed menstruation alter cancer risk in females? Discuss.

COMMON TECHNIQUES FOR ASSESSING BODY COMPOSITION

Direct Assessment

List the two approaches to the direct assessment of body composition.

1.

2.

Indirect Assessment

List seven indirect body composition assessment procedures.

1.   5.

2.   6.

3.   7.

4.

Hydrostatic Weighing: Archimedes' Principle

Describe Archimedes' procedure for assessing the composition of the king's crown.

State Archimedes' principle of buoyant force as related to body volume.

Validity of Hydrostatic Weighing for Estimating Body Fat

Describe Behnke's experimental evidence for validating the hydrostatic weighing method for body composition assessment.

Possible Limitations

List one assumption in using body density for body composition assessment.

Computing Body Density

What is the body volume of someone who weighs 50 kg when weighed in air but only 2 kg when submerged underwater?

Computing Body Fat Percentage

Write the formulas for computing body density and body fat percentage with the Siri equation.

• Body density =

• Percent fat =

Compute the body fat percentage for a person whose body density is $1.0742 \text{ g} \cdot \text{cm}^{-3}$.

Possible Limitations for Density Assumptions
Limitations of Density Assumptions

Describe how the assumption underlying the density of the body's fat and fat-free mass could cause errors in estimating fat percentage from whole-body density.

Write the equations for calculating the body fat percentage from density for blacks.

Computing the Mass of Fat

Give the formula for computing fat mass.

Fat mass =

Compute the fat mass for a person who weighs 65 kg and has a fat percentage of 22.

Computing Fat-Free Body Mass

Give the formula for computing fat-free body mass.

Fat-free body mass =

Compute the fat-free body mass for a person who weighs 65 kg and who has a fat percentage of 22.

Measurement of Body Volume

List two methods for determining whole-body volume.

1.

2.

Water Displacement
Hydrostatic Weighing

In both water displacement and hydrostatic weighing, why is it important to know the subject's residual lung volume?

During underwater weighing, which of the underwater weight scores is most appropriate?

Variations with Menstruation

Under most normal conditions, are variations in total body water related to the phase of the menstrual cycle and cause "errors" in body volume determinations?

Calculating Body Composition from Body Mass, Body Volume, and Residual Lung Volume

Calculate body density, body fat percentage, fat mass, and fat-free mass for a person who weighs 65 kg in air and 1.5 kg underwater (water density = 0.996) and has a residual lung volume of 1.3 L. (Show your work.)

- Body density
- % fat
- Fat mass
- Fat-free mass

Fatfold and Girth Measurements

Measurement of Subcutaneous Fatfolds

The Caliper

How much tension is exerted at the tips of the skinfold calipers?

The Sites

List five common sites for measuring fatfolds.

1.

2.

3.

4.

5.

Usefulness of Fatfold Scores

Give two ways to use fatfold scores when assessing body composition.

1.

2.

Fatfolds and Age

Does the same fatfold score for a person at age 15 and at age 40 reflect the same percentage of total body fat? Explain.

User Beware

Describe a major drawback of using fatfolds to assess total body fat.

Measurement of Girths
Usefulness of Girth Measurements

Compute the body fat percentage and fat-free body mass of a 35-year-old woman who weighs 70.4 kg and has the following girth measurements: abdomen = 82.6 cm; right thigh = 57.8 cm; right calf = 44.5 cm.

- Percent body fat

- Fat-free body mass

List two advantages of girth measurements over fatfolds to assess total body fat.

1.

2.

Target Body Fat from Changes in Abdominal Girth

Calculate your body fat percentage from abdominal girth using the method described in the text.

Bioelectric Impedance Analysis (BIA)

How accurate is the BIA method compared to the fatfold method?

List one factor that affects the accuracy of BIA measurements.

Near-Infrared Interactance (NIR)

Describe the basis of NIR measurements for body composition assessment.

Questionable Validity of NIR

Do objective data support the use of NIR for the assessment of body composition?

Ultrasound Assessment of Fat
Arm X-Ray Assessment of Fat

Give one advantage of the ultrasound and x-ray indirect methods for body composition assessment.

- Ultrasound

- X-Ray

Computed Tomography, Magnetic Resonance Imaging, and Dual-Energy X-Ray Absorptiometry

Computed Tomography (CT)

What is the relationship between CT scans and abdominal adipose tissue area?

Magnetic Resonance Imaging (MRI)

What is the validity of MRI scanning for determining body fatness?

Dual-Energy X-Ray Absorptiometry (DEXA)

Describe the relationship between fat percentage determined by DEXA and fat percentage determined by densitometry.

DEXA and Body Composition in Anorexia Nervosa

Describe the difference in bone mineral density between anorectics and normals.

What Is Average for Percent Body Fat?

Give the "average" values for body fat percentage for young and older adult men and women. (*Hint: Refer to Table 27.5 in your textbook.*)

- Young males

- Older males

- Young females

- Older females

Representative Samples Are Lacking

Give one explanation for the observed change in body fat percentage with increasing age.

Desirable Body Mass

Write the equation to compute desirable body mass.

A 20-year-old man weighs 89 kg and has 22% body fat. If this man reduces his body fat to a desired 12% level, what will his new body mass be, and how much total fat mass will he have lost? Assume all weight lost is fat.

- Desirable body mass

- Desirable fat loss

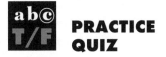 **PRACTICE QUIZ**

MULTIPLE CHOICE

1. **Once underwater weight is known, it is possible to compute all of the following except:**
   a. body density
   b. body fat percentage
   c. fat-free body mass
   d. approximate number of fat cells
   e. c and d

2. **What is the main limitation of height-weight tables?**
   a. they do not allow for differences in bone structure
   b. they do not consider a person's age
   c. they give no indication of the composition of the body, especially fat and lean
   d. they are based on old normative data
   e. none of the above

3. **According to Behnke's model for the reference man and reference woman:**
   a. a woman may jeopardize her health if her body fat falls below 22%
   b. a man may jeopardize his health if his body fat falls below 8%
   c. the average quantity of essential fat for men is about 3% of body mass
   d. the average quantity of storage fat for women is about 26% of body mass.
   e. a and c

4. **Very lean female athletes often experience secondary amenorrhea; this is indirect verification of Behnke's concept of:**
   a. minimal weight
   b. storage fat
   c. energy drain
   d. lean body mass
   e. none of the above

5. **Among young adults, the average body fat percentage is ___ for men and ___ for women.**
   a. 10%, 25%
   b. 15%, 25%
   c. 20%, 30%
   d. 25%, 35%

6. **What percentage of body fat is cited as the critical level for the onset of menstruation in females?**
   a. 15%
   b. 17%
   c. 19%
   d. 21%
   e. none of the above

7. **When calculating body volume with hydrostatic weighing, what must be subtracted from the measured body volume?**
   a. residual lung volume
   b. vital capacity
   c. expiratory lung volume
   d. inspiratory lung volume
   e. total lung capacity

8. **Which of the following limits the use of fatfolds to predict body fat percentage?**
   a. the person taking the measurements must be experienced
   b. for obese people the thickness of the fatfold often exceeds the caliper's jaws
   c. the particular caliper used may contribute to measurement error
   d. variations in prediction equations contribute to error
   e. all of the above

9. **All of the following affect the accuracy of bioelectric impedance analysis except:**
   a. overhydration
   b. skin temperature
   c. dehydration
   d. weight of the individual
   e. a, b, and d

10. **DEXA, CT, MRI, and BIA are all methods to estimate:**
    a. total body water
    b. body composition
    c. body temperature
    d. subcutaneous body fat
    e. none of the above

TRUE/FALSE

1. _____ The three major structural components of the body are body mass, lean body mass, and fat percentage.

2. _____ The error in predicting an individual's body fat percentage from fatfold or girth equations is generally within 2.5 to 4.0 fat units from the body fat percentage determined by hydrostatic weighing.

3. _____ Desirable body mass is computed as fat-free body mass minus desired fat percentage.

4. _____ The existing equations to calculate body composition from body density in whites would tend to overestimate the fat-free body mass when applied to blacks.

5. _____ The essential fat percentages are 8% for men and 15% for women.

6. _____ Girth measurements provide meaningful information concerning body fat and its distribution.

7. _____ As one ages, a greater quantity of fat is deposited as subcutaneous fat than as internal fat.

8. _____ Magnetic resonance imaging provides valuable information about the body's tissue compartments.

9. _____ Changes in body composition with age could occur partly because of the age-related decrease in bone density.

10. _____ The Siri equation is used to calculate body density.

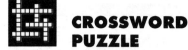

CROSSWORD PUZZLE

ACROSS

5 Irregular menstrual cycle
9 These equations consider age when predicting body fat
11 Body mass, kg ÷ stature, m² (abbr.)
13 Body's external surface area (abbr.)
15 Internal fat in relation to subcutaneous fat increases with ____
16 This component of body's lipids serves as an energy depot
17 Muscle mass plus a small percentage of essential fat stored chiefly within the CNS, bone marrow, and internal organs (abbr.)
18 Mass per unit volume
19 Body mass devoid of extractable fat (abbr.)
21 Body composition assessment technique using high-frequency sound
22 $0.90 \text{ g} \cdot \text{cm}^{-3}$ is the density of this tissue
25 Ratio of an object's mass to the mass of equivalent volume of water
29 Discovered principle of water displacement
32 Condition in which body mass is greater than some standard, usually the mean body mass for a given stature
33 Body composition technique using roentgenograms
34 Additional fat stores in females important for childbearing and other hormone-related functions

DOWN

1 Risk for this disease is lower in female athletes with delayed-onset menstruation
2 _____ weighing is a technique to assess body volume

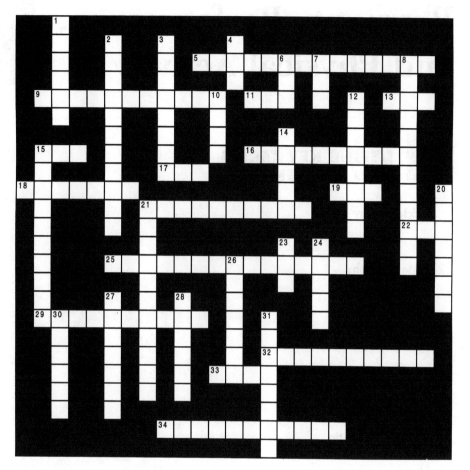

3 Lung volume subtracted from underwater weight to determine body volume
4 Body composition technique that measures electrical flow in body's (abbr.)
6 Body composition technique using magnetic imaging (abbr.)
7 Body composition technique using infrared light (abbr.)
8 Lipids in bone marrow, heart, lungs, liver, spleen, kidneys, intestines, muscles, and lipid-rich tissues in the CNS
10 Dual x-ray absorptiometry (abbr.)
12 Too little fat for frame size
14 Reference ____ averages 25 to 27% body fat
15 Absence of menses
20 Double thickness of skin plus fat

21 Condition in which body mass is less than some standard, usually average body mass for a given stature
23 The reference ____ averages 15% body fat
24 Another term for circumference measurements
26 Instrument to measure thickness of fat at selected body sites
27 Lower limit of body mass for women that includes about 14% essential fat
28 Navy physician who pioneered work on body composition
30 There are _____ differences in density of body's fat-free component
31 Upward, vertical thrust exerted on an object immersed in water

See page 373 for Crossword Puzzle Solution.

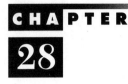

CHAPTER 28

Physique, Performance, and Physical Activity

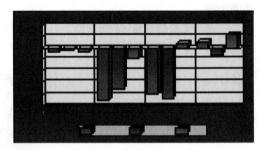

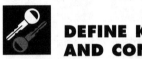 **DEFINE KEY TERMS AND CONCEPTS**

1. Ectomorphy

2. Mesomorphy

3. Endomorphy

4. Somatotyping

5. Lean-to-fat ratio

6. Making weight

7. Weight loss recommendations for wrestlers

8. Ponderal (mass) equivalents

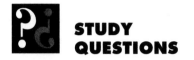

STUDY QUESTIONS

PHYSIQUE OF CHAMPION ATHLETES

List the three body types.

1.

2.

3.

Olympic and Elite Athletes

Describe major differences in physique components between different types of Olympic athletes. (*Hint: Refer to Tables 28.1, 28.2, and 28.3 in your textbook.*)

Sex Differences

Outline the sex differences in body fat percentage for elite performers in three different sport categories.

1.

2.

3.

World Records

Indicate the sex differences in world record running speeds for three different distances.

1.

2.

3.

Fat-Free to Fat Ratio

Give the highest fat-free to fat ratios for male and female elite athletes.

Sex	Sport Category
• Male	
• Female	

Body Fat Percentage Grouped by Sport Category

List six classifications of sport activities based on their particular characteristics and requirements. (*Hint: Refer to Figure 28.5 in your textbook.*)

1.   4.

2.   5.

3.   6.

Racial Differences

Discuss racial differences in the physique of elite athletes.

Field Event Athletes

Which group of athletes have the largest overall body size?

Female Long-Distance Runners
Male Long-Distance Runners

Compare representative values for body mass, stature, and body fat percentage for elite male and female distance runners and untrained counterparts.

	Male Runners	Untrained Males	Female Runners	Untrained Females
• Body mass				
• Stature				
• Percent fat				

Triathletes

Summarize the body composition characteristics of elite male and female triathletes.

- Male

- Female

Football Players

What are the similarities and differences in body composition between professional football players and elite collegiate competitors?

- Similarities

- Differences

Maximal Running Performance and Body Composition

Discuss the relationship between body composition and 50-yd maximal sprint performance.

High School Wrestlers

What is the recommendation of the ACSM concerning the lower acceptable level of body fat for high school wrestlers?

Physical Characteristics of High School Wrestlers

Give the mean (± SD) for body fat percentage of Nebraska high school wrestlers.

Weight Loss Recommendations for Wrestlers

Give an objective basis for making prudent weight loss recommendations for high school wrestlers.

Weight Lifters and Body Builders
Men

Women

Men versus Women

Compare the body fat percentage and excess muscle of male competitive body builders, weight lifters, and power lifters.

	Body Fat %	Excess Muscle
• Body builders		
• Weight lifters		
• Power lifters		

Can women change their muscle size on a relative basis to the same extent as men?

Comparative Data: Analysis of Muscular and Nonmuscular Components

Summarize the major differences between the muscular and nonmuscular components for the following groups:

- Professional ballet dancers
- Champion male and female body builders
- College-age males
- Twelfth-grade Caucasian males and females
- Entering and graduating classes of Amherst College (1882–1886)

EFFECTS OF EXERCISE TRAINING ON BODY COMPOSITION

Ten-Week Jogging Program

What is the average body weight and body fat loss resulting from a 10-week jogging program for an average adult man?

Walking-Running for Different Durations

What effect does exercise duration have on fat loss with exercise training?

Walking, Running, and Bicycling

Is there a selective effect of running, walking, or cycling on body composition changes?

Resistance Training

In what way can resistance training favorably affect body composition?

Frequency of Training

What is the role of training frequency in altering body composition?

EFFECTS OF DIET AND EXERCISE ON BODY COMPOSITION DURING WEIGHT LOSS

What is an important advantage of utilizing regular exercise in a weight loss program?

Gaining Weight

Give a prudent recommendation to an athlete desiring to gain weight.

Is There an Upper Limit to Fat-Free Body Mass?

What is the largest fat-free body mass reported in the literature for an athlete?

- Fat-free mass
- Athletic group

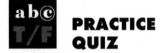 **PRACTICE QUIZ**

MULTIPLE CHOICE

1. **What is the lower acceptable limit of body fat percentage recommended for high school wrestlers?**
   a. 3–5
   b. 5–7
   c. 7–9
   d. 9–11
   e. none of the above

2. **Visual appraisal of body shape is called:**
   a. somatotyping
   b. androgyny
   c. densitometry
   d. angiography
   e. visual dynamics

3. **Ectomorphy refers to:**
   a. muscular body type
   b. fat body type
   c. normal body type
   d. thin body type
   e. none of the above

4. **Endomorphy refers to:**
   a. muscular body type
   b. fat body type
   c. normal body type
   d. thin body type
   e. none of the above

5. **Mesomorphy refers to:**
   a. muscular body type
   b. fat body type
   c. normal body type
   d. thin body type
   e. none of the above

6. **The most striking aspect of the body composition of female Olympic athletes is:**
   a. their relatively low body fat values, averaging about 13%
   b. their relatively high body fat values, averaging about 18%
   c. the wide diversity of their body fat levels
   d. their similarity in body fat levels to normal, nonathletic females
   e. their extremely low lean-to-fat ratios

7. **On average, professional football players have:**
   a. less body fat than top collegiate football players
   b. more body fat than top collegiate football players
   c. about the same body fat as top collegiate football players
   d. excessive amounts of lean tissue compared to top collegiate football players
   e. low lean-to-fat ratios

8. **Male weight lifters and body builders have an average body fat percentage:**
   a. less than 11%
   b. less than 8%
   c. less than 5%
   d. equal to their essential fat level
   e. two times greater than their fat mass

9. **In terms of reducing body fat, the most effective approach is:**
   a. diet only
   b. exercise only
   c. diet in combination with exercise
   d. exercise in combination with behavior therapy
   e. psychotherapy

10. **Compared to weight loss with diet plus exercise, when body mass is reduced by diet only there is:**
   a. less loss of lean tissue
   b. a greater loss of body fat
   c. less body water loss
   d. greater loss of lean tissue and less fat loss
   e. an increase in the RDA for vitamins

TRUE/FALSE

1. _____ The most striking compositional characteristic of the female body builder is her lean-to-fat ratio of 4:1.

2. _____ Heavy muscular overload supported by a prudent diet is an effective means to increase muscle mass.

3. _____ Thirty minutes of moderately strenuous running, bicycling, or circuit resistance exercise, or at least 60 minutes of walking, stimulates body fat loss.

4. _____ The threshold energy expenditure to stimulate body fat loss with exercise is about 300 kcal per day.

5. _____ Body composition assessment reveals that athletes generally have physique characteristics unique to their specific sport.

6. _____ An extra energy intake of 700 to 1000 kcal per day can support a weekly gain of 0.5 to 1.0 kg in lean tissue and training energy requirements.

7. _____ Champion long-distance female runners have body fat levels similar to those of nonathletic females.

8. _____ For female Olympic athletes in general, the most striking observation is their relatively high body fat values.

9. _____ Body fat percentage and aerobic capacity of triathletes are similar to values reported for other endurance athletes in single endurance sports.

10. _____ Women can never increase their muscle size to the same extent as men, even when muscle mass is scaled to a body size factor.

CROSSWORD PUZZLE

ACROSS

1   Elite athletes in this sport have relatively short arms and legs for their stature

4   Technique to describe body size and shape in terms of muscular and nonmuscular components

7   Body build condition characterized by a rounded body shape and predominance of fat

8   Athletes who compete in three different modes of exercise in succession

11 Combination of these two contributes most effectively to fat loss

13 Body build condition characterized by well-developed musculature

14 This group of female athletes has the highest lean-to-fat ratio

15 Body typing that assigns a characteristic shape and physical appearance

DOWN

2   Adding this to a weight-loss program most favorably affects the composition of the weight lost

3   Lower limit of body fat percentage proposed as the lowest acceptable level for safe wrestling competition

5   Dimension of body build characterized by a tall, thin, and linear body

6   The physique of male and female triathletes is most similar to these single-sport athletes

9   In terms of body composition, marathon runners and gymnasts have the highest ____ __ ___ ratio among men

10 This strength measure is not a good indication of excessive lean body mass loss among wrestlers

12 Classification of hormones that increase lean body mass

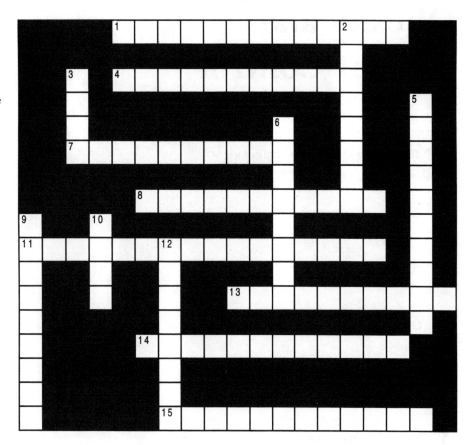

Obesity and Weight Control

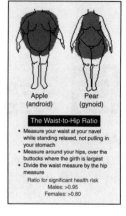

Apple (android) Pear (gynoid)

The Waist-to-Hip Ratio
* Measure your waist at your navel while standing relaxed, not pulling in your stomach
* Measure around your hips, over the buttocks where the girth is largest
* Divide the waist measure by the hip measure

Ratio for significant health risk
Males: >0.95
Females: >0.80

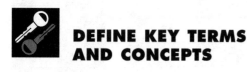

DEFINE KEY TERMS AND CONCEPTS

1. Obesity

2. "Creeping obesity"

3. Ob gene

4. Obesity-producing environment

5. Familial aggregation

6. Percentage fat standards for overfatness

7. Regional fat distribution

8. Waist-to-hip girth ratio

9. Android-type obesity

10. Gynoid-type obesity

11. **Adipocyte**

12. **Fat cell hypertrophy**

13. **Fat cell hyperplasia**

14. **Fat cell biopsy**

15. **Preadipocyte pool**

16. **Energy balance equation**

17. **Ketogenic diets**

18. **Set-point theory**

19. **Yo-yo effect**

20. **3500 kcal**

21. **High-protein diets**

22. **VLCD**

23. **Surgical procedures**

24. **Protein-sparing modified fast**

25. **Dose-response**

26. **Recovery "afterglow"**

27. **Spot reduction**

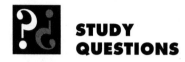

STUDY QUESTIONS

OBESITY

What percentage of American males and females are currently on weight-loss programs?

- Males

- Females

What percentage of the adult American population is considered to be overweight?

Obesity Often Is a Long-Term Process

Discuss the trend for weight gain in adult men and women as they age.

Obesity Is Not Necessarily Related to Overeating

List five factors that predispose a person to excessive weight gain.

1.

2.

3.

4.

5.

Genetics Plays a Role

How much of the variation in weight gain among individuals can be accounted for by genetic factors?

A Mutant Gene?

Explain the role of the mutant "obese" gene in the development of obesity.

Physical Activity: An Important Component

Discuss how increases in body fat with age can be more a function of physical inactivity than age itself.

Health Risks of Obesity

The Culprit: Body Weight or Body Fat?

Is excess body weight or excess body fat more strongly related to heart disease risk?

Overweight in Adolescence Predicts Adverse Health Effects

Coronary heart disease risk during the adult years is increased how many times by being obese as an adolescent?

Specific Risks of Excess Fat: Being Overweight Shortens One's Life

List six health risks of obesity.

1.   4.

2.   5.

3.   6.

Criteria for Obesity: How Fat is Too Fat?

Percent Body Fat

What body fat percentage indicates borderline obesity in adult men and women?

• Men

• Women

Criterion for Children

Give an objective measure to assess excess fat in children.

Regional Fat Distribution

Describe two types of body fat distribution.

1.

2.

Adipocyte Size and Number: Hypertrophy versus Hyperplasia

Describe two ways that fat cells increase in the body.

1.

2.

Varieties of Human Obesities

What is the criterion for identifying severe clinical obesity in males and females?

• Males

• Females

Adipose Cellularity

Comparison of Cellularity in the Normal and Obese

Give average values for fat cell size and fat cell number in obese and nonobese adults.

	Obese	Nonobese

- Cell number
- Cell size

Effects of Weight Reduction

When a person <u>reduces</u> body mass, what happens to fat cell size and fat cell number?

- Fat cell size
- Fat cell number

Effects of Weight Gain

When a person <u>increases</u> body mass, what generally happens to fat cell size and fat cell number?

- Fat cell size
- Fat cell number

The Possibility of Making New Ones

What happens to adipocyte development during massive weight gain in adulthood?

Adipocyte Development

Human Studies

Cell Size

Describe the general pattern for the growth in adipocytes size in humans from birth to adulthood.

Cell Number

Indicate three general stages during which adipocyte number develops in humans.

1.

2.

3.

Can Adipose Cellularity Be Modified?

How much maternal weight gain during pregnancy generally results in increased fatness of the offspring?

Influence of Nutrition

Based on animal research, when is the "critical" period when adipose tissue cellularity could be modified?

Influence of Physical Activity

Discuss the relative merits of physical activity in modifying adipose tissue.

WEIGHT CONTROL

Energy Balance: Input versus Output

Write the energy balance equation.

List two ways to unbalance the energy balance equation in the direction of weight loss.

1.

2.

Dieting for Weight Control

What would be considered a prudent daily caloric deficit for weight loss?

Very Difficult on a Long-Term Basis

Summarize the general trend for long-term weight loss success.

Setpoint Theory: A Case Against Dieting

Summarize the main premise of the setpoint theory with regard to body fat accumulation.

Resting Metabolism Is Lowered

How much does dieting lower RMR?

Weight Cycling: Going No Place Fast

List two possible negative aspects of weight cycling.

1.

2.

Extremes of Dieting

Ketogenic Diets

Describe the rationale for a ketogenic diet for weight loss.

High-Protein Diets

Describe the rationale for a high-protein diet for weight loss.

Semistarvation Diets

List four negative aspects of very low-calorie diets (VLCDs).

1.

2.

3.

4.

Exercise for Weight Control

Not Simply a Problem of Gluttony

Cite specific evidence that obesity does not necessarily result from excessive food intake.

Increased Energy Output Worth Considering

Misconception 1. Exercise and Food Intake

Discuss whether all levels of increased physical activity have a stimulating effect on food intake.

Misconception 2. Caloric Stress of Physical Activity

Are the calorie-expending effects of exercise cumulative?

The Recovery "Afterglow"

Give approximate values for the recovery "afterglow" following submaximum exercise lasting less than 80 minutes. Is this amount large enough to make a significant difference in terms of weight loss?

Exercise Is Effective

How long would it take to burn 13.6 kg of body fat assuming a daily caloric deficit of 300 kcal?

A Dose-Response Relationship

Describe the concept of dose-response for the role of increased physical activity for weight loss.

Some General Guidelines for an Exercise-Weight Loss Program

List two important points to consider when formulating an exercise program for weight loss.

1.

2.

Diet plus Exercise: The Ideal Combination

Why is exercise plus diet the ideal combination for weight loss?

A Reality Check

List three long-term lifestyle changes needed for successful weight control.

1.

2.

3.

Some Factors That Affect Weight Loss

Early Weight Loss Is Largely Water

Outline the dynamics of body water loss as a percentage of weight loss during dieting.

Maintain Adequate Hydration

Discuss the effect of hydration level on body fat loss during weight loss.

Longer-Term Deficit Promotes Fat Loss

What is the trend for the caloric equivalent for each pound of weight lost as a weight-loss program progresses?

Spot Reduction: Does It Work?

Can specific exercises promote fat loss at specific body sites? Explain.

Where on the Body Does Fat Reduction Occur?

What body area tends to be the most resistant to weight loss?

A Possible Sex Difference?

Explain why men may be more responsive than women to the effects of exercise on weight loss.

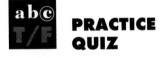 **PRACTICE QUIZ**

MULTIPLE CHOICE

1. **Which of the following statements are <u>true</u>?**
   a. the actual number of fat cells decreases with severe dietary restriction
   b. increases in body fat in previously nonobese adults generally occur by filling existing fat cells
   c. new fat cells can develop with further weight gain among the massively obese
   d. a and c
   e. b and c

2. **Documented health risks of obesity include:**
   a. coronary heart disease
   b. low blood pressure
   c. hyperthyroidism
   d. exercise-induced bronchospasm
   e. a and b

3. **Fat cell number in humans probably increases significantly:**
   a. during the first trimester of pregnancy
   b. during the last trimester of pregnancy
   c. during the first year of life
   d. b and c
   e. all of the above

4. **Severe dieting is generally inadvisable for prudent weight loss because:**
   a. it increases water retention and causes edema
   b. significant lean tissue is lost
   c. obese people do not eat in great excess, so true gluttony is often not the problem
   d. b and c
   e. all of the above

5. **If you burn 10 kcal per minute, you will have burned the calories in 1 pound of body fat in about:**
   a. 500 minutes
   b. 6 hours
   c. 3 hours
   d. 200 minutes
   e. none of the above

6. **This enzyme helps to govern the body's pattern of fat distribution:**
   a. hexokinase
   b. lipoprotein lipase
   c. dehydrogenase
   d. acetyl-CoA
   e. insulin

7. **This type of obesity poses the greater health risk:**
   a. abdominal obesity
   b. peripheral obesity
   c. gynoid-type obesity
   d. mastoid-type obesity
   e. a and c

8. **How many extra kcal will lead to the accumulation of 1 pound of body fat?**
   a. 2500
   b. 3500
   c. 4500
   d. 5500
   e. 6000

9. **Even when extremely obese people lose body fat, they have difficulty achieving permanent fat loss because:**
   a. they still have an excessive number of fat cells
   b. they have a decreased level of lipoprotein lipase
   c. they maintain their increased level of resting metabolism
   d. their sensitivity to insulin increases
   e. none of the above

10. **The limit of weekly weight loss recommended for long-term success is:**
    a. 0–1 lb
    b. 1–2 lb
    c. 3–4 lb
    d. 4–5 lb
    e. 5–6 lb

TRUE/FALSE

1. _____ The average adult gains weight during middle age despite a progressive decrease in food intake.

2. _____ Research indicates there is no general genetic link to susceptibility to obesity.

3. _____ Diets that restrict water intake cause greater weight loss but not greater fat loss.

4. _____ The calorie-expending effects of exercise are cumulative.

5. _____ Combining exercise with a low-calorie diet helps conserve the body's lean tissue.

6. _____ The chances for adult obesity are increased threefold when obesity begins in childhood.

7. _____ With weight loss, the number of fat cells actually decreases.

8. _____ All individuals essentially have the same physiological "set point" for body weight.

9. _____ Localized exercise of a specific body area will selectively increase fat loss from that area.

10. _____ Resistance training, along with a well-balanced diet, can increase muscle mass and strength.

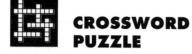

CROSSWORD PUZZLE

ACROSS

1 Significant increase in number of adipocytes

6 Male-pattern obesity

7 Key to weight loss is to _____ the energy balance equation

11 Another term for obesity

14 Excessive amount of body fat, usually > 30% for women, > 20% for men

15 Repetitive bouts of dieting, each followed by subsequent weight gain

16 University researcher (name starts with letter H) who pioneered studies in fat cellularity

20 Fat-storing enzyme

25 _____-to-hip ratio is important health indicator

26 Word describing distribution of fat over the body

29 Describes relationship between quantity of exercise and amount of weight loss

DOWN

2 Theory that the body physiologically tries to maintain a particular level of body fat

3 Patterning where fat accumulates in lower body regions

4 Percentage body fat is an important _____ for obesity

5 Opposite of gain or increase

8 Synonym for fat tissue

9 3500 kcal in 1 lb of ____ fat

10 _____ cycling is another term for yo-yo dieting

12 Synonym for lipid

13 Localized fat loss with exercise

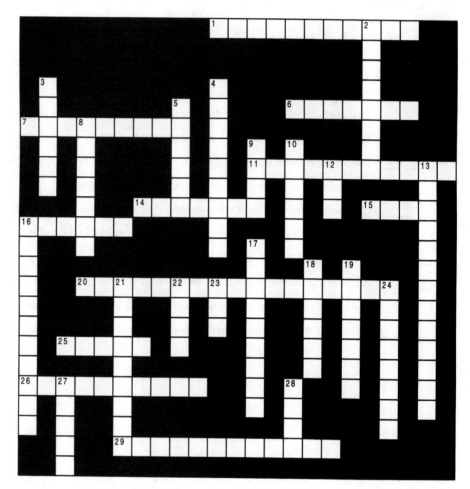

16 Most adult weight gain is due to this change in adipocytes

17 Obesity often begins in this stage of life

18 Sampling of small amounts of fat from subcutaneous depots

19 Excellent exercise mode for weight control

21 LBM is _____ when weight loss is accompanied by exercise (word begins with letter p)

22 NIH views even low levels of excess body fat to be a health ____

23 The upper limit for recommended weekly pounds of weight loss

24 When this is part of a weight-loss program, more of the weight lost is fat

27 Area of the body where fat may be more easily lost

28 It is probably not necessary for adults to ____ weight as they grow older

See page 374 for Crossword Puzzle Solution.

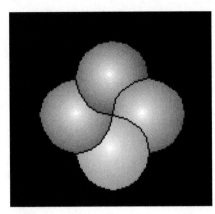

Exercise, Aging, and Cardiovascular Health

 DEFINE KEY WORDS AND CONCEPTS

1. Epidemiology

2. Physical activity epidemiology

3. Physical activity

4. Exercise

5. Physical fitness

6. Health

7. Longevity

8. Health-related physical fitness

9. Healthy People 2000

10. Most prevalent exercise complications

11. **Denervation muscle atrophy**

12. **Estimated HRmax** =

13. **Cross-sectional data**

14. **Longitudinal data**

15. **Harvard alumni study**

16. **Ischemic**

17. **Thrombus**

18. **Myocardial infarction**

19. **Non-modifiable CHD risks**

20. **"Big four" CHD risks**

21. **Angina pectoris**

22. **Modifiable CHD risks**

23. **Gender advantage in CHD risk**

24. **Hyperlipidemia**

25. **Hyperlipoproteinemia**

26. High-density lipoproteins

27. Low-density lipoproteins

28. Cigarette smoking and CHD risk

29. RISKO

30. Exercise stress tests

31. Multistage exercise testing

32. QRS complex

33. PVC

34. Ventricular fibrillation

35. Hypertensive exercise response

36. Hypotensive exercise response

37. Bruce test

38. Balke test

39. Stress test sensitivity

40. True-positive

41. **False-negative**

42. **True-negative**

43. **False-positive**

44. **Exercise prescription**

45. **Unsupervised exercise programs**

46. **Supervised exercise programs**

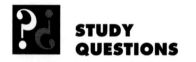 **STUDY QUESTIONS**

PHYSICAL ACTIVITY IN THE POPULATION
Physical Activity Epidemiology
What is the goal of epidemiology?

Terminology
Distinguish between the terms *physical activity* and *exercise*.

Participation in Physical Activity
List four methods to assess physical activity.

1.

2.

3.

4.

Describe the average level of exercise participation for the American male and female.

• Male

• Female

Is Exercising Safe?

What is the risk of dying suddenly during exercise?

What is the most prevalent complication caused by exercise?

What two factors increase the likelihood of an exercise-related catastrophe?

1.

2.

AGING AND PHYSIOLOGIC FUNCTION

Age Trends

Draw a generalized curve that relates the level of body functions to chronological age. (*Hint: Refer to Figure 30.3 in your textbook.*)

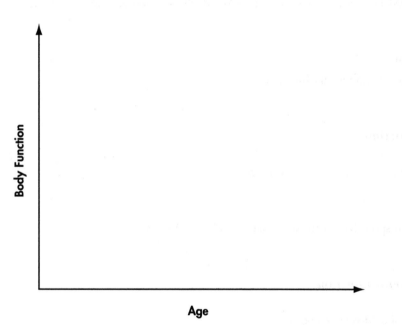

Some Differences in Exercise Physiology between Children and Adults

List four physiologic and performance differences in exercise between children and adults.

1.

2.

3.

4.

Muscular Strength

How much does muscular strength decline by age 70?

Decrease in Muscle Mass

Reduced muscle mass is a primary factor responsible for what age-associated decrease in physiologic function?

Strength Trainability among the Elderly

How much can the elderly increase their strength with a proper resistance training program? (*Hint: Refer to Figure 30.6 in your textbook.*)

Neural Function

What general effect does aging have on the nervous system?

Discuss whether a physically active lifestyle can delay the decline of neural function with age.

Pulmonary Function

Describe how aging affects pulmonary function.

Cardiovascular Function
Aerobic Capacity

How much does $\dot{V}O_2$max generally decline with age?

What factor could be responsible for the age-related decline in $\dot{V}O_2$max?

Central and Peripheral Function
Heart Rate

Estimate the HRmax of a 70-year-old person.

Cardiac Output

List two factors responsible for the age-associated reduction in cardiac output.

1.

2.

The decreased stroke volume with aging reflects what diminished aspect(s) of myocardial function?

Local Factors
What factors are likely responsible for the reduction in peripheral blood flow capacity with aging?

Lifestyle or Aging?
Estimate the contribution of lifestyle and aging to the decline in cardiovascular function with aging.

- Lifestyle

- Aging

Endurance Performance Capacity
Are world records for the marathon age dependent? Explain.

Aerobic Trainability among the Elderly
What physiologic adaptations cause the increase in $\dot{V}O_2max$ in response to aerobic training for elderly men and women?

- Men

- Women

Body Composition
How much weight will the average 20-year-old man gain by age 60?

Describe the effects of resistance training on fat-free body mass in the elderly.

Bone Mass
What is the average decrease in bone mass for a typical 60-year-old woman?

Trainability and Age
List three variables that affect the magnitude of loss in physiologic function with aging.

1.

2.

3.

Are there any negative aspects to regular exercise training for the healthy elderly?

PHYSICAL ACTIVITY, HEALTH, AND LONGEVITY
Exercise and Longevity
Enhanced Quality to a Longer Life: A Study of Harvard Alumni
Describe the major findings of the study of Harvard alumni.

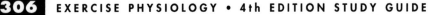

Epidemiological Evidence

Give the summary findings of the critique of 43 studies of the relationship between physical activity and CHD risk.

Describe the type of physical activity needed to achieve the largest improvement in health benefits for previously sedentary men and women.

Improved Fitness: A Little Goes A Long Way

Describe the major findings of the experimental study described in Figure 30.14 of your textbook.

Does a Change in Fitness Improve One's Health Outlook?

How much can a sedentary man expect to reduce his risk of dying by initiating a regular program of moderate to vigorous physical activity?

CORONARY HEART DISEASE

Changes on the Cellular Level

List three early signs of coronary heart disease.

1.

2.

3.

Still an Epidemic

How much has the incidence of CHD declined since 1970?

How much obstruction must take place in the arteries before CHD can be clinically detected?

Coronary Heart Disease Risk Factors

List ten CHD risk factors.

1.	6.
2.	7.
3.	8.
4.	9.
5.	10.

List three CHD risk factors that are "predetermined," and three that are "treatable" by lifestyle modification.

Predetermined Factors	Treatable Factors
1.	1.
2.	2.
3.	3.

Age, Sex, and Heredity

At what age do the chances of dying from CHD increase progressively and dramatically for men and for women? (*Hint: refer to Figure 30.18.*)

- Men

- Women

Blood Lipid Abnormalities

List the current standards for desirable levels of total cholesterol and levels above which adults should seek treatment. (*Hint: Refer to Table 30.3 in your textbook.*)

- Desirable

- Treatment required

How much does a cholesterol level of 230 mg·dL^{-1} raise the risk for CHD?

List four different lipoproteins. (*Hint: Refer to Table 30.4 in your textbook.*)

1.

2.

3.

4.

Regular Exercise

Regular aerobic exercise exerts its greatest effect on which lipoprotein?

Obesity

Discuss the effect of weight loss on blood lipid levels.

Cigarette Smoking

What is the risk of death from heart disease for smokers compared to nonsmokers?

Physical Activity

The relative risk of a fatal heart attack among the sedentary is how much greater compared to physically active adults?

Mechanisms of Protection

List six ways in which physical activity may operate to protect against CHD.

1.

2.

3.

4.

5.

6.

Interaction of CHD Risk Factors

Which CHD risk factor seems to be the most "common root" of the other CHD risk factors?

Risk Factors in Children

What are the two most common CHD risk factors in children aged 7 to 12 years?

PRUDENT PRE-EXERCISE EVALUATION

Exercise Stress Testing

List the two main purposes for exercise stress testing.

1.

2.

What are the two most common modalities for exercise stress testing?

1.

2.

What clinical evaluation should always precede the exercise stress test?

Why Be Stress Tested?

List five reasons to include stress testing in the overall CHD evaluation.

1.

2.

3.

4.

5.

Who Should Be Stress Tested?

How do the American College of Sports Medicine guidelines for stress testing differ for adults under and over the age of 35?

Exercise-Induced Indicators of CHD

Angina Pectoris

Describe the most prominent symptom of angina pectoris during exercise.

Electrocardiographic Disorders

Draw and label a normal and an abnormal ECG tracing. (*Hint: Refer to Figure 30.22 in your textbook.*)

• Normal

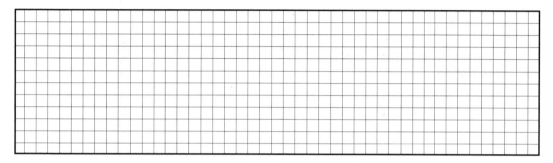

• Abnormal

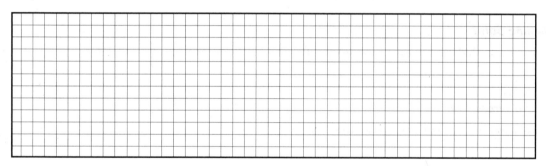

Cardiac Rhythm Abnormalities

List three common cardiac rhythm abnormalities.

1.

2.

3.

Other Indices of CHD

List three non-electrocardiographic indices of possible CHD.

1.

2.

3.

Stress Test Protocols

The _____ is the most common exercise mode for stress testing.

The Bruce and Balke Treadmill Tests

Give one difference between the Bruce and Balke stress test protocols.

Bicycle Ergometer Tests

Give two advantages of using a bicycle ergometer as a stress test device.

1.

2.

List two different types of bicycle ergometers.

1.

2.

Arm-Crank Ergometers

Arm-crank $\dot{V}O_2$max values are about _____ % lower than those observed during treadmill running.

Guidelines for Stress Testing

List seven reasons for terminating an exercise stress test.

1.   5.

2.   6.

3.   7.

4.

Is Stress Testing Safe?

What is the risk of death during an exercise stress test for men who show clinical signs of CHD?

Outcomes of a Stress Test

List four possible outcomes from an exercise stress test.

1.

2.

3.

4.

Which two excercise stress test outcomes are most prevalent?

Exercise Prescription

List six factors to consider when planning an exercise prescription.

1.   4.

2.   5.

3.   6.

Practical Illustration

Summarize the information in Figure 30.23 that can be applied to an exercise prescription.

Improvements in CHD Patients

What physiological adaptations indicate that exercise training reduces the work of the heart in CHD patients?

The Program

What factor increases adherence to preventive and rehabilitative exercise programs?

Level of Supervision

In what instances do medical personnel need to be present during exercise training? (*Hint: Refer to Table 30.8 in your textbook.*)

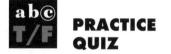

PRACTICE QUIZ

MULTIPLE CHOICE

1. **Regular physical activity can:**
   a. lower blood pressure
   b. lower blood lipids
   c. normalize the blood clotting mechanism
   d. improve blood supply to the myocardium
   e. all of the above

2. **Which declines the most with increasing age?**
   a. nerve conduction velocity
   b. joint flexibility
   c. lean body mass
   d. liver function
   e. kidney function

3. **Reduced muscle mass with aging:**
   a. explains the age-associated increases in total body density
   b. explains the age-associated strength decrease
   c. reflects loss of total muscle carbon
   d. reflects hypertrophy of individual muscle fibers
   e. all of the above

4. **The following formula is used to predict maximum heart rate in beats per minute:**
   a. max HR = 200 + age (years)
   b. max HR = 220 − age (years)
   c. max HR = age (years) + 200
   d. max HR = age (years) + 220
   e. max HR = age (years) + max HR − rest HR

5. **What percentage of total deaths in the United States are caused by diseases of the heart and blood vessels?**
   a. 25%
   b. 50%
   c. 65%
   d. 75%
   e. 85%

6. **Which statement is <u>true</u> of cardiovascular disease in men and women?**
    a. men are more likely to have heart attacks than women during middle age
    b. women are more likely to have a second heart attack than men
    c. women who have bypass surgery are more likely to survive than men
    d. hyperglycemia affects men more than women
    e. none of the above

7. **The desirable cholesterol level for young adults is:**
    a. < 150 mg/dL
    b. < 180 mg/dL
    c. 200 mg/dL
    d. 220 mg/dL
    e. none of the above

8. **Regular exercise can:**
    a. improve myocardial circulation and metabolism
    b. enhance contractile properties of the myocardium
    c. normalize the blood lipid profile
    d. reduce the work of the heart
    e. all of the above

9. **It is important to include stress testing in a medical evaluation to:**
    a. screen for possible "silent" coronary disease
    b. reproduce and document exercise-related chest symptoms
    c. detect an abnormal blood pressure response
    d. monitor responses to various therapeutic interventions
    e. all of the above

10. **Which is <u>not</u> an exercise-induced indicator of coronary heart disease?**
    a. $\dot{V}O_2max$
    b. angina pectoris
    c. ECG abnormalities
    d. extreme changes in blood pressure
    e. PVCs

TRUE/FALSE

1. _____ The chances of sudden death during exercise are greater than during rest.

2. _____ Children have a lower economy during weight-bearing exercise than adults.

3. _____ There are no additional health or longevity benefits beyond weekly exercise of 3500 kcal.

4. _____ Increased CHD occurrence for women in later years is related to a loss of estrogen following menopause.

5. _____ Low-density lipoproteins help transport cholesterol to the liver, where it is metabolized and then excreted in the bile.

6. _____ Regular aerobic exercise elevates high-density lipoprotein levels.

7. _____ Diabetes is often called the "silent killer" because it generally progresses unnoticed for decades.

8. _____ A medical evaluation is advised before any major increase in exercise for all adults above 25 years of age.

9. _____ A depressed S-T segment of an ECG is an indicator of coronary heart disease.

10. _____ A true-positive stress test means that the test results are correct in diagnosing a person with heart disease (the stress test is a success).

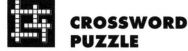 **CROSSWORD PUZZLE**

ACROSS

1 High blood lipid levels

5 Alumni from this school were studied for factors related to mortality

7 This circulation supplies blood to the heart

8 Cholesterol is transported in blood as a lipo_____

10 At any age, active adults have lower levels of body ____ than less active counterparts

11 Most prevalent killer of men and women (abbr.)

13 Degenerative process that causes coronary artery narrowing

15 Bad cholesterol (abbr.)

16 Pain caused by inadequate oxygen supply to myocardium

18 _____ flexibility declines 20 to 30% from 30 to 80 years of age

20 Circulating blood clot

23 Undesirable ventricular beat (abbr.)

24 About 6 of every 100 of this sex die from CHD between ages 55 and 65

25 Unmodifiable CHD risk factor

DOWN

2 The _____ blood pressure reading should not exceed 90 mm Hg

3 Inadequate oxygen supply

4 Exercise test to evaluate myocardial function and oxygen supply

6 Personality type probably at risk for heart disease

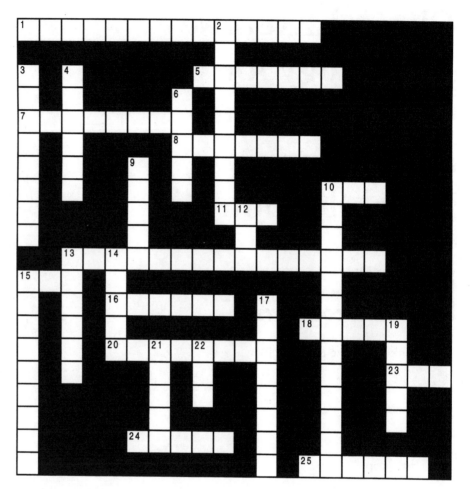

9 Coronary ____ describes individuals at greater than normal risk for CHD

10 Test results are abnormal without disease

12 Good cholesterol (abbr.)

13 Harvard group studied by epidemiologists

14 _____ attack is a popular term for myocardial infarction

15 While regular moderate exercise may improve health and well-being, it has little effect on _____

17 Higher of the blood pressure readings

19 "Easy-going" personality type

21 A _____ of total cholesterol to HDL cholesterol greater than 4.5 indicates high CHD risk

22 This sex dies younger

See page 374 for Crossword Puzzle Solution.

Clinical Exercise Physiology for Cancer, Cardiovascular, and Pulmonary Rehabilitation

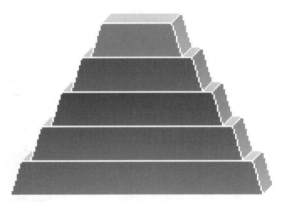

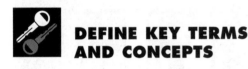 **DEFINE KEY TERMS AND CONCEPTS**

1. Clinical exercise physiologist

2. Disability

3. Handicap

4. WHO definition of physical fitness

5. Oncology

6. Functional status

7. ATHS

8. Walk-through angina

9. Coronary occlusion

10. Pericarditis

11. CHF

12. Pulmonary congestion

13. Aneurysm

14. Stenosis

15. Regurgitation

16. Prolapse

17. Endocarditis

18. MVP

19. Arrhythmias

20. Ectopic

21. Sinus tachycardia

22. Sinus bradycardia

23. Heart auscultation

24. **CPK**

25. **LDH**

26. **SGOT**

27. **Echocardiography**

28. **Thallium imaging**

29. **Ventriculography**

30. **Cardiac catheterization**

31. **Coronary angiography**

32. **RLD**

33. **Lung compliance**

34. **COPD**

35. **Emphysema**

36. **Cystic fibrosis**

37. **Dyspnea**

38. **Positive sweat electrolyte (chloride) test**

39. **Roentgenogram**

40. CT scanning

41. MRI

42. Mild lung disease

43. Moderate lung disease

44. Severe lung disease

STUDY QUESTIONS

THE EXERCISE PHYSIOLOGIST IN THE CLINICAL SETTING

Describe the primary focus of the clinical exercise physiologist.

SPORTS MEDICINE AND EXERCISE PHYSIOLOGY: A VITAL LINK

List two activities of the clinical exercise physiologist along with other members of the health care team.

1.

2.

PREVALENCE AND TYPES OF DISABILITIES

List three different disabilities that adversely affect functional capacity.

1.

2.

3.

ONCOLOGY

List three of the most prevalent forms of cancer.

1.

2.

3.

Give the overall goal of the exercise specialist in cancer treatment.

Possible Mechanisms of Exercise Effects on Cancer

State two hypotheses of how exercise affects cancer.

1.

2.

Exercise Prescription and Cancer

Considering the small amount of objective data that exists on exercise prescription and cancer, describe a prudent approach to exercising for cancer patients.

Initially, is interval or continuous training best for the cancer patient?

The Specific Case of Breast Cancer and Regular Exercise

List three primary risk factors for breast cancer.

1.

2.

3.

List two areas in which regular aerobic exercise can help breast cancer patients.

1.

2.

CARDIOVASCULAR DISEASES

Overview and Scope of Cardiovascular Disabilities

List three categories of heart disease that lead to functional disabilities. (*Hint: Refer to Table 31.4 in your textbook.*)

1.

2.

3.

List four different terms that generally refer to myocardial degenerative disease.

1.

2.

3.

4.

Diseases of the Heart Muscle

Outline the steps in the pathogenesis of CHD.

1.

2.

3.

4.

5.

List three major disorders caused by a reduced myocardial blood supply.

1.

2.

3.

Angina Pectoris

Anginal pain is believed to result from _____.

List three symptoms of angina pectoris.

1.

2.

3.

Myocardial Infarction (MI, Heart Attack)

Describe the major symptom of a person having an acute MI.

Pericarditis

List four usual symptoms of pericarditis.

1.

2.

3.

4.

Congestive Heart Failure (CHF or Chronic Decompensation)

List two common symptoms of CHF.

1.

2.

Aneurysm

Describe the common symptoms of an aneurysm.

Diseases Affecting the Heart Valves

List three heart valve abnormalities.

  1.

  2.

  3.

Endocarditis

Describe the symptoms of endocarditis.

Congenital Malformations

Congenital malformations of the heart occur about _____ times in every 100 births.

Diseases of the Cardiac Nervous System

List three diseases of the heart's electrical conduction system.

  1.

  2.

  3.

Cardiac Disease Assessment

Patient History

List two typical symptoms in the differential diagnosis of chest pain.

  1.

  2.

Physical Examination

List the four vital signs.

  1.

  2.

  3.

  4.

Heart Auscultation

List two heart abnormalities that are readily discovered by heart auscultation.

  1.

  2.

Laboratory Tests

List five laboratory tests for CHD assessment.

1.

2.

3.

4.

5.

Noninvasive Physiological Tests

List two prevalent noninvasive tests for cardiac dysfunction.

1.

2.

Echocardiography

What are the major advantages of echocardiography?

Graded Exercise Stress Test (GXT)

What is the main purpose of performing a GXT in the clinical setting?

Invasive Physiological Tests

List three types of invasive tests used for CHD diagnosis. Give one major purpose of each.

	Test	Purpose
1.		
2.		
3.		

Classification of Patients for Cardiac Rehabilitation

Give the usual first sign or symptom of CHD.

List three symptoms of advanced CHD.

1.

2.

3.

Which clinical test is generally used to classify patients for differential rehabilitation?

Phases of Cardiac Rehabilitation

List three important aspects of a successful cardiac rehabilitation program.

1.

2.

3.

List three phases of a cardiac rehabilitation program. (*Hint: Refer to Table 31.11 in your textbook.*)

1.

2.

3.

The Exercise Prescription

Which aspect of the exercise prescription is the most difficult to determine?

List two "systems" for determining training intensity.

1.

2.

Resistance Exercise Can Be Beneficial

What is the best type of resistance exercise for the CHD patient?

List two benefits of resistance training for the CHD patient.

1.

2.

Cardiac Medications

List six classifications of common cardiac drugs.

1.

2.

3.

4.

5.

6.

PULMONARY DISEASES

List two major classifications of pulmonary abnormalities.

1.

2.

Restrictive Lung Dysfunction (RLD)

What are the two major characteristics of RLD?

1.

2.

Explain what is meant by "lung compliance."

List five major types of RLD. (*Hint: Refer to Table 31.15 in your textbook.*)

1.

2.

3.

4.

5.

Chronic Obstructive Pulmonary Disease (COPD)

List three of the classic symptoms of COPD

1.

2.

3.

Chronic Bronchitis

Describe some of the symptoms and characteristics of a patient with chronic bronchitis.

Emphysema

Describe the characteristics and cause of the "emphysemic look."

• Characteristics

• Cause

Cystic Fibrosis (CF)

What is the objective diagnosis for CF?

Pulmonary Assessments

List five major pulmonary assessment procedures.

1.

2.

3.

4.

5.

Pulmonary Rehabilitation and Exercise Prescription

List five goals of pulmonary rehabilitation.

1.

2.

3.

4.

5.

Describe the perceived dyspnea scale.

How does the exercise prescription differ between patients with moderate and severe lung disease?

Pulmonary Medications

List three common pulmonary drugs and their action.

	Drug	Action
1.		
2.		
3.		

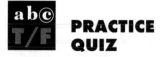 **PRACTICE QUIZ**

MULTIPLE CHOICE

1. **The highest incidence of cancer is noted for the:**
   a. breasts, lungs, bowel, and uterus
   b. skin, lungs, pancreas, and kidney
   c. skin, lungs, and intestines
   d. breasts and skin
   e. myocardium

2. **Disability refers to having a:**
    a. defined handicap
    b. diminished functional capacity
    c. physical performance limitation
    d. particular disease
    e. none of the above

3. **Exercise:**
    a. has no effect on lowering cancer risk
    b. has no effect on lowering cancer risk but is important in cancer rehabilitation
    c. plays an important role in cancer risk reduction by increasing levels of anti-inflammatory cytokines
    d. decreases cancer risk by increasing antioxidant tolerance
    e. c and d

4. **Exercise as a therapy for breast cancer:**
    a. can decrease levels of depression and anxiety
    b. usually has little effect on psychosocial variables
    c. can increase plasma cytokines, which help healing
    d. is beneficial only for older women
    e. a and d

5. **Diseases of the myocardium include:**
    a. angina pectoris, myocardial infarction, pericarditis, congestive heart failure, and aneurysms
    b. stenosis, regurgitation, and prolapse
    c. dysrhythmias and endocarditis
    d. prolapse and endocarditis
    e. none of the above

6. **Most angina pain is located in the area of the ____ and lasts for less than ____ minutes:**
    a. left shoulder and down inside of left arm, 5
    b. right shoulder and head, 20
    c. abdominal area, 5
    d. abdominal area and legs, 20
    e. back and hips, 5

7. **A myocardial infarction results from:**
    a. increases in the heart's H^+ ion concentration, which decreases contractility
    b. decreases in the pulmonary blood flow due to reduced alveolar Po_2
    c. deprivation of blood (oxygen) to a portion of the myocardium
    d. inflammation of the heart's pericardium
    e. decreases in the hormones epinephrine and norepinephrine

8. **Increased levels of ____ , ____ , and ____ can verify the presence or absence of an acute MI:**
    a. CP, SDH, SGOT
    b. LDH, PFK, CP
    c. ADP, SDH, PK
    d. CPK, LDH, SGOT
    e. none of the above

9. **The most difficult yet important aspect of the exercise prescription involves the determination of the:**
    a. exercise duration
    b. patient's initial functional capacity
    c. exercise intensity
    d. exercise frequency
    e. patient's maximal MET capacity

10. **Cystic fibrosis is diagnosed by:**
    a. a depressed S-T segment of the ECG
    b. a positive sweat electrolyte (chloride)
    c. decreased residual lung volume
    d. decreased vital capacity during moderate exercise
    e. a and b

TRUE/FALSE

1. _____ Bradycardia refers to slowing of the heart rate.

2. _____ Tachycardia refers to slowing of the heart rate.

3. _____ Sinus bradycardia occurs normally in endurance athletes and young adults.

4. _____ Valvular stenosis refers to constriction or narrowing of the heart valves.

5. _____ COPD is normally diagnosed by changes in pulmonary function tests.

6. _____ COPD is common in sedentary nonsmokers who eat high-fat foods.

7. _____ Aerobic exercise can be beneficial for cystic fibrosis patients.

8. _____ For pulmonary disease patients, exercise is important for improving respiratory muscle function.

9. _____ A person with advanced emphysema often has a normal-appearing chest on visual inspection.

10. _____ MRI scans are of limited use in diagnosing pulmonary disease.

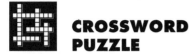 **CROSSWORD PUZZLE**

ACROSS

1 _____ diseases are leading cause of death in industrialized nations

4 _____ pulmonary disease impedes air flow

6 When chronic, considered one of three major COPDs

7 Type of imaging of limited use in pulmonary assessment (abbr.)

11 Prolapse affects this heart valve

12 Imaging technique for left ventricle dynamics

16 Pericarditis is inflammation of _____ myocardial lining

18 Type of scanning using translation-rotation process (abbr.)

19 _____ pectoris is a Latin term for chest pain

21 Endurance athletes often display _____ bradycardia

24 Lack of blood (oxygen) to tissues

26 Change in lung volume in relation to pressure differentials

DOWN

2 COPD associated with this personal behavior

3 Diet high in _____ elevates breast cancer risk

5 _____ exercise physiologist works in health care

8 Sinus tachycardia is _____ HR greater than 100 beats/min.

9 DLCO measure of pulmonary _____ capacity

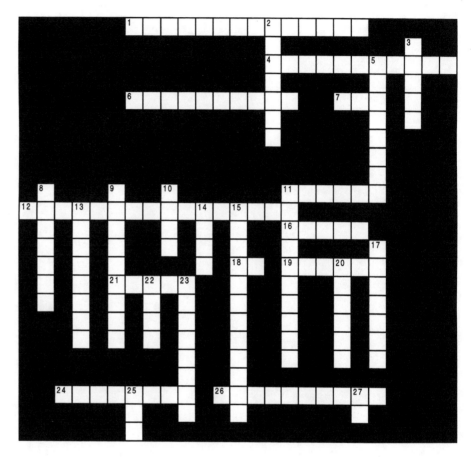

10 _____ bloater: a person with severe chronic bronchitis

11 Heart muscle

13 _____ imaging evaluates myocardial perfusion

14 Angiography considered _____ standard to evaluate coronary blood flow

15 Listening to heart sounds

17 Light level of resistance used with strength training in _____ rehabilitation

20 Regular exercise may affect _____ system to protect against cancer

22 One out of _____ women contracts breast cancer

23 Damage to _____ muscle can elevate serum CPK

25 Tracing of heart's electrical activity (abbr.)

27 Inherited form of COPD (abbr.)

See page 374 for Crossword Puzzle Solution.

SECTION 2

SELF-ASSESSMENT TESTS

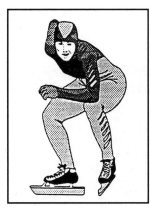

Physical Activity Readiness (PAR-Q)

COMPLETE THE FOLLOWING Physical Activity Readiness Questionnaire (The PAR-Q[a]) to get a general idea of whether you are physically ready to exercise.

PAR-Q is designed to help you help yourself. Many health benefits are associated with regular exercise, and the completion of PAR-Q is a sensible first step if you are planning to increase your physical activity. For most people, physical activity should not pose any problem or health hazard. PAR-Q has been designed to identify the small number of adults for whom physical activity might be inappropriate, or those who should have medical advice concerning the type of activity most suitable for them.

COMMON SENSE IS YOUR BEST GUIDE IN ANSWERING THESE QUESTIONS. READ EACH QUESTION CAREFULLY AND CHECK YES OR NO IF IT APPLIES TO YOU.

YES _____ NO _____ 1. Has your doctor ever said you have heart trouble?

YES _____ NO _____ 2. Do you frequently have pains in your heart and chest?

YES _____ NO _____ 3. Do you often feel faint or have spells of severe dizziness?

YES _____ NO _____ 4. Has a doctor ever said your blood pressure was too high?

YES _____ NO _____ 5. Has your doctor told you that you have a bone or joint problem that has been aggravated by exercise, or might be made worse with exercise?

YES _____ NO _____ 6. Is there a good physical reason not mentioned here why you should not follow an activity program even if you wanted to?

YES _____ NO _____ 7. Are you over age 65 and not accustomed to vigorous exercise?

IF YOU ANSWERED YES TO ONE OR MORE QUESTIONS

If you have not recently done so, consult with your personal physician by telephone or in person **BEFORE** increasing your physical activity and/or taking a fitness test. Show your doctor a copy of this quiz. After medical evaluation, seek advice from your physician as to your suitability for:

- Unrestricted physical activity, probably on a gradually increasing basis
- Restricted or supervised activity to meet your specific needs, at least on an initial basis. Check in your community for special programs or services

[a]PAR-Q was developed by the British Columbia Ministry of Health. Conceptualized and critiqued by the Multidisciplinary Advisory Board on Exercise (MABE). Reference: PAR-Q Validation Report, British Columbia Ministry of Health, May 1978.

IF YOU ANSWERED NO TO ALL QUESTIONS

If you answered PAR-Q accurately, you have reasonable assurance of your present suitability for:

- A *graduated exercise program:* a gradual increase in proper exercise promotes good fitness development while minimizing or eliminating discomfort

- *An exercise test:* simple tests of fitness (such as the Canadian Home Fitness Test) or more complex types may be undertaken if you so desire

- *Postpone exercising:* if you have a temporary minor illness, such as a common cold, postpone any exercise program

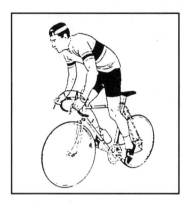

Revised **Physical Activity Readiness Questionnaire (rPar-Q)**

ONE LIMITATION OF the original PAR-Q was that a relatively large number (about 20%) of potential exercisers failed the test—and many of these exclusions were unnecessary as subsequent evaluation of these men and women showed that they were apparently healthy. Consequently, to reduce the number of unnecessary exclusions (false-positives) the revised PAR-Q (rPar-Q) was developed. This revision is a recommended method for determining the exercise readiness of apparently healthy middle-aged adults with no more than one major risk factor for coronary heart disease.

YES_____ NO_____ 1. Has a doctor said that you have a heart condition and recommended only medically supervised activity?

YES_____ NO_____ 2. Do you have chest pain brought on by physical activity?

YES_____ NO_____ 3. Have you developed chest pain in the past month?

YES_____ NO_____ 4. Do you tend to lose consciousness or fall over as a result of dizziness?

YES_____ NO_____ 5. Do you have a bone or joint that could be aggravated by the proposed physical activity?

YES_____ NO_____ 6. Has a doctor ever recommended medication for your blood pressure or a heart condition?

YES_____ NO_____ 7. Are you aware through your own experience, or a doctor's advice, of any other physical reason against your exercising without medical supervision?

NOTE: Postpone testing if you have a temporary illness like a common cold, or are not feeling well.

IF YOU ANSWERED YES TO ONE OR MORE QUESTIONS

If you have not recently done so, consult with your personal physician by telephone or in person **BEFORE** increasing your physical activity and/or taking a fitness test. Show your doctor a copy of this quiz. After medical evaluation, seek advice from your physician as to your suitability for:

- Unrestricted physical activity, probably on a gradually increasing basis.

- Restricted or supervised activity to meet your specific needs, at least on an initial basis. Check in your community for special programs or services.

(From: Shephard, R. J., et al.: The Canadian Home Fitness Test: Update. Sports Med, 1:359, 1991.)

Eating Smart
Assessment

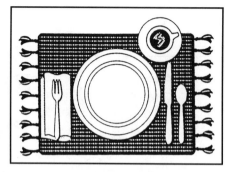

LET'S SEE HOW "SMART" you are in terms of the quality of your food intake. Complete the *Eating Smart Assessment* and get a broad view of the diversity of your diet, especially its content of fat- and fiber-rich foods. A high rating means that you're on the right track in terms of prudent nutrition to help you fight the battle against heart disease and certain cancers.

OILS AND FATS: butter, margarine, shortening, mayonnaise, sour cream, lard, oil		POINTS
I always add these foods in cooking and/or at the table		0
I occasionally add these to foods in cooking and/or at the table		1
I rarely add these foods in cooking and/or at the table		2

DAIRY PRODUCTS: milk, yogurt, cheese, ice cream		POINTS
I drink whole milk		0
I drink 1 or 2% fat-free milk		1
I seldom eat frozen desserts or ice cream		2
I eat ice cream almost every day		0
Instead of ice cream, I eat ice milk, low-fat frozen yogurt and sherbet		1
I eat only fruit ices, seldom eat frozen dairy desserts		2
I eat mostly high-fat cheese (jack, cheddar, colby, Swiss, cream)		0
I eat both low- and high-fat cheeses		1
I eat mostly low-fat cheeses (2% cottage, skim milk, mozzarella)		2

(Source: American Cancer Society, Rev. 1989, pp. 2–5)

334

SNACKS: potato/corn chips, nuts, buttered popcorn, candy bars POINTS

I eat these every day.. _____ 0

I eat some of these occasionally.. _____ 1

I seldom or never eat these snacks .... _____ 2

BAKED GOODS: pies, cakes, cookies, sweet rolls, doughnuts POINTS

I eat them 5 or more times a week .... _____ 0

I eat them 2–4 times a week .... _____ 1

I seldom eat baked goods or eat only low-fat baked goods .... _____ 2

POULTRY AND FISH: (If you do not eat meat, fish, or poultry, give yourself 2 points) POINTS

I rarely eat these foods... _____ 0

I eat them 1–2 times a week .... _____ 1

I eat them 3 or more times a week .... _____ 2

LOW-FAT MEATS: extra lean hamburger, round steak, pork loin, roast, tenderloin, chuck roast. (If you do not eat meat, fish, or poultry, give yourself 2 points) POINTS

I rarely eat these foods... _____ 0

I occasionally eat these foods... _____ 1

I eat mostly fat-trimmed red meats... _____ 2

HIGH-FAT MEATS: luncheon meats, bacon, hot dogs, sausage, steak, regular and lean ground beef. (If you do not eat meat, fish, or poultry, give yourself 2 points) POINTS

I eat these every day... _____ 0

I occasionally eat these foods... _____ 1

I rarely eat these foods... _____ 2

CURED AND SMOKED MEAT AND FISH: luncheon meats, hot dogs, bacon, ham and other smoked or pickled meats and fish. (If you do not eat meat, fish, or poultry, give yourself 2 points) POINTS

I eat these foods 4 or more times a week .... _____ 0

I eat some of these foods 1–3 times a week .... _____ 1

I seldom eat these foods... _____ 2

LEGUMES: dried beans, peas (kidney, navy, lima, pinto, garbanzo, split-pea, lentil)	POINTS
I eat legumes less than once a week	_____ 0
I eat legumes 1–2 times a week	_____ 1
I eat legumes 3 or more times a week	_____ 2

WHOLE GRAINS AND CEREAL: whole grain breads, brown rice, pasta, grain cereals	POINTS
I seldom eat these foods	_____ 0
I eat these foods 1–2 times a day	_____ 1
I eat these foods 4 or more times daily	_____ 2

VITAMIN-C RICH FRUITS AND VEGETABLES: citrus fruits, juices, green peppers, berries	POINTS
I seldom eat these foods	_____ 0
I eat these foods 3–5 times a week	_____ 1
I eat these foods 1–2 times a day	_____ 2

DARK GREEN AND DEEP YELLOW FRUITS AND VEGETABLES: broccoli, greens, carrots, peaches (dark green and yellow fruits and vegetables contain beta carotene that your body turns into vitamin A. Vitamin A helps protect against certain types of cancer-causing substances)	POINTS
I seldom eat these foods	_____ 0
I eat these foods 1–2 times a week	_____ 1
I eat these foods 3–4 times a week	_____ 2

VEGETABLES OF THE CABBAGE FAMILY: broccoli, cabbage, brussels sprouts, cauliflower	POINTS
I seldom eat these foods	_____ 0
I eat these foods 1–2 times a week	_____ 1
I eat these foods 3–4 times a week	_____ 2

ALCOHOL:	POINTS
I drink more than 2 oz daily	_____ 0
I drink every week, but not daily	_____ 1
I occasionally or never drink alcohol	_____ 2

YOUR BODY WEIGHT:		POINTS
I am more than 20 lb over my ideal weight	_____	0
I am 10–20 lb over my ideal weight	_____	1
I am within 10 lb of my ideal weight...	_____	2

ADD UP YOUR TOTAL POINTS HERE   total points

YOUR EATING SMART RATING

0–12 Points: A Warning Signal

Your diet is too high in fat and too low in fiber-rich foods. Assess your eating habits to see where you could make improvements.

13–17 Points: Not Bad

You still have a way to go. Review your quiz to identify those areas in which you rate poorly, then make the necessary adjustments.

18–36 Points: Good For You, You're Eating Smart

You should feel very good about yourself. You have been careful to limit your fats and eat a varied diet. Keep up the good habits and continue to look for ways to improve.

Your Weight and Heart Disease I.Q.

THE FOLLOWING STATEMENTS are either **true** or **false.** The statements test your knowledge of overweight and heart disease. The correct answers can be found on the next page. A complete discussion of each topic can also be found in your textbook.

(From the National Heart, Lung, and Blood Institute, National Institutes of Health)

TRUE/FALSE

1. _____ Being overweight puts you at risk for heart disease.

2. _____ If you are overweight, losing weight helps lower your high blood cholesterol and high blood pressure.

3. _____ Quitting smoking is healthy, but it commonly leads to excessive weight gain that increases your risk for heart disease.

4. _____ An overweight person with high blood pressure should pay more attention to a low-sodium diet than to weight reduction.

5. _____ A reduced intake of sodium or salt does not always lower high blood pressure to normal.

6. _____ The best way to lose weight is to eat fewer calories and to increase exercise.

7. _____ Skipping meals is a good way to cut down on calories.

8. _____ Foods high in complex carbohydrates (starch and fiber) are good choices when you are trying to lose weight.

9. _____ The single most important change most people can make to lose weight is to avoid sugar.

10. _____ Polyunsaturated fat has the same number of calories as saturated fat.

11. _____ Overweight children are very likely to become overweight adults.

ANSWERS TO YOUR WEIGHT AND HEART DISEASE I.Q. TEST

1. True.
Being overweight increases your risk for high blood cholesterol and high blood pressure. Even if you do not have high cholesterol or high blood pressure, being overweight may increase your risk for heart disease. Where you carry extra weight also may affect your risk. Weight carried at your waist or trunk seems to be associated with an increased risk for heart disease in many people.

2. True.
If you are overweight, even moderate reductions in weight, such as 5 to 10%, can produce substantial reduction in blood pressure. Moderate weight loss may also reduce your LDL-cholesterol and increase your HDL-cholesterol.

3. False.
The average weight gain after quitting smoking is 5 lb. The proportion of ex-smokers who gain large amounts of weight

338

(>20 lb) is relatively small. Even if you gain weight when you stop smoking, you should change your eating and exercise habits to lose weight rather than starting to smoke again. Smokers who quit smoking decrease their risk for heart disease by more than 50%!

4. False.

Weight loss, if you are overweight, may reduce your blood pressure even if you don't reduce the amount of sodium consumed. Weight loss is recommended for all overweight people who have high blood pressure. Even if weight loss does not reduce blood pressure to normal, it may help you cut back on your blood pressure medications.

5. True.

While a high sodium or salt intake plays a key role in maintaining high blood pressure, there is no easy way to determine who will benefit from consuming less sodium and salt. Also, a high sodium or salt intake may limit how well certain high blood pressure medications work.

6. True.

Eating fewer calories and exercising more is the best way to lose weight and keep it off. A steady weight loss of 1–2 lb/week is safe, and the weight is more likely to stay off. Losing weight, if you are overweight, may also help reduce your blood pressure and raise your HDL-cholesterol.

7. False.

To cut calories, some people regularly skip meals, snacks, or caloric drinks. If you do this, your body thinks that it is starving even if your intake is not reduced to a low amount. Your body will try to save energy by slowing its metabolism. This makes losing weight harder and may even add body fat.

8. True.

Contrary to popular belief, foods high in complex carbohydrates are lower in calories than foods high in fat. In addition, complex carbohydrates are good sources of vitamins, minerals, and fiber.

9. False.

Sugar has not been found to cause obesity; however, many foods high in sugar are also high in fat. Fat has more than twice the calories as the same amount of protein or carbohydrate.

10. True.

All fats—polyunsaturated, monounsaturated, and saturated—have the same number of calories. All calories count regardless of their source. Fats are the richest sources of calories; thus eating less total fat will help reduce the total number of calories consumed daily.

11. False.

Obesity in childhood does increase the likelihood of adult obesity, but most overweight children will not become obese. Several factors influence whether an overweight child becomes an overweight adult. These include age of onset of overweight, degree of childhood and family history of overweight, and dietary and activity habits.

YOUR SCORE

10–11 CORRECT: Congratulations! You know a lot about weight and heart disease. Share this information with your family and friends.

8–9 CORRECT: Very good.

<8 CORRECT: Go over the answers and try to learn more about weight and heart disease. Refer to Chapter 29 and 30 of your textbook.

Healthy Heart I.Q.

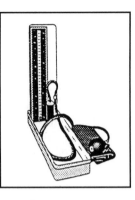

THE FOLLOWING STATEMENTS are either **true** or **false**. The statements test your knowledge about heart disease and its risk factors. The correct answers are on the next page.

(From the National Heart, Lung, and Blood Institute, National Institutes of Health)

TRUE/FALSE

1. _____ The risk factors for heart disease that you *can do something about* are: high blood pressure, high blood cholesterol, smoking, obesity, and physical inactivity.

2. _____ A stroke is often the first symptom of high blood pressure, and a heart attack is often the first symptom of high blood cholesterol.

3. _____ A blood pressure greater than or equal to 140/90 mm Hg is generally considered high.

4. _____ High blood pressure affects the same number of blacks as it does whites.

5. _____ The best ways to treat and control high blood pressure are to control your weight, exercise, eat less salt, restrict alcohol intake, and take your prescribed high blood pressure medicine.

6. _____ A blood cholesterol level of 240 mg/dL is desirable for adults.

7. _____ The most effective dietary way to lower your blood cholesterol is to eat foods low in cholesterol.

8. _____ Lowering blood cholesterol levels can help people who have already had a heart attack.

9. _____ Only children from families at high risk of heart disease need to check their blood cholesterol levels.

10. _____ Smoking is a major risk factor for four of the five leading causes of death, including heart attack, stroke, cancer, and lung disease such as emphysema and bronchitis.

11. _____ If you have had a heart attack, quitting smoking can help reduce your chances of having a second attack.

12. _____ Someone who has smoked for 30 to 40 years probably will not be able to quit smoking.

13. _____ Heart disease is the leading killer of men and women in the United States.

ANSWERS TO YOUR HEALTHY HEART I.Q. TEST

1. True.

High blood pressure, smoking, and high cholesterol are the three most important risk factors. On average, each factor doubles your chance of developing heart disease. Thus, a person who has all three risk factors is 8 times more likely to develop heart disease than someone who has none. Obesity increases the likelihood of developing high blood cholesterol and high blood pressure. Increased activity decreases heart disease risk since exercisers are more likely to cut down or stop smoking.

2. True.

A person with high blood pressure or high blood cholesterol may feel fine and look great, and there are often no signs that anything is wrong.

3. True.

A blood pressure of 140/90 mm Hg or greater is classified as high. If the lower number is 85 or greater, this is considered a high risk.

4. False.

High blood pressure is more common in blacks than whites, and affects 40 out of every 100 black adults compared to 25 out of every 100 whites. With aging, high blood pressure is more severe among blacks than among whites.

5. True.

Lifestyle changes can help keep blood pressure levels normal even into advanced age, and are important in treating and preventing high blood pressure.

6. False.

A total blood cholesterol of under 200 mg/dL is desirable and puts you at a lower risk for heart disease. A level of 200–239 mg/dL is considered borderline high and usually increases your risk for heart disease. All adults 20 years of age or older should have their cholesterol checked at least every 5 years.

7. False.

Reducing cholesterol is important; however, eating foods low in saturated fat is the most effective dietary way to lower cholesterol levels along with eating less total fat and cholesterol.

8. True.

People who have had one heart attack are at much higher risk for a second attack. Reducing cholesterol can slow down (and in some cases even reverse) and reduce the chances of a second attack.

9. True.

Children from "high" risk families should have their cholesterol checked at least every other year.

10. True.

Heavy smokers are 2 to 4 times more likely to have a heart attack than non-smokers. The heart attack death rate among all smokers is 70% greater than non-smokers. The risk of dying of lung cancer is 22 times higher for male smokers than non-smokers, and 12 times higher for female smokers than female non-smokers. Eighty percent of all deaths from lung disease are due directly to smoking.

11. True.

One year after quitting, ex-smokers cut their extra risk by about half or more, and eventually the risk returns to normal in healthy ex-smokers.

12. False.

Older smokers are more likely to succeed at quitting smoking than younger smokers.

13. True.

Heart disease is the #1 killer in the U.S. Approximately 489,000 Americans died of heart disease in 1990, and approximately half of these deaths were women.

YOUR SCORE

12–13 CORRECT: Congratulations! You know a lot about heart disease. Share this information with your family and friends.

10–11 CORRECT: Very good.

< 10: CORRECT: Go over the answers and try to learn more about weight and heart disease. Refer to Chapters 29 and 30 of your textbook.

Assessment of Energy and Nutrient Intake:
Three-Day Dietary Survey

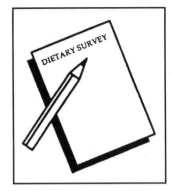

YOUR THREE-DAY DIETARY SURVEY is a relatively simple yet accurate method to determine the nutritional quality and total calories of the food consumed each day. The secret is to keep a daily log of food intake for any three days that represent your normal eating pattern.

Experiments have shown that calculations of caloric intake made from records of daily food consumption are usually within 10% of the number of calories actually consumed. For example, suppose the caloric value of your daily food intake was directly measured in a bomb calorimeter and averaged 2130 kcal. If you kept a three-day dietary history and estimated your caloric intake, the daily value would likely be within 10% of the actual value, or between 1920 kcal and 2350 kcal. As long as you maintained a careful record, the degree of accuracy for daily determinations would be within acceptable limits.

Before recording your daily caloric intake over the three-day period, you should become familiar with "honest" calorie counting. This requires four items for measuring food: a plastic ruler, a standard measuring cup, measuring spoons, and an inexpensive balance or weighing scale. You can purchase these items at most hardware stores. Second, you should familiarize yourself with the nutritional and caloric values of foods by consulting food labels and Section 4 of this Study Guide. Listed under "Specialty and Fast-Food Items" in the food listings are the nutritional values for items sold at fast-food chain stores.

Measure or weigh each of the food items in your diet. This is the only reliable way to obtain an accurate estimate of the size of a food portion. If you elect to use Section 4 of this Study Guide to estimate the nutritional and kcal values, you only need to weigh each food item. If you use a supplementary calorie-counting guide, this may require the measuring cup, spoons, and ruler.

FOOD CATEGORIES

Meat and Fish

Measure the portion of meat or fish by thickness, length, and width, or record weight on the scale.

Vegetables, Potatoes, Rice, Cereals, Salads

Measure the portion in a measuring cup or record weight on the scale.

Cream or Sugar Added to Coffee or Tea

Measure with measuring spoons before adding to the drink, or record weight on the scale.

Fluids and Bottled Drinks

Check the labels for volume or empty the container into the measuring cup. If you weigh the fluid, be sure to subtract the weight of the cup or glass. Sugar-free soft drinks usually have kcal values listed on their labels.

Cookies, Cakes, Pies

For these items, measure the diameter and thickness with a ruler, or weigh on the scale. Evaluate frosting or sauces separately.

Fruites

Cut them in half before eating and measure the diameters, or weigh them on the scale. For fruits that must be peeled or have rinds or cores, be sure the weight of the non-edible portion is subtracted from the total weight of the food. Do this for items such as oranges, apples, and bananas.

Jam, Salad Dressing, Catsup, Mayonnaise

Measure the condiment with the measuring spoon or weigh the portion on the scale.

DIRECTIONS FOR COMPUTING YOUR THREE-DAY DIETARY SURVEY

Step 1.

Prepare a table (similar to Table E.1) indicating the intake of food items during a day. Include the amount (g or oz); caloric value; and carbohydrate, lipid, and protein content; the minerals Ca and Fe; and vitamins C, B_1 (thiamine), and B_2 (riboflavin); fiber; and cholesterol.

Step 2.

Be sure to list <u>each</u> food you consume for breakfast, lunch, dinner, between-meal eating, and snacks. Include food items that are used in preparing the meal (e.g., butter, oils, margarine, bread crumbs, egg coating, etc.).

Step 3.

Weigh, measure or approximate the size of each portion of food that you eat. Record these values on your daily record chart (e.g., 3 oz of salad oil, 1/8 piece of 8″ diameter apple pie, etc.).

Step 4.

Record your daily calorie and nutrient intake on a chart similar to Table E.1, which was recorded for a 21-year-old college student. Record the daily totals for the caloric and nutrient headings on the "Daily and Average Daily Summary Chart" (Table E.2). When you've completed your three-day survey, compute the three-day total by adding up the values for days 1, 2, and 3; then divide by 3 to determine the daily average of each nutrient category.

Step 5.

Using each of the average daily nutrient values, calculate the percent of the RDA consumed for that particular nutrient and graph your results as shown in Figure E.1. An example for calculating the percent of the RDA is shown in Table E.3, along with the specific RDA values for men and women.

Step 6.

Be as accurate and honest as possible. <u>Do not</u> include unusual or atypical days in your dietary survey (e.g., days that you are sick, special occasions such as birthdays, or eating out at restaurants unless that is normal for you).

Step 7.

Remember that the protein RDA is equal to 0.8 g protein per kilogram of body weight (1 kg = 2.2 lb).

Step 8.

Compute the percentage of your total calories supplied from carbohydrate, lipid, and protein.

For example, if total average daily caloric intake is 2450 kcal/day, and 1600 kcal are from carbohydrates, the daily percentage of total calories from carbohydrates is: 1600/2450 × 100 = 65%

Step 9.

While there is no specific RDA for lipid or carbohydrate, a prudent recommendation is that lipid should not exceed more than 30% of your total caloric intake; for active men and women, carbohydrates should be approximately 60% of the total calories ingested. Thus, in computing the percentage of "RDA" for graphing purposes in Figures E.1, you should assume that:

a. "RDA" for lipid is 30% of total calories
b. "RDA" for carbohydrate is 60% of total calories

For example, if 50% of your average daily calories comes from lipid, you are taking in 167% of the recommended value ("RDA") for this nutrient: [50% divided by 30% (recommended percentage) × 100 = 167%]

Step 10.

As was the case for lipid and carbohydrate, there is no RDA for average daily caloric intake. Any recommendation for energy intake needs to be based on one's present status for body fat as well as current daily energy expenditure. However, average values for daily caloric intake have been published for the typical young adult and equal about 2100 kcal for young women and 3000 kcal for young men. Thus, for graphing purposes in Figure E.1, you can evaluate your average daily caloric intake against the "average" values for your sex and age.

For example, if you are a 20-year-old female and you consume an average of 2400 kcal daily, your energy intake would be equal to 114% of the average ("RDA") for your age and sex. [2400 kcal divided by 2100 kcal (average) × 100 = 114%]. This does not mean that you need to go on a diet and reduce food intake to bring you in line with the average U.S. value. To the contrary, your higher-than-average caloric intake may be required to power your active lifestyle that contributes to maintaining a desirable body mass and body composition.

If you eat a food item not listed in Section 4, try to make an intelligent guess as to its composition and amount consumed. It is better to overestimate the amount of food consumed than to underestimate or to make no estimation at all. If you go to a restaurant for dinner, or to a friend's house where it may be inappropriate to measure the food, then omit this day from the counting procedure and resume record keeping the following day.

Because the purpose of keeping records for three days is to obtain an accurate appraisal of the average daily energy and nutrient intake, record-keeping is extremely important. **Be sure to record everything you eat.** If you are not completely honest, you are wasting your time. Most people find it easier to keep accurate records if they record food items while preparing a meal or immediately afterwards when eating snack items.

TABLE E.1.
SAMPLE ONE-DAY CALORIC AND NUTRIENT INTAKE FOR A 21-YEAR-OLD COLLEGE STUDENT

Food Item	Amount	kcal	Protein (g)	CHO (g)	Lipid (g)	Ca (mg)	Fe (mg)	Fiber (g)	Cholesterol (mg)	Thiam[a] (mg)	Ribofl[a] (mg)
BREAKFAST											
Eggs, hard boiled	2 (2 oz ea)	160	14.1	1.4	11.2	55.2	1.9	0.0	452	0.06	0.53
Orange juice	8 oz	104	0.9	86.4	0.5	72.4	0.8	0.9	0.0	0.20	0.06
Corn flakes	1 cup/1 oz	110	2.3	24.4	0.5	1.0	1.8	0.6	0.0	0.37	0.42
Skim milk	8 oz	80	7.8	10.6	0.6	279.2	0.1	0.0	3.7	0.08	0.32
SNACK											
None											
LUNCH											
Tuna fish (oil pack)	2 oz	112	16.5	0.0	68.0	7.8	0.8	0.0	10.0	0.02	0.06
White bread (toast)	2 pieces	168	5.3	31.4	2.5	81.2	1.8	1.3	0.0	0.24	0.21
Mayonnaise	1 oz	203	0.3	0.8	22.6	5.7	0.2	0.0	16.8	0.01	0.01
Skim milk	8 oz	80	7.8	10.6	0.6	279.2	0.1	0.0	3.7	0.08	0.32
Plums	4 (2 oz ea)	128	1.8	29.5	1.4	10.3	0.2	4.4	0.0	0.10	0.22
SNACK											
Chocolate milkshake	8 oz	288	7.7	46.4	8.4	256	0.7	0.3	29.6	0.13	0.55
Dinner											
Sirloin steak, lean	8 oz	456	64.8	0.0	20.2	18.6	5.8	0.0	173.6	0.21	0.47
French fries, veg. oil	6 oz	540	6.8	67.2	28.1	34.2	1.3	3.4	0.0	0.30	0.05
Cole slaw	4 oz	80	1.4	14.1	3.0	51.2	0.7	2.3	9.2	0.08	0.07
Italian bread	2 oz	156	5.1	32.0	1.0	9.4	1.5	0.9	0.0	0.23	0.13
Light beer	8 oz	96	0.6	8.8	0.0	11.2	0.1	0.5	0.0	0.02	0.06
SNACK											
Yogurt, whole milk	6 oz	102	5.9	7.9	5.5	205.8	0.1	0.0	22.1	0.05	0.24
Daily Total		2863	149.1	371.5	174.1	1378.4	17.2	14.6	720.7	2.18	3.72

[a]Thiam, thiamin; Ribofl, riboflavin.

TABLE E.2.

DAILY AND AVERAGE DAILY SUMMARY CHART OF THE INTAKE OF CALORIES AND SPECIFIC FOOD NUTRIENTS

Day	kcal	Protein[a] (g)	Lipid[a] (g)	Carbo[a] (g)	Ca (mg)	Fe (mg)	Thiamine (mg)	Riboflavin (mg)	Fiber (g)	Cholesterol (mg)
#1										
#2										
#3										
Three-day total										
Average Daily Value[b]										

[a]Use the following caloric transformations to convert your average daily grams of carbohydrate (CHO), lipid, and protein to average daily calories:

1 g CHO = 4 kcal
1 g Lipid = 9 kcal
1 g Protein = 4 kcal

[b]The Average Daily Value is used to determine the percentage of the RDA for your graph. See Table E.1 for sample calculations. Figure E.1 is a bar graph showing the nutrient values as a percentage of the average or recommended value for each item.

TABLE E.3.

RDA VALUES FOR SELECTED NUTRIENTS INCLUDING SAMPLE COMPUTATIONS FOR DERIVING THE PERCENT OF RDA FROM YOUR DIETARY SURVEY. VALUES LISTED IN THE TABLE ARE 100% VALUES FOR PURPOSES OF GRAPHING YOUR DIETARY SURVEY

MEN							
Age	kcal[a]	Protein (g/kg)	Ca (mg)	Fe (mg)	Thiamine (mg)	Riboflavin (mg)	Fiber[a] (g)	Cholesterol[a] (mg)
---	---	---	---	---	---	---	---	---
19–22	3000	0.8	1200	10	1.5	1.7	30	300
23–50	2700	0.8	800	10	1.5	1.7	30	300

WOMEN							
Age	kcal[a]	Protein (g/kg)	Ca (mg)	Fe (mg)	Thiamine (mg)	Riboflavin (mg)	Fiber[a] (g)	Cholesterol[a] (mg)
---	---	---	---	---	---	---	---	---
19–22	2100	0.8	1200	15	1.1	1.3	30	300
23–50	2000	0.8	800	15	1.1	1.3	30	300

Source: Recommended Dietary Allowances, Revised 1989. Washington, DC: Food and Nutrition Board, National Academy of Sciences– National Research Council, 1989.

[a]There is no RDA for daily caloric intake or for the intake of fiber or cholesterol. Values for caloric intake represent an average for adult Americans, while fiber and cholesterol values are recommended as being prudent for maintaining good health.

HOW TO DETERMINE THE PERCENTAGE OF THE RDA FROM YOUR DIETARY SURVEY

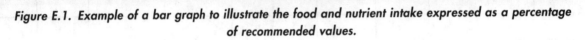

Example # 1: Percentage of RDA for protein for a 70-kg
person
Daily protein intake = 68 g
RDA = (70 kg × 0.8 g/kg) = 56 g
% of RDA = 56/68 × 100 = 121%

Example #2: Percentage of RDA for iron (female)
Daily iron intake = 7.5 mg
RDA = 15 mg
% of R

Figure E.1. Example of a bar graph to illustrate the food and nutrient intake expressed as a percentage of recommended values.

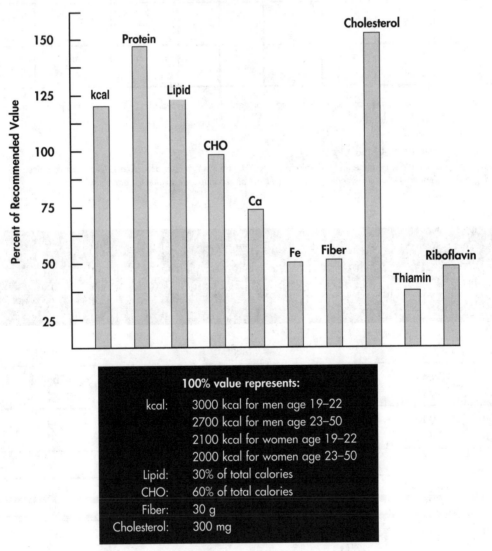

F

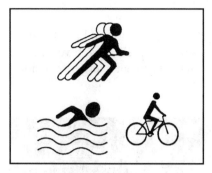

Assessment of Physical Activity: Three-Day Activity Recall

ANY HOPE OF CHANGING the pattern and quantity of daily physical activity must be predicated on an accurate appraisal of the daily energy expenditure.

Step 1.

Determine your daily pattern of physical activity, including such minimal daily requirements as sleeping, eating, sitting in class, and bathing. An activity profile can be constructed by keeping a *daily log* for three days of the actual time allotted to the various activities that represent your usual pattern of activity. To illustrate the procedure, Table F.1 shows a fairly detailed activity profile for a college professor during a typical day of summer vacation. This record includes a description of the activity, its duration, and the calories expended during the activity. For this professor, if it were not for the hour and a half devoted to his daily run, his total daily energy expenditure would be just slightly above average.

Step 2.

(a) Determine your Basal Metabolic Rate (BMR) in kcal/h as follows:

> **MEN:**
> BMR (kcal/h) = 38 kcal/m^2/h^a × surface area (m^2)^b
>
> **WOMEN:**
> BMR (kcal/h) = 35 kcal/m^2/h^a × surface area (m^2)^b

^{a}*For added precision, determine BMR (kcal/m^2/h) for your age and sex from Figure 9.3 in your textbook.*
^{b}*Surface area (m^2) is determined from stature and body mass from Figure 9.4 in your textbook.*

(b) Divide the BMR value in kcal/h obtained in Step 2(a) by 60 to compute the BMR value per minute. This value will be used to represent your energy expenditure per minute during sleep.

> **EXAMPLE OF BMR CALCULATIONS**
> **DATA: MALE**
>
> Age, 40 y
> Stature, 182 cm (72 in)
> Body mass, 86.4 kg (190 lb)
> Body surface area (from Figure 9.4) = 2.09 m^2
> kcal/m^2/h (from Fig. 9.3) = 37.2
>
> **CALCULATIONS**
> a. kcal/h = 37.2 × 2.09 = 77.7
> b. kcal/min = 77.7/60 = 1.3

Step 3.

Determine the energy expenditure in kcal/min for each of the activities listed in your profile. For sleep use the BMR computed in Step 2b. These values are listed in Section 4 of this Study Guide. The values are gross values that include the resting energy value. If an activity is not included, choose an activity most similar to the one you list.

Step 4.

Multiply the energy expenditure value from the table by the number of minutes spent in each activity.

Step 5.

Sum the total energy expenditure for each activity, including the value for sleep, to arrive at your <u>total</u> energy expenditure for the day.

Step 6.

Repeat steps 2 through 5 for each of the three days. Obtain the average daily energy expenditure for the three-day period by summing the total calories expended over the three-day period and divide by 3.

HOW TO INTERPRET YOUR AVERAGE DAILY ENERGY EXPENDITURE

There is no norm or desirable standard for the number of calories you should expend during a day. Many factors are involved, including body size, age, sex, and—most importantly—level of physical activity. The average daily energy expenditure is 3000 kcal for men and 2100 kcal for women between the ages of 19 and 22 years. If you are not gaining or losing body weight, then your energy expenditure equals your energy intake.

TABLE F.1.

DETAILED RECORD OF PHYSICAL ACTIVITY FOR ONE DAY FOR A UNIVERSITY PROFESSOR

Activity	Begin Time	End Time	Total Minutes	Similar Activity Section 4	kcal/min	Total kcal
Wake, bathroom use	6:45AM	6:53AM	8	Standing quietly	2.3	18.4
Go back to bed	6:53	7:30	38	BMR	1.3	48.1
Eat breakfast	7:30	7:50	10	Eating, sitting	2.0	40.0
Use bathroom	7:50	8:00	10	Standing quietly	2.3	23.0
Dress	8:00	8:06	6	Standing quietly	2.3	13.8
Drive to school	8:06	8:17	11	Sitting quietly	2.0	22.0
Walk to office	8:17	8:25	8	Walking, normal pace	6.9	55.8
Work in office, pick up mail	8:25	10:00	95	Writing, sitting	2.5	237.5
Up/down stairs	10:00	10:10	10	11 min 30 sec pace	11.7	117.0
Work in office	10:10	12:10PM	120	Writing, sitting	2.5	300.0
Go to locker	12:10PM	12:12	2	Walking, normal pace	6.9	13.8
Get dressed	12:12	12:16	4	Standing quietly	2.3	9.2
Walk to track	12:16	12:20	4	Walk, normal pace	6.9	27.6
Wait for friend	12:20	12:30	10	Standing quietly	2.3	23.0
Run to park, back	12:30	2:00	90	8-min mile pace	17.2	1553.0
Walk to locker	2:00	2:04	4	Walk, normal pace	6.9	27.6
Shower, dress	2:04	2:20	16	Quiet standing	2.3	36.8
Walk to office	2:20	2:24	4	Walk, normal pace	6.9	27.6
Meeting/lunch	2:24	3:00	36	Eating, sitting	2.0	72.0
Work in office	3:00	5:05	125	Writing, sitting	2.5	312.5
Walk to library	5:05	5:12	7	Walk, normal pace	6.9	48.3
Work in library	5:12	6:05	53	Writing, sitting	2.5	132.5
Walk to dean	6:05	6:10	5	Walk, normal pace	6.9	34.5
Meeting, dean	6:10	6:35	25	Writing, sitting	2.5	62.5
Walk to office	6:35	6:43	8	Walk, normal pace	6.9	55.2
Walk to car	6:43	6:51	8	Walk, normal pace	6.9	55.2
Drive home	6:51	7:03	12	Sitting quietly	1.8	21.6
Change clothes	7:03	7:07	4	Standing quietly	2.3	9.2
Wash-up	7:07	7:11	4	Standing quietly	2.3	9.2
Cook dinner	7:11	8:00	49	Cooking	4.1	200.9
Watch TV	8:00	8:30	30	Sitting quietly	1.8	54.0
Eat dinner	8:30	9:00	30	Eating, sitting	2.0	60.0
Mail letter	9:00	9:05	5	Walk, normal pace	6.9	34.5
Listen to stereo	9:05	9:30	25	Sitting quietly	1.8	45.0
Watch TV	9:30	10:30	60	Sitting quietly	1.8	108.0
Wash-up	10:30	10:38	8	Standing quietly	2.3	18.4
Read in bed	10:38	11:15	37	Lying at ease	1.9	70.3

DAILY TOTAL = 4583

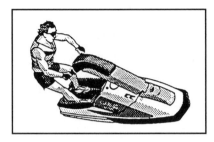

Assessment of Health-Related Physical Fitness

THE TREND IN FITNESS assessment over the past 20 years has been to deemphasize physical fitness tests that stress motor performance and athletic fitness (i.e., tests of speed, power, balance, and agility). Today's trend is to focus on those measures that assess *functional capacity* and also reflect various aspects of overall good health or disease prevention, or both. The four components of health-related physical fitness that are commonly evaluated include aerobic power (cardiorespiratory fitness), body composition, abdom-

inal muscular strength and endurance, and lower back and hamstring flexibility. An upper-extremity measure of muscular strength also is often included, although it is not directly related to health status.

A person's performance on each of the test items of health-related physical fitness is not fixed but can be significantly improved through a program of regular exercise and weight control.

TEST COMPONENT #1: LOWER-BACK FLEXIBILITY

A. Rationale

A substantial amount of clinical evidence indicates that maintenance of trunk, hip, lower back, and posterior thigh flexibility is important in the prevention and alleviation of lower-back pain and tension. Back disorders are associated with weak muscles in the abdominal area and limited range of motion of the lower spine. There also is reduced elasticity of the hamstring muscles at the back of the upper leg. The importance of lower-back flexibility as a health-related fitness measure is further supported by the fact that physicians frequently prescribe specific trunk and thigh flexibility stretches for their patients with lower-back problems, or for individuals who desire to prevent the occurrence of such problems.

B. Lower-Back Flexibility Assessment Test: The Sit and Reach Test

Sit on a mat with your legs extended. Your feet should rest against the base of a box on which a yardstick is mounted with the 9 inch (23 cm) mark on the near side of the box (see Fig. G.1). After a general warm-up that includes stretching of the lower back and posterior thighs, slowly reach forward with both hands as far as possible and hold the position momentarily. Record the distance reached on the yardstick by your fingertips. Use the best of four trials as your flexibility score.

Figure G.1. Sit and reach flexibility test.

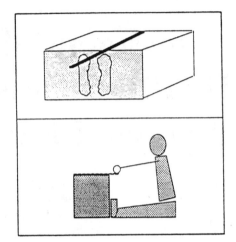

C. How Do You Rate on Lower-Back Flexibility?

Compare your results with the normative data in Table G.1.

TABLE G.1.

NORMS FOR THE SIT AND REACH (cm) FOR YOUNG ADULT MEN AND WOMEN

Percentile	Men				Women			
	18 y	19 y	20 y	21 y	18 y	19 y	20 y	21 y
99	50	49	49	50	52	52	51	50
95	45	45	46	45	47	47	46	46
90	42	43	43	42	46	45	45	44
85	41	42	41	41	44	43	43	43
80	40	40	41	40	43	42	42	42
75	39	39	40	39	42	41	41	42
70	38	38	39	38	40	41	39	40
65	37	37	38	36	40	40	38	39
60	36	36	37	35	39	38	38	38
55	35	35	36	35	38	38	37	37
50	34	34	35	33	38	37	37	36
45	34	33	34	32	37	36	36	36
40	32	32	33	31	36	36	35	35
35	31	31	32	31	35	34	34	34
30	30	29	31	30	34	33	33	33
25	29	28	30	28	33	32	32	32
20	27	27	27	27	32	31	31	31
15	25	26	25	25	30	29	30	29
10	23	23	22	24	29	27	28	27
5	19	19	18	20	26	23	24	25

From: Norms for College Students: Health Related Physical Fitness Test. Reston, Va, American Alliance for Health, Physical Education, Recreation, and Dance, 1985.

TEST COMPONENT #2: BODY FAT PERCENTAGE

A. Rationale

Body composition is defined as the relative percentage of fat and fat-free body mass. An excessive accumulation of body fat significantly hinders the ability to perform tasks requiring speed, endurance, and coordination. Additionally, research indicates that an excess amount of body fat is an associative and/or contributing factor to four categories of health hazards: (a) disturbance of normal body functions, (b) increased risk of disease (e.g., hypertension, high cholesterol, diabetes, coronary heart disease), (c) exacerbation of existing disease states, and (d) adverse psychological effects.

B. Body Fat Percentage Assessment Test: Measurement of Fatfolds

Evaluation of body fat can be made by different indirect procedures. These can include *girths* or *fatfolds* measured at specific body sites. In the *Exercise Physiology* textbook we describe how to use girth measurements to estimate percentage body fat. In this section we describe the alternative method using fatfolds. The fatfold measurements are:

> **MEN:** Chest, Abdomen, Thigh
> **WOMEN:** Triceps, Suprailium, Thigh

Measurements at each site are taken in accordance with standard procedures. The exact anatomical sites for each fatfold measurement are described in your textbook in Chapter 27.

Abdomen (*Men only*): Vertical fold measured 1 inch to the right of the umbilicus.

Chest (*Men only*): A diagonal fold taken one-half of the distance between the anterior axillary line and the nipple.

Suprailium (*Women only*): Slightly oblique fold just above the crest of the hip bone. The fold is lifted to follow the natural diagonal line at this point.

Thigh (*Men and Women*): Vertical fold measured at the anterior midline of the thigh, midway between the knee cap and the hip.

Triceps (*Women only*): Vertical fold measured at the posterior midline of the upper arm halfway between the tip of the shoulder and the tip of the elbow. The elbow should be extended and relaxed.

TABLE G.2.

PERCENT FAT ESTIMATES FOR MEN. SUM OF CHEST, ABDOMINAL, AND THIGH FATFOLDS

Sum Fatfolds (mm)	AGE TO THE LAST YEAR			
	Under 22	23 to 27	28 to 32	33 to 37
8–10	1.3	1.8	2.3	2.9
11–13	2.2	2.8	3.3	3.9
14–16	3.2	3.8	4.3	4.8
17–19	4.2	4.7	5.3	5.8
20–22	5.1	5.7	6.2	6.8
23–25	6.1	6.6	7.2	7.7
26–28	7.0	7.6	8.1	8.7
29–31	8.0	8.5	9.1	9.6
32–34	8.9	9.4	10.0	10.5
35–37	9.8	10.4	10.9	11.5
38–40	10.7	11.3	11.8	12.4
41–43	11.6	12.2	12.7	13.3
44–46	12.0	13.1	13.6	14.2
47–49	13.4	13.9	14.5	15.1
50–52	14.3	14.8	15.4	15.9
53–55	15.1	15.7	16.2	16.8
56–58	16.0	16.5	17.1	17.7
59–61	16.9	17.4	17.9	18.5
62–64	17.6	18.2	18.8	19.4
65–67	18.5	19.0	19.6	20.2
68–70	19.3	19.9	20.4	21.0
71–73	20.1	20.7	21.2	21.8
74–76	20.9	21.5	22.0	22.6
77–79	21.7	22.2	22.8	23.4
80–82	22.4	23.0	23.6	24.2
83–85	23.2	23.8	24.4	25.0
86–88	24.0	24.5	25.1	25.7
89–91	24.7	25.3	25.9	25.5
92–94	25.4	26.0	26.6	27.2
95–97	26.1	26.7	27.3	27.9
98–100	26.9	27.4	28.0	28.6
101–103	27.5	28.1	28.7	29.3
104–106	28.2	28.8	29.4	30.0
107–109	28.9	29.5	30.1	30.7
110–112	29.6	30.2	30.8	31.4
113–115	30.2	30.8	31.4	32.0
116–118	30.9	31.5	32.1	32.7
119–121	31.5	32.1	32.7	33.3
122–124	32.1	32.7	33.3	33.9
125–127	32.7	33.3	33.9	34.9

From: Jackson, A. S. and Pollock, M. L. Practical Assessment of Body Composition. Phys. Sportsmed., 13 (5): 76, 1985. Reproduced with permission of McGraw-Hill, Inc.

TABLE G.3.

PERCENT FAT ESTIMATES FOR WOMEN. SUM OF TRICEPS, SUPRAILIUM, AND THIGH FATFOLDS

Sum Fatfolds (mm)	AGE TO THE LAST YEAR			
	Under 22	23 to 27	28 to 32	33 to 37
23–25	9.7	9.9	10.2	10.4
26–28	11.0	11.2	11.5	11.7
29–31	12.3	12.5	12.8	13.0
32–34	13.6	13.8	14.0	14.3
35–37	14.8	15.0	15.3	15.5
38–40	16.0	16.3	16.5	16.7
41–43	17.2	17.4	17.7	17.9
44–46	18.3	18.6	18.8	19.1
47–49	19.5	19.7	20.0	20.2
50–52	20.6	20.8	21.1	21.3
53–55	21.7	21.9	22.1	22.4
56–58	22.7	23.0	23.2	23.4
59–61	23.7	24.0	24.2	24.5
62–64	24.7	25.0	25.2	25.5
65–67	25.7	25.9	26.2	26.4
68–70	26.6	26.9	27.1	27.4
71–73	27.5	27.8	28.0	28.3
74–76	28.4	28.7	28.9	29.2
77–79	29.3	29.5	29.8	30.0
80–82	30.1	30.4	30.6	30.9
83–85	30.9	31.2	31.4	31.7
86–88	31.7	32.0	32.2	32.5
89–91	32.5	32.7	33.0	33.2
92–94	33.2	33.4	33.7	33.9
95–97	33.9	34.1	34.4	34.6
98–100	34.6	34.8	35.1	35.3
101–103	35.3	35.4	35.7	35.9
104–106	35.8	36.1	36.3	36.6
107–109	36.4	36.7	36.9	37.1
110–112	37.0	37.2	37.5	37.7
113–115	37.5	37.8	38.0	38.2
116–118	38.0	38.3	38.5	38.8
119–121	38.5	38.7	39.0	39.2
122–124	39.0	39.2	39.4	39.7
125–127	39.4	39.6	39.9	40.1
128–130	39.8	40.0	40.3	40.5

From: Jackson, A. S. and Pollock, M. L. Practical Assessment of Body Composition. Phys. Sportsmed. 13 (5): 76, 1985. Reproduced with permission of McGraw-Hill, Inc.

Compute your body fat percentage from the sum of the three fatfold measures as indicated in Table G.2 (men) or Table G.3 (women). Then see how you rate by determining your percent body fat percentile using Table G.4.

TABLE G.4.

PERCENTILE NORMS FOR PERCENT BODY FAT FOR MEN AND WOMEN[a]

Percentile	Males	Females
95	6.7	16.8
90	8.1	18.1
85	9.8	19.8
80	10.8	20.8
75	11.6	21.6
70	12.4	22.4
65	13.1	23.1
60	13.7	23.7
55	14.4	24.4
50	15.0	25.0
45	15.6	25.6
40	16.3	26.3
35	16.9	26.9
30	17.6	27.6
25	18.4	28.4
20	19.2	29.2
15	20.2	30.2
10	21.9	31.9

From McArdle, W. D., et al.: Exercise Physiology: Energy, Nutrition, and Human Performance. 3rd Edition. Philadelphia: Lea & Febiger, 1991.

[a]Normative standards are based on an average body fat for males of 15% and 25% for females with one standard deviation of ± 5% body fat for both sexes.

TEST COMPONENT #3: AEROBIC/CARDIOVASCULAR FUNCTION

A. Rationale

Enhanced aerobic-cardiovascular function permits higher levels of extended energy expenditure and physical working capacity, and also facilitates recovery. Also, lack of regular exercise (with a reduced aerobic fitness) has been linked to an increased risk of heart disease.

B. Aerobic-Cardiovascular Assessment Test: The 1-Mile Run

Aerobic-cardiovascular performance during exercise can be measured by a running performance over a distance of 1 mile. Warm up for several minutes, then run/walk as rapidly as possible for 1 mile, and record your time to the nearest second. This test can be performed on a quarter-mile (440-yd) track.

C. How Do You Rate on Aerobic-Cardiovascular Function?

Compare your mile run times with the normative data in Table G.5.

TABLE G.5.

PERCENTILE NORMS FOR THE MILE RUN (MIN:SEC) FOR AGE AND SEX

Percentile	Men (age, y)				Women (age, y)			
	18	19	20	21	18	19	20	21
99	4:57	5:00	4:33	4:38	5:33	5:27	5:16	6:26
95	5:29	5:30	5:21	5:28	7:01	6:56	7:00	7:02
90	5:43	5:42	5:40	5:47	7:28	7:22	7:21	7:21
85	5:55	5:55	5:46	6:01	7:47	7:45	7:41	7:35
80	6:05	6:04	5:59	6:09	8:01	8:00	7:59	7:47
75	6:13	6:09	6:08	6:15	8:15	8:13	8:15	8:01
70	6:21	6:15	6:15	6:22	8:31	8:25	8:30	8:09
65	6:28	6:25	6:23	6:31	8:48	8:34	8:40	8:16
60	6:35	6:32	6:30	6:39	8:59	8:52	8:56	8:30
55	6:40	6:39	6:35	6:47	9:06	9:01	9:07	8:40
50	6:48	6:45	6:43	6:53	9:23	9:13	9:20	8:57
45	6:55	6:53	6:51	6:57	9:35	9:26	9:29	9:04
40	7:03	7:01	6:56	7:02	9:49	9:41	9:43	9:24
35	7:10	7:09	7:09	7:09	10:01	10:00	9:45	9:51
30	7:17	7:15	7:19	7:20	10:16	10:07	10:10	10:02
25	7:29	7:27	7:29	7:34	10:35	10:25	10:28	10:30
20	7:45	7:45	7:41	7:49	10:50	11:00	10:45	11:00
15	8:05	8:00	7:56	8:07	11:17	11:18	11:00	11:20
10	8:33	8:30	8:30	8:29	12:00	12:00	11:30	12:13
5	9:40	9:31	9:48	9:22	13:01	13:05	12:39	12:57

From: Norms for College Students: Health Related Physical Fitness Test. Reston, VA, American Alliance For Health, Physical Education, Recreation, and Dance, 1985.

TEST COMPONENT #4: ABDOMINAL MUSCULAR STRENGTH AND ENDURANCE

A. Rationale

Abdominal muscular strength and endurance are important in stabilizing the torso while performing diverse physical tasks involving effort. From a health-related fitness perspective, the functional capacity of this muscle group is of considerable importance to the maintenance of proper posture and spinal alignment, and to provide muscular support to reduce lower back strain. Clinical evidence implicates weak muscles of the abdominal wall as a major cause of lower back pain; strengthening these muscles is consistently recommended in both preventive and rehabilitative back programs.

B. Abdominal Muscular Strength and Endurance Assessment: The Modified Sit-Up Test

Lie on your back with your knees flexed, feet flat on floor, and heels between 12 and 18 inches from the buttocks (see Fig. G.2). Cross your arms over your chest with the hands on opposite shoulders. Have a partner hold your feet to keep them in touch with the floor. Curl to the sitting position; arm contact with the chest must be maintained, and the chin should remain tucked to the chest. The sit-up is completed when your elbows touch your thighs. Return to the starting position until your mid-back contacts the floor.

Your partner gives the signal **"Ready, Go."** The test is started on the word **"Go"** and ceases on the word **"Stop."** Your score is the number of correctly executed sit-ups performed in 60 seconds. If necessary, you can rest during the test.

C. How Do You Rate on Abdominal Muscular Strength and Endurance?

Compare your abdominal muscular strength and endurance with the normative data in Table G.6.

Figure G.2. Example of the modified sit-up.

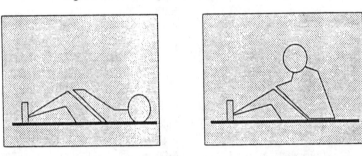

TABLE G.6.

PERCENTILE NORMS FOR 1-MINUTE TIMED SIT-UPS FOR AGE AND SEX

	Men (age, y)				Women (age, y)			
Percentile	18	19	20	21	18	19	20	21
99	70	69	65	67	61	62	63	67
95	62	60	54	61	54	52	53	54
90	57	57	55	55	49	48	49	51
85	55	55	52	54	46	45	46	47
80	53	52	52	52	44	43	44	46
75	51	50	50	50	42	41	42	45
70	50	49	49	48	40	40	41	42
65	48	48	48	47	39	39	40	40
60	47	46	47	45	38	38	38	39
55	46	45	46	44	37	37	37	37

TABLE G.6.—continued

Percentile	Men (age, y)				Women (age, y)			
	18	19	20	21	18	19	20	21
45	43	43	44	42	34	35	35	35
40	42	42	43	41	33	33	34	34
35	41	41	41	41	32	32	33	33
30	40	40	40	40	31	31	31	31
25	39	39	39	39	30	30	30	30
20	37	36	37	37	29	29	30	29
15	36	35	35	36	27	27	28	26
10	34	33	33	34	25	25	25	25
5	30	30	30	31	21	22	22	21

From: Norms For College Students: Health Related Physical Fitness Test. Reston, VA, American Alliance For Health, Physical Education, Recreation, and Dance, 1985.

TEST COMPONENT #5: UPPER-BODY MUSCULAR STRENGTH

A. Rationale

While not a bona fide health-related fitness component, upper-body strength (shoulders, chest, upper arms) is required for the performance of many sport, recreational, and occupational tasks. The 1-RM bench press measures the maximum weight pushed from the bench press position to full extension of the arms, and is used as a measure of upper-body strength. The test is scored as a ratio of weight pushed divided by your body weight.

B. Upper-Body Muscular Strength Assessment: The 1-RM Bench Press Ratio Test

Equipment includes either a barbell set with a bench, or a fixed bench press station on a single or multi-station apparatus. Determining the maximum weight you can lift in one repetition involves trial and error. Find a weight you can press two or three times. Add increments of 10 pounds and attempt the lift again. Add increments of 5 or 10 pounds (with rest between lifts) until you determine the maximum amount you can lift one time.

C. How Do You Rate on Upper-Body Muscular Strength?

Compare your results with the normative standards in Table G.7 that have been developed in our university strength and conditioning classes.

TABLE G.7.

UPPER-BODY BENCH PRESS TO BODY WEIGHT RATIO NORMS (WEIGHT PUSHED [lb] DIVIDED BY BODY WEIGHT [lb])

Percentile	Female (age, y)		Male (age, y)	
	18–20	20–29	18–20	20–29
99	>0.90	>1.06	>1.70	>1.60
95	0.86	1.00	1.58	1.55
90	0.83	0.92	1.42	1.44
85	0.80	0.88	1.38	1.30
80	0.75	0.83	1.32	1.29
75	0.72	0.79	1.26	1.26
70	0.68	0.76	1.24	1.20
65	0.70	0.74	1.20	1.14
60	0.67	0.70	1.16	1.11
55	0.64	0.68	1.14	1.07
50	0.63	0.64	1.11	1.06
45	0.61	0.61	1.08	1.00
40	0.60	0.59	1.06	0.97
35	0.58	0.57	1.00	0.96
30	0.55	0.56	0.98	0.90
25	0.54	0.54	0.90	0.85
20	0.53	0.51	0.86	0.82
15	0.52	0.47	0.82	0.80
10	0.47	0.46	0.81	0.72
5	0.41	0.42	0.76	0.70
1	<0.39	<0.40	<0.68	<0.65

YOUR OVERALL HEALTH-RELATED FITNESS PROFILE

Create a bar graph to visually display your percentile ranking on each component of your health-related fitness. Because scores on each item are not strongly related to each other (i.e., people with good muscular strength do not necessarily score high in aerobic fitness or flexibility, etc.) it is unusual for individuals to rank high on all items.

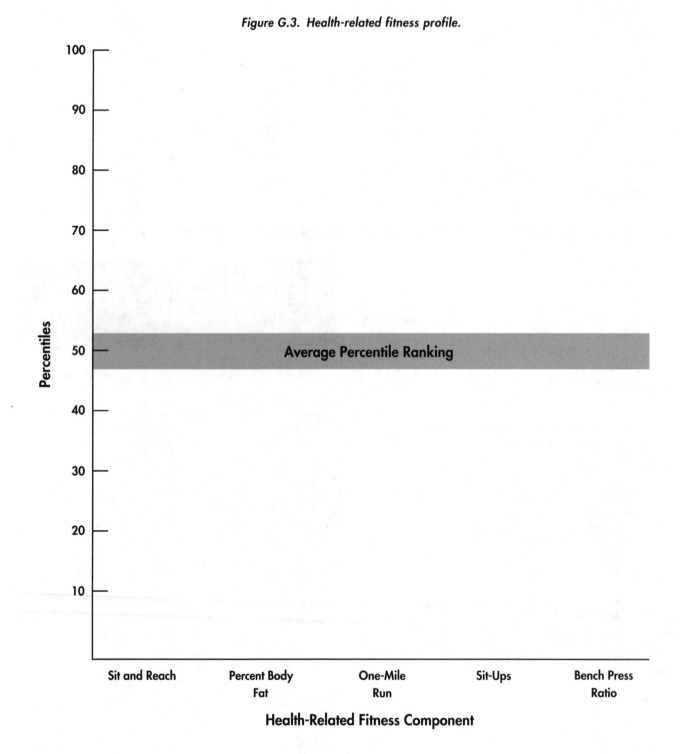

Figure G.3. Health-related fitness profile.

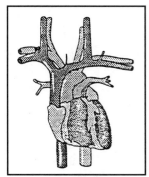

Assessment of Heart Disease Risk (RISKO)

THE ASSESSMENT OF HEART disease risk factors provides some idea of your chances for developing heart disease. The chart on the next page is modified from a more elaborate version generated from 35 years of research on the natural history of heart disease in Framingham, Massachusetts. RISKO is appropriate for adult men and women of all ages. While a RISKO score is certainly not a substitute for a regular medical checkup, the information is helpful in providing insight as to potential areas for concern. Many of these telltale characteristics are habits (or the result of habits) that can be controlled. It certainly would be beneficial to identify risk factors at an early age to thwart the escalation of silent heart disease so prevalent in our highly mechanized, sedentary society.

Assign the appropriate numerical value that represents your present status for each category. Find the box applicable to you and circle the number in it. For example, if you are 19 years old, circle the number "1 pt" in the box labeled 10 to 20 years. After checking all the rows, add the circled numbers. The total number of points is your risk score. Refer to the **Relative Risk Category** to see how you rank. While there is nothing you can do about your age, sex, and heredity, other risks such as high blood pressure, tension, cigarette smoking, serum cholesterol, diet, lack of exercise, and obesity can be modified if not totally eliminated!

EXPLANATION OF RISK VARIABLES

Heredity

Count parents, brothers, and sisters who have had a heart attack or stroke.

Smoking

If you inhale deeply and smoke a cigarette way down, add one point to your score. Do not subtract because you think you do not inhale or smoke only a half inch on a cigarette.

Exercise

Lower your score one point if you exercise regularly and frequently.

Cholesterol–Saturated Fat Intake

A cholesterol blood level is best. If you have not had a blood test recently, then estimate honestly the percentage of solid fats you eat. These are usually of animal origin like lard, cream, butter, and beef and lamb fat. If you eat much saturated fat, your cholesterol level will probably be high.

Blood Pressure

If you have no recent reading but have passed an insurance or general medical examination, chances are you have a systolic blood pressure level (upper reading) of 140 or less.

Sex

This takes into account the fact that men have from 6 to 10 times more heart attacks than women of childbearing age.

HEREDITY	No known history of heart disease	1 relative with cardiovascular disease over age 60	2 relatives with cardiovascular disease over age 60	1 relative with cardiovascular disease under age 60	2 relatives with cardiovascualr disease under age 60	3 relatives with cardiovascular disease under age 60
	1 pt	**2 pts**	**3 pts**	**4 pts**	**6 pts**	**8 pts**
AGE	10 to 20	21 to 30	31 to 40	41 to 50	51 to 60	61 and over
	1 pt	**2 pts**	**3 pts**	**4 pts**	**6 pts**	**8 pts**
CHOLESTEROL OR DIETARY FAT %	Cholesterol below 180 mg/dL; diet contains no animal or solid fats	Cholesterol 180–205 mg/dL; diet contains 10% animal or solid fats	Cholesterol 206–230 mg/dL; diet contains 20% animal or solid fats	Cholesterol 231–255 mg/dL; diet contains 30% animal or solid fats	Cholesterol 256–280 mg/dL; diet contains 40% animal or solid fats	Cholesterol 281–300 mg/dL; diet contains 50% animal or solid fats
	1 pt	**2 pts**	**3 pts**	**4 pts**	**5 pts**	**7 pts**
SEX	Female under age 40	Female age 40 to 50	Female over age 50	Male	Stocky male	Bald stocky male
	1 pt	**2 pts**	**3 pts**	**4 pts**	**6 pts**	**7 pts**
EXERCISE	Intensive occupational and recreational exertion	Moderate occupational and recreational exertion	Sedentary work and intense recreational exertion	Sedentary occupational and moderate recreational exertion	Sedentary work and light recreational exertion	Complete lack of all exercise
	1 pt	**2 pts**	**3 pts**	**5 pts**	**6 pts**	**3 pts**
BLOOD PRESSURE	100 upper reading	120 upper reading	140 upper reading	160 upper reading	180 upper reading	200 or more upper reading
	1 pt	**2 pts**	**3 pts**	**4 pts**	**6 pts**	**8 pts**
TOBACCO SMOKING	Non-user	Cigar and/or pipe	10 cigarettes or less per day	20 cigarettes per day	30 cigarettes per day	40 cigarettes per day
	0 pts	**1 pt**	**3 pts**	**4 pts**	**6 pts**	**8 pts**
BODY WEIGHT	+5 lb below standard weight	−5 to +5 lb of standard weight	6 to 20 lb overweight	21 to 35 lb overweight	36 to 50 lb overweight	51 to 65 lb overweight
	0 pts	**1 pt**	**2 pts**	**3 pts**	**5 pts**	**7 pts**

SCORE	RELATIVE RISK CATEGORY
6 to 11	Risk well below average
12 to 17	Risk below average
18 to 24	Average risk

SCORE	RELATIVE RISK CATEGORY
25 to 31	Moderate risk
32 to 40	High risk
41 to 62	Very high risk, see a doctor

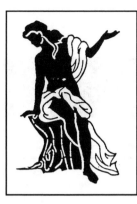

Desirable Body Weight and Body Fat Distribution

THERE ARE A NUMBER of different methods used to determine desirable body weight. We present four of the most common methods. **Method One** is based on the popular Height-Weight Charts. **Method Two** is based on your Body Mass Index, which is computed as the ratio of your body weight to height squared. **Method Three** determines your desirable body weight based on your percent body fat. **Method Four** does not determine your desirable body weight, but rather provides an estimate of your desirable body fat distribution based on the ratio of your waist girth to your hip girth.

METHOD ONE: HEIGHT-WEIGHT TABLES

1. Determine your height to the nearest half-inch.
2. Determine your body weight to the nearest one half-pound.
3. Review Table I.1 that presents weight-for-height for males and females.
4. Determine your desirable weight range as the midpoint and the low-end value of the listed weight range. The upper value of your desirable weight range would be your current body weight minus the midpoint of the desirable weight range from Table I.1. The low end of your desirable weight range would be your current body weight minus the low end of your desirable weight range from Table I.1.

CALCULATIONS

_____ Height (in)

_____ Body Weight (lb)

_____ Desirable Body Weight Range (From Table I.1)

_____	**Minus** _____	**Equals** _____
Current Body Weight	Midpoint of Desirable Range	Upper Value of Desirable Range

_____	**Minus** _____	**Equals** _____
Current Body Weight	Low End of Desirable Range	Lower Value of Desirable Range

TABLE I.1.

USE WITH METHOD ONE. WEIGHT RANGES FOR HEIGHT FOR MALES AND FEMALES

Height (without shoes)		Weight—Males		Weight—Females	
cm	ft-in	kg	lb	kg	lb
146	4'9"			48–54	106–118
149	4'10"			48–54	106–120
151	4'11"			50–56	110–123
154	5'0"			51–57	112–126
156	5'1"	57–62	126–136	52–59	115–129
159	5'2"	58–63	128–138	54–60	118–132
162	5'3"	59–64	130–140	55–61	121–135
164	5'4"	60–65	132–143	56–63	124–138
167	5'5"	61–66	134–146	58–64	127–141
169	5'6"	62–68	137–149	59–65	130–144
172	5'7"	64–69	140–152	60–67	133–147
174	5'8"	65–70	143–155	62–68	136–150
177	5'9"	66–72	146–158	63–69	139–153
179	5'10"	68–73	149–161	64–71	142–156
182	5'11"	69–75	152–165		
185	6'0"	70–77	166–169		
187	6'1"	72–78	168–173		
190	6'2"	73–80	162–177		
192	6'3"	76–83	166–182		

METHOD TWO: BODY MASS INDEX (BMI)

1. Determine your height in meters. (Multiply your height in inches by 0.0254 to determine your height in meters.)
2. Determine your body weight in kilograms. (Divide your body weight in pounds by 2.205 to determine your weight in kilograms.)
3. Determine your BMI as weight (in kilograms) divided by height (in meters) squared.

4. Determine the desirable body weight corresponding to the upper and lower limits of the desirable BMI values as:

$$\text{Desirable Body Weight (kg)} = \text{BMI} \times [\text{Height (m)}]^2$$

The suggested BMI ranges for females is 21.3 to 22.1, and for males it is 21.9 to 22.4. BMI values above 27.8 for men and 27.3 for women have been associated with increased incidence rates of high blood pressure, diabetes, and coronary heart disease. The American Dietetic Association, in its position statement on nutrition and physical fitness, states that a BMI of 30 or more is classified as obese.

CALCULATIONS

_____ Height, m (in $\times$ 0.0254 = m)

_____ Body Weight, kg (lb/2.205 = kg)

_____ BMI = Body Weight, kg/(Height, m)^2

_____ Body Weight at Upper End of Desirable BMI Range
Males: Body Weight, kg = 22.4 $\times$ (Height, m)^2
Females: Body Weight, kg = 22.1 $\times$ (Height, m)^2

_____ Body Weight at Lower End of Desirable BMI Range
Males: Body Weight, kg = 21.9 $\times$ (Height, m)^2
Females: Body Weight, kg = 21.3 $\times$ (Height, m)^2

EXAMPLE

Male: **Height** = 5'9" (1.753 m); **Weight** = 170 lb (77.1 kg); **BMI** = 25.089 kg/m^2 (77.1/1.753^2)
Desirable Body Weight at Upper End of Desirable BMI Range = (22.4 $\times$ 1.753^2) = 68.84 kg (151.8 lb)
Desirable Body Weight at Lower End of Desirable BMI Range = (21.9 $\times$ 1.753^2) = 67.30 kg (148.4 lb)

In this example, this person should lose 19 to 22 lb to bring his body weight into the desirable upper range of BMI values.

METHOD THREE: FAT-FREE BODY MASS (FFM)

For this method you will need to determine your percentage body fat. You can do this by using either the fatfold, girth, or underwater weighing method. Refer to Chapter 27 in your textbook on how to do these calculations when using girth measures. Also, self-assessment test G in this Study Guide presents the methods for predicting your percentage body fat by the fatfold technique.

STEP 1.

Determine your body fat percentage from fatfold, girths, or other method

STEP 2.

Determine your body's fat weight as body weight times body fat percentage expressed as a decimal (25% body fat would be 0.25)

STEP 3.

Determine your fat-free body mass as body mass minus fat weight

STEP 4.

Indicate the body percentage fat that you desire

STEP 5.

Determine your desired body weight as:

$$\text{Desired Body Weight} = \frac{\text{FFM}}{1.00 - \text{Desired \% Body Fat}}$$
$$\text{(expressed as a decimal)}$$

CALCULATIONS

_____ Percentage body fat from skinfolds, girths, or other method

_____ Body fat weight, kg = body weight $\times$ decimal %body fat

_____ FFM, kg = body weight minus fat weight

_____ Desired body weight at desired %body fat = (FFM/1.00 − desired %body fat)

EXAMPLE

Body weight	= 190 lb (86.17 kg)
Percent body fat	= 19%
Fat weight	= 36.1 lb (16.37 kg)
FFM	= 153.9 lb (69.80 kg)
Desired body weight	= 153.9 lb/(1.00 − 0.15)
	= 153.9 lb/0.85
	= 181.1 lb (82.1 kg)
Recommended fat	= 190 lb − 181.1 lb fat loss
Loss	= 8.9 lb (4.04 kg)

METHOD FOUR: WAIST-TO-HIP RATIO (WHR)

The waist-to-hip girth ratio (WHR) is a measure of regional fat distribution. It is obtained by measuring the waist girth (average of the girth at the natural waist and at the umbilicus) and the hip girth (largest girth around the hips or buttocks). Wear tight clothing or no clothing. Do not compress the skin while taking the measurements. The significance of the WHR as a health risk is discussed in Chapter 29 of your textbook.

STEP 1.

Determine your waist girth in centimeters

STEP 2.

Determine your hip girth in centimeters

STEP 3.

Determine your waist-to-hip girth ratio (waist girth/hip girth) (round to 2 significant digits; e.g., 0.90)

STEP 4.

Compare your results with the recommendations below

CALCULATIONS

_____ Waist girth (average of girth at waist and girth at navel)

_____ Hip girth (widest girth around hips)

_____ WHR (average waist girth/hip girth)

EXAMPLE

FEMALE

1. Natural waist girth = 90.6 cm
2. Umbilicus girth = 64.5 cm
3. Average waist girth = (90.6 + 64.5/2) = 77.55 cm
4. Hip girth = 86.5 cm
5. WHR = 77.5 cm/86.5 cm = 0.90
6. Risk = Higher risk

WAIST-TO-HIP GIRTH RATIO RISK RATINGS

	Males	Females
Higher risk	>0.90	>0.85
Moderately high risk	0.90–0.95	0.80–0.85
Lower risk	<0.90	<0.80

SECTION 3

ANSWERS TO CHAPTER QUIZZES

CROSSWORD PUZZLE SOLUTIONS

ANSWERS TO CHAPTER QUIZZES

CHAPTER 1

Multiple Choice	True/False
1. c	1. T
2. a	2. T
3. c	3. T
4. c	4. F
5. a	5. F
6. a	6. F
7. b	7. F
8. b	8. F
9. d	9. T
10. e	10. T

CHAPTER 2

Multiple Choice	True/False
1. b	2. T
2. a	2. F
3. b	3. T
4. c	4. T
5. a	5. T
6. b	6. F
7. a	7. T
8. a	8. F
9. a	9. F
10. a	10. T

CHAPTER 3

Multiple Choice	True/False
1. b	1. T
2. b	2. F
3. b	3. F
4. d	4. F
5. e	5. T
6. a	6. T
7. a	7. T
8. b	8. F
9. a	9. F
10. a	10. T

CHAPTER 4

Multiple Choice	True/False
1. b	1. T
2. c	2. T
3. d	3. T
4. e	4. F
5. a	5. T
6. b	6. F
7. c	7. T
8. a	8. T
9. a	9. T
10. a	10. T

CHAPTER 5

Multiple Choice	True/False
1. c	1. F
2. d	2. T
3. e	3. F
4. a	4. F
5. b	5. F
6. c	6. T
7. d	7. T
8. d	8. T
9. a	9. F
10. c	10. T

CHAPTER 6

Multiple Choice	True/False
1. b	1. F
2. a	2. T
3. b	3. T
4. a	4. F
5. d	5. F
6. c	6. F
7. e	7. F
8. c	8. T
9. a	9. T
10. a	10. T

CHAPTER 7

Multiple Choice	True/False
1. b	1. T
2. a	2. F
3. a	3. F
4. d	4. F
5. e	5. T
6. b	6. F
7. d	7. T
8. b	8. F
9. a	9. F
10. d	10. T

CHAPTER 8

Multiple Choice	True/False
1. c	1. T
2. b	2. F
3. b	3. F
4. a	4. T
5. e	5. T
6. c	6. T
7. a	7. T
8. b	8. F
9. c	9. T
10. b	10. F

CHAPTER 9

Multiple Choice	True/False
1. c	1. T
2. b	2. F
3. b	3. F
4. e	4. F
5. e	5. T
6. c	6. T
7. c	7. F
8. a	8. F
9. a	9. T
10. d	10. F

CHAPTER 10

Multiple Choice	True/False
1. c	1. T
2. a	2. T
3. b	3. F
4. e	4. F
5. c	5. T
6. e	6. T
7. d	7. F
8. a	8. F
9. a	9. T
10. d	10. F

CHAPTER 11

Multiple Choice	True/False
1. a	1. T
2. b	2. F
3. d	3. F
4. e	4. T
5. b	5. F
6. e	6. T
7. a	7. T
8. e	8. T
9. c	9. F
10. a	10. T

CHAPTER 12

Multiple Choice	True/False
1. c	1. F
2. b	2. T
3. e	3. F
4. b	4. T
5. b	5. F
6. ac	6. T
7. c	7. T
8. a	8. F
9. d	9. T
10. d	10. F

CHAPTER 13

Multiple Choice	True/False
1. c	1. F
2. b	2. T
3. e	3. T
4. b	4. T
5. b	5. F
6. c	6. T
7. c	7. T
8. a	8. T
9. d	9. T
10. d	10. F

CHAPTER 14

Multiple Choice	True/False
1. a	1. T
2. b	2. T
3. c	3. T
4. d	4. F
5. d	5. T
6. a	6. T
7. b	7. T
8. c	8. T
9. e	9. T
10. d	10. F

CHAPTER 15

Multiple Choice	True/False
1. c	1. T
2. d	2. F
3. a	3. F
4. c	4. F
5. d	5. T
6. b	6. F
7. e	7. T
8. d	8. T
9. c	9. T
10. d	10. F

CHAPTER 16

Multiple Choice	True/False
1. a	1. F
2. d	2. T
3. c	3. T
4. e	4. F
5. b	5. T
6. d	6. F
7. e	7. T
8. b	8. T
9. d	9. T
10. c	10. F

CHAPTER 17

Multiple Choice		True/False	
1.	b	1.	T
2.	d	2.	F
3.	a	3.	F
4.	b	4.	F
5.	d	5.	F
6.	b	6.	T
7.	d	7.	T
8.	a	8.	F
9.	d	9.	T
10.	d	10.	T

CHAPTER 18

Multiple Choice		True/False	
1.	c	1.	T
2.	c	2.	F
3.	c	3.	T
4.	c	4.	T
5.	a	5.	T
6.	a	6.	F
7.	c	7.	F
8.	b	8.	T
9.	c	9.	F
10.	a	10.	T

CHAPTER 19

Multiple Choice		True/False	
1.	c	2.	T
2.	c	2.	F
3.	c	3.	F
4.	c	4.	T
5.	a	5.	T
6.	b	6.	F
7.	c	7.	F
8.	b	8.	F
9.	c	9.	F
10.	d	10.	F

CHAPTER 20

Multiple Choice		True/False	
1.	d	1.	T
2.	e	2.	F
3.	a	3.	T
4.	c	4.	T
5.	b	5.	F
6.	b	6.	F
7.	d	7.	T
8.	e	8.	T
9.	b	9.	T
10.	a	10.	T

CHAPTER 21

Multiple Choice		True/False	
1.	c	1.	T
2.	a	2.	F
3.	e	3.	T
4.	c	4.	F
5.	c	5.	T
6.	a	6.	F
7.	d	7.	T
8.	e	8.	T
9.	b	9.	F
10.	c	10.	F

CHAPTER 22

Multiple Choice		True/False	
1.	c	1.	T
2.	a	2.	T
3.	a	3.	T
4.	c	4.	T
5.	a	5.	F
6.	b	6.	T
7.	b	7.	F
8.	c	8.	F
9.	a	9.	T
10.	b	10.	T

CHAPTER 23

Multiple Choice		True/False	
1.	a	1.	F
2.	a	2.	F
3.	d	3.	T
4.	a	4.	T
5.	c	5.	F
6.	c	6.	T
7.	d	7.	F
8.	e	8.	F
9.	e	9.	F
10.	a	10.	T

CHAPTER 24

Multiple Choice		True/False	
1.	c	1.	T
2.	e	2.	T
3.	a	3.	F
4.	e	4.	F
5.	d	5.	F
6.	b	6.	T
7.	c	7.	T
8.	a	8.	F
9.	b	9.	F
10.	a	10.	T

CHAPTER 25

Multiple Choice		True/False	
1.	b	1.	T
2.	c	2.	T
3.	d	3.	T
4.	c	4.	F
5.	b	5.	T
6.	e	6.	F
7.	e	7.	T
8.	a	8.	F
9.	e	9.	T
10.	e	10.	T

CHAPTER 26

Multiple Choice		True/False	
1.	d	1.	T
2.	c	2.	T
3.	a	3.	T
4.	a	4.	F
5.	a	5.	T
6.	d	6.	T
7.	b	7.	F
8.	a	8.	T
9.	b	9.	F
10.	c	10.	F

CHAPTER 27

Multiple Choice		True/False	
1.	d	1.	T
2.	c	2.	T
3.	c	3.	F
4.	a	4.	T
5.	b	5.	F
6.	b	6.	T
7.	a	7.	F
8.	e	8.	T
9.	d	9.	T
10.	b	10.	F

CHAPTER 28

Multiple Choice		True/False	
1.	b	1.	F
2.	a	2.	T
3.	d	3.	T
4.	b	4.	T
5.	a	5.	T
6.	a	6.	T
7.	c	7.	F
8.	a	8.	F
9.	c	9.	T
10.	d	10.	F

CHAPTER 29

Multiple Choice		True/False	
1.	e	1.	T
2.	a	2.	F
3.	d	3.	T
4.	d	4.	T
5.	b	5.	T
6.	b	6.	T
7.	a	7.	F
8.	b	8.	F
9.	a	9.	F
10.	b	10.	T

CHAPTER 30

Multiple Choice		True/False	
1.	e	1.	T
2.	b	2.	T
3.	b	3.	T
4.	b	4.	T
5.	b	5.	F
6.	b	6.	T
7.	b	7.	F
8.	e	8.	F
9.	e	9.	T
10.	a	10.	T

CHAPTER 31

Multiple Choice		True/False	
1.	a	1.	T
2.	b	2.	F
3.	c	3.	T
4.	a	4.	T
5.	a	5.	T
6.	a	6.	F
7.	c	7.	T
8.	d	8.	T
9.	c	9.	T
10.	b	10.	T

CROSSWORD PUZZLE SOLUTIONS

CHAPTER 1

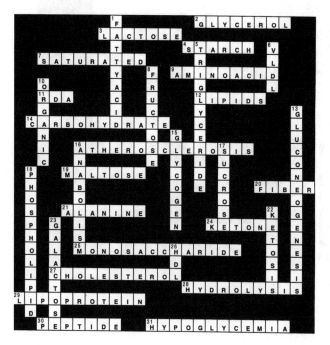

CHAPTER 2

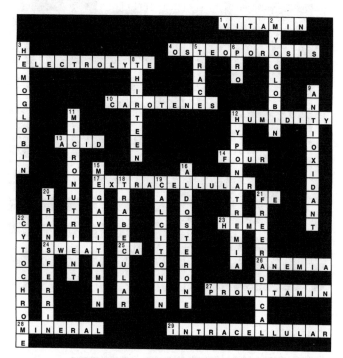

CHAPTER 3

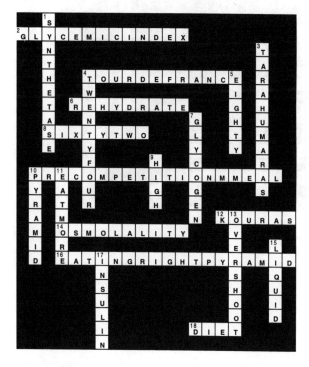

CHAPTER 4

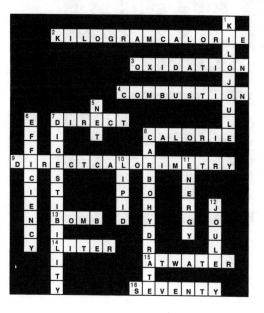

CHAPTER 5

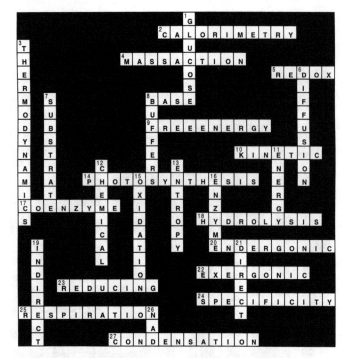

CHAPTER 6

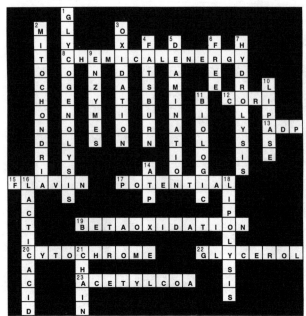

CHAPTER 7

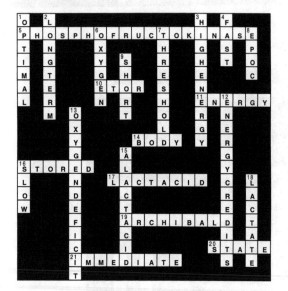

CHAPTER 8

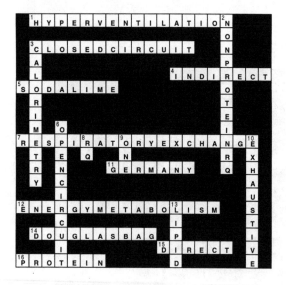

CHAPTER 9

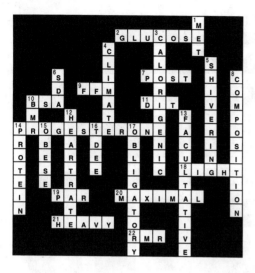

CHAPTER 10

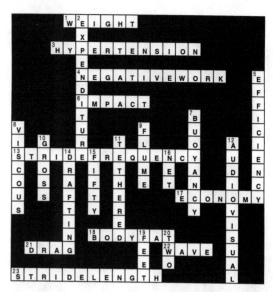

CHAPTER 11

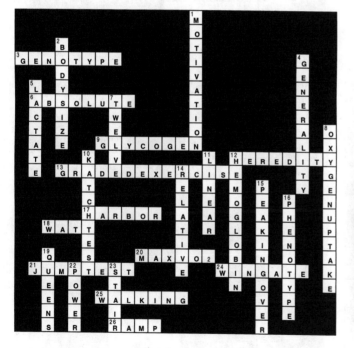

CHAPTER 12

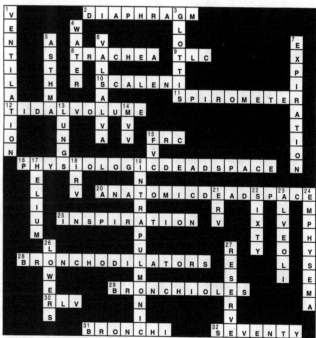

CHAPTER 13

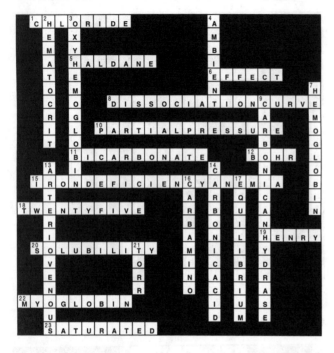

CHAPTER 14

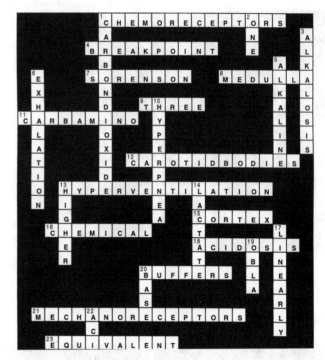

CHAPTER 15

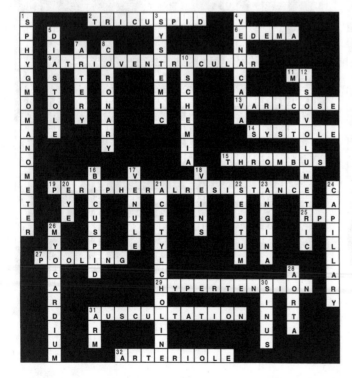

CHAPTER 16

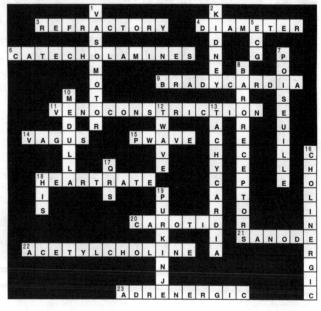

CHAPTER 17

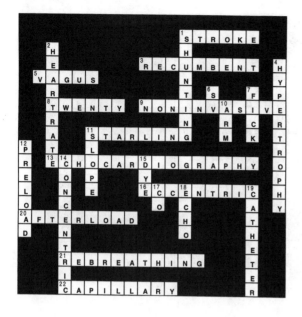

CHAPTER 18

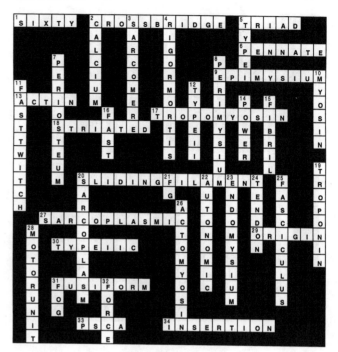

CHAPTER 19

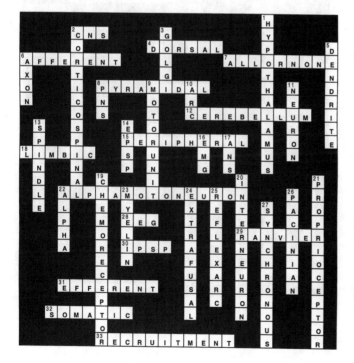

CHAPTER 20

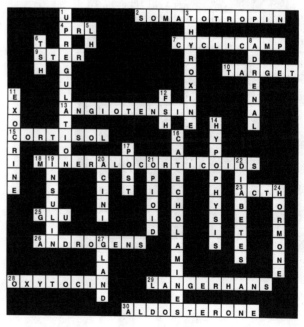

CHAPTER 21

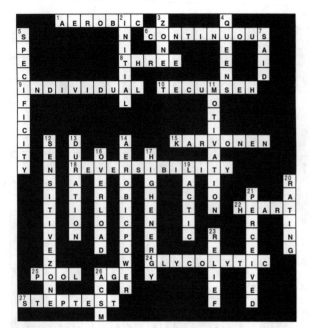

CHAPTER 22

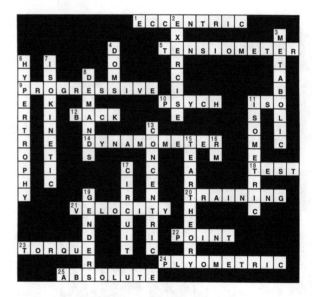

CHAPTER 23

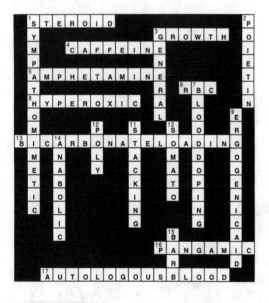

CHAPTER 24

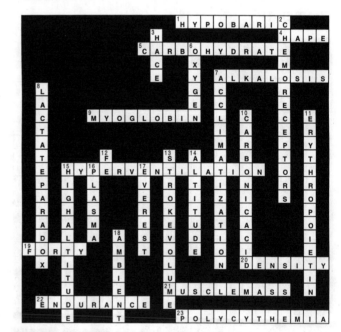

CHAPTER 25

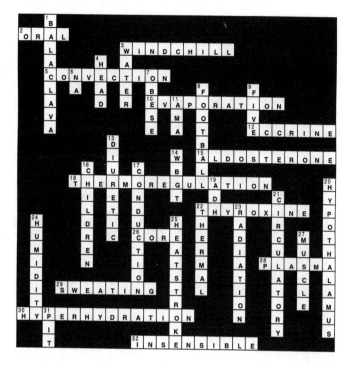

CHAPTER 26

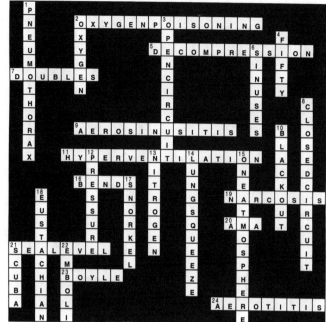

CHAPTER 27

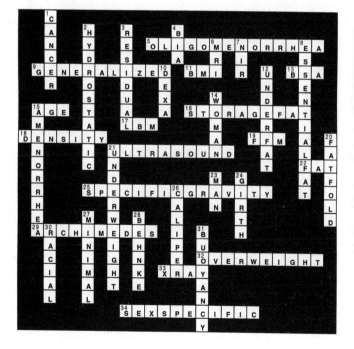

CHAPTER 28

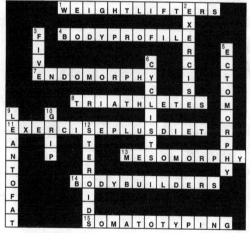

CHAPTER 29

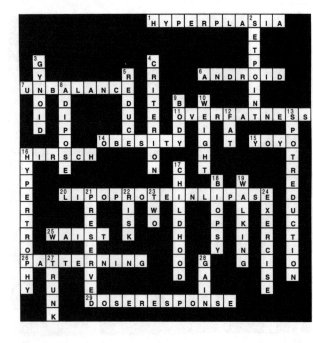

CHAPTER 30

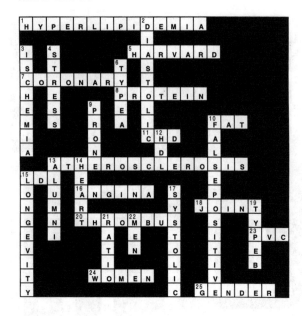

CHAPTER 31

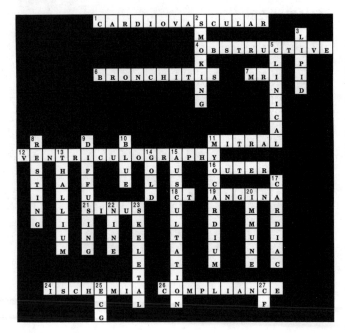

SECTION 4

APPENDIXES

Energy Expenditure in Household, Occupational, Recreational, and Sports Activities[a,b]

HOW TO USE APPENDIX A

Refer to the column that comes closest to your present body mass. Multiply the number in this column by the number of minutes you spend in the activity. Suppose that an individual weighing 62.3 kg (137 lb) spends 30 minutes playing a casual game of billiards. To determine the energy cost of participation, multiply the caloric value per minute (2.6 kcal) by 30 to obtain the 30-minute gross expenditure of 78 kcal. If the same individual does aerobic dance for 45 minutes, the **gross** (value includes resting energy expenditure) energy expended would be calculated as 6.4 kcal × 45 minutes, or 288 kcal.

[a] All values for energy expenditure are in kilocalories per minute.
[b] Copyright © 1996 by Frank I. Katch, Victor L. Katch, and William D. McArdle, and Fitness Technologies, Inc. P.O. Box 430, Amherst, MA 01004. No part of this appendix may be reproduced in any manner without written permission from the copyright holders.

YOUR BODY WEIGHT

Activity	kg lb	47 104	50 110	53 117	56 123	59 130	62 137	65 143	68 150
Archery		3.1	3.3	3.4	3.6	3.8	4.0	4.2	4.4
Backpacking									
without load		5.7	6.1	6.4	6.8	7.1	7.5	7.9	8.2
with 11 pound load		6.1	6.5	6.8	7.2	7.6	8.0	8.4	8.8
with 22 pound load		6.6	7.0	7.4	7.8	8.3	8.7	9.1	9.5
with 44 pound load		7.0	7.4	7.8	8.2	8.7	9.1	9.6	10.0
Badminton									
leisure		4.6	4.9	5.1	5.4	5.7	6.0	6.3	6.6
tournament		7.0	7.3	7.7	8.1	8.6	9.0	9.4	9.9
Baking, general (F)		1.6	1.8	1.9	2.0	2.1	2.2	2.3	2.4
Baseball									
fielder		2.8	3.0	3.2	3.4	3.6	3.8	4.0	4.1
pitcher		4.2	4.5	4.8	5.0	5.3	5.6	5.9	6.2
Basketball									
competition		7.1	7.4	7.9	8.3	8.7	9.2	9.6	10.1
practice		6.5	6.9	7.3	7.7	8.1	8.6	9.0	9.4
Baton twirling		6.3	6.8	7.3	7.6	8.1	8.5	8.9	9.3
Billiards ("pool")		2.0	2.1	2.2	2.4	2.5	2.6	2.7	2.9
Bookbinding		1.8	1.9	2.0	2.1	2.2	2.4	2.5	2.6
Bowling		4.4	4.8	5.2	5.4	5.7	6.0	6.3	6.6
Boxing									
in ring, match		10.4	11.1	11.8	12.4	13.1	13.8	14.4	15.1
sparring, practice		6.5	6.9	7.3	7.7	8.1	8.6	9.0	9.4
Calisthenics, warm-ups		3.4	3.7	4.0	4.2	4.4	4.7	4.9	5.1
Canoeing									
leisure (2.5 mph)		2.1	2.2	2.3	2.5	2.6	2.7	2.9	3.0
racing ("fast")		4.8	5.2	5.5	5.8	6.1	6.4	6.7	7.0
Car washing		3.3	3.5	3.7	3.9	4.1	4.3	4.5	4.8
Card playing		1.2	1.3	1.3	1.4	1.5	1.6	1.6	1.7
Carpentry, general		2.4	2.6	2.8	2.9	3.1	3.2	3.4	3.5
Carpet sweeping (F)		2.2	2.3	2.4	2.5	2.7	2.8	2.9	3.1
Carpet sweeping (M)		2.3	2.4	2.5	2.7	2.8	3.0	3.1	3.3
Circuit resistance training									
Free weights		4.0	4.3	4.5	4.8	5.0	5.3	5.5	5.8
Hydra-Fitness		6.2	6.6	7.0	7.4	7.8	8.2	8.6	9.0
Nautilus		4.3	4.6	4.9	5.2	5.5	5.8	6.0	6.3
Universal		5.3	5.8	6.2	6.5	6.9	7.2	7.5	7.9
Cleaning (F)		2.9	3.1	3.3	3.5	3.7	3.8	4.0	4.2
Cleaning (M)		2.7	2.9	3.1	3.2	3.4	3.6	3.8	3.9
Coal mining									
drilling coal, rock		4.4	4.7	5.0	5.3	5.5	5.8	6.1	6.4
erecting supports		4.1	4.4	4.7	4.9	5.2	5.5	5.7	6.0
shoveling coal		5.1	5.4	5.7	6.0	6.4	6.7	7.0	7.3
Cooking (F)		2.1	2.3	2.4	2.5	2.7	2.8	2.9	3.1
Cooking (M)		2.3	2.4	2.5	2.7	2.8	3.0	3.1	3.3

Note: Symbols (M) and (F) denote experiments for males and females, respectively.

Copyright © 1996 by Frank I. Katch, Victor L. Katch and William D. McArdle, and Fitness Technologies, Inc., P.O. Box 430, Amherst, MA 01004. fax (313) 662-8153

No part of this appendix may be reproduced in any manner without written permission from the copyright holders.

| 71 | 74 | 77 | 80 | 83 | 86 | 89 | 92 | 95 | 98 |
157	163	170	176	183	190	196	203	209	216
4.6	4.8	5.0	5.2	5.4	5.6	5.8	6.0	6.2	6.4
8.6	9.0	9.3	9.7	10.0	10.4	10.8	11.1	11.5	11.9
9.2	9.5	9.9	10.3	10.7	11.1	11.5	11.9	12.3	12.6
9.9	10.4	10.8	11.2	11.6	12.0	12.5	12.9	13.3	13.7
10.4	10.9	11.3	11.8	12.2	12.6	13.1	13.5	14.0	14.4
6.9	7.2	7.5	7.8	8.1	8.3	8.6	8.9	9.2	9.5
10.4	10.8	11.2	11.6	12.1	12.5	12.9	13.4	13.8	14.3
2.5	2.6	2.7	2.8	2.9	3.0	3.1	3.2	3.3	3.4
4.3	4.5	4.7	4.9	5.1	5.2	5.4	5.6	5.8	6.0
6.4	6.7	7.0	7.2	7.5	7.8	8.0	8.3	8.6	8.9
10.5	10.9	11.4	11.8	12.3	12.7	13.1	13.6	14.0	14.5
9.8	10.2	10.6	11.0	11.5	11.9	12.3	12.7	13.1	13.5
9.5	9.7	9.9	10.1	10.4	10.6	10.8	11.0	11.2	11.4
3.0	3.1	3.2	3.4	3.5	3.6	3.7	3.9	4.0	4.1
2.7	2.8	2.9	3.0	3.2	3.3	3.4	3.5	3.6	3.7
6.9	7.2	7.5	7.7	8.1	8.4	8.6	8.9	9.2	9.5
15.8	16.4	17.1	17.8	18.4	19.1	19.8	20.4	21.1	21.8
9.8	10.2	10.6	11.0	11.5	11.9	12.3	12.7	13.1	13.5
5.3	5.5	5.8	6.0	6.2	6.5	6.7	6.9	7.1	7.3
3.1	3.3	3.4	3.5	3.7	3.8	3.9	4.0	4.2	4.3
7.3	7.6	7.9	8.2	8.5	8.9	9.2	9.5	9.8	10.1
5.0	5.2	5.5	5.7	5.7	5.9	6.1	6.3	6.5	6.9
1.8	1.9	1.9	2.0	2.1	2.2	2.2	2.3	2.4	2.5
3.7	3.8	4.0	4.2	4.3	4.5	4.6	4.8	4.9	5.1
3.2	3.3	3.5	3.6	3.7	3.9	4.0	4.1	4.3	4.4
3.4	3.6	3.7	3.8	4.0	4.1	4.3	4.4	4.6	4.7
6.1	6.3	6.6	6.8	7.1	7.4	7.6	7.9	8.1	8.4
9.4	9.7	10.2	10.5	10.9	11.4	11.7	12.1	12.5	12.9
6.6	6.8	7.1	7.4	7.7	8.0	8.2	8.5	8.8	9.1
8.3	8.6	8.9	9.3	9.6	10.0	10.3	10.7	11.0	11.4
4.4	4.6	4.8	5.0	5.1	5.3	5.5	5.7	5.9	6.1
4.1	4.3	4.5	4.6	4.8	5.0	5.2	5.3	5.5	5.7
6.7	7.0	7.2	7.5	7.8	8.1	8.4	8.6	8.9	9.2
6.2	6.5	6.8	7.0	7.3	7.6	7.8	8.1	8.4	8.6
7.7	8.0	8.3	8.6	9.0	9.3	9.6	9.9	10.3	10.6
3.2	3.3	3.5	3.6	3.7	3.9	4.0	4.1	4.3	4.4
3.4	3.6	3.7	3.8	4.0	4.1	4.3	4.4	4.6	4.7

YOUR BODY WEIGHT—*continued*

Activity	kg lb	47 104	50 110	53 117	56 123	59 130	62 137	65 143	68 150
Cricket									
batting		3.9	4.2	4.4	4.6	4.9	5.1	5.4	5.6
bowling		4.2	4.5	4.8	5.0	5.3	5.6	5.9	6.1
fielding		3.7	3.9	4.1	4.3	4.8	4.8	5.0	5.3
Croquet		2.8	3.0	3.1	3.3	3.5	3.7	3.8	4.0
Cycling									
leisure, 5.5 mph		3.0	3.2	3.4	3.6	3.8	4.0	4.2	4.4
leisure, 9.4 mph		4.8	5.0	5.3	5.6	5.9	6.2	6.5	6.8
racing, fast		8.0	8.5	9.0	9.5	10.0	10.5	11.0	11.5
Dancing									
aerobic, easy		4.3	4.8	5.2	5.6	5.9	6.2	6.4	6.7
aerobic, medium		4.8	5.2	5.5	5.8	6.1	6.4	6.7	7.0
aerobic, intense		6.3	6.7	7.1	7.5	7.9	8.3	8.7	9.2
ballroom		2.4	2.6	2.7	2.9	3.0	3.2	3.3	3.5
choreographed		5.0	5.2	5.5	5.8	6.1	6.4	6.7	7.0
"twist," "lambada"		8.0	8.4	8.9	9.4	9.9	10.4	10.9	11.4
modern		3.4	3.6	3.8	4.0	4.3	4.5	4.7	4.9
Digging trenches		6.8	7.3	7.7	8.1	8.6	9.0	9.4	9.9
Drawing (standing)		1.7	1.8	1.9	2.0	2.1	2.2	2.3	2.4
Eating (sitting)		1.1	1.2	1.2	1.3	1.4	1.4	1.5	1.6
Electrical work		2.7	2.9	3.1	3.2	3.4	3.6	3.8	3.9
Farming									
barn cleaning		6.3	6.8	7.2	7.6	8.0	8.4	8.8	9.2
driving harvester		1.9	2.0	2.1	2.2	2.4	2.5	2.6	2.7
driving tractor		1.8	1.9	2.0	2.1	2.2	2.3	2.4	2.5
feeding cattle		4.2	4.3	4.5	4.8	5.0	5.3	5.5	5.8
feeding animals		3.1	3.3	3.4	3.6	3.8	4.0	4.2	4.4
forking straw bales		6.7	6.9	7.3	7.7	8.1	8.6	9.0	9.4
milking by hand		2.5	2.7	2.9	3.0	3.2	3.3	3.5	3.7
milking by machine		1.1	1.2	1.2	1.3	1.4	1.4	1.5	1.6
shoveling grain		4.2	4.3	4.5	4.8	5.0	5.3	5.5	5.8
Fencing									
competition		7.2	7.6	8.1	8.5	9.0	9.4	9.9	10.8
practice		3.6	3.9	4.2	4.4	4.6	4.9	5.1	5.3
Field hockey		6.5	6.7	7.1	7.5	7.9	8.3	8.7	9.1
Fishing		3.0	3.1	3.3	3.5	3.7	3.8	4.0	4.2
Food shopping (F)		3.0	3.1	3.3	3.5	3.7	3.8	4.0	4.2
Football, competition		6.2	6.6	7.0	7.4	7.8	8.2	8.6	9.0
Forestry									
ax chopping, fast		14.0	14.9	15.7	16.6	17.5	18.4	19.3	20.2
ax chopping, slow		4.0	4.3	4.5	4.8	5.0	5.3	5.5	5.8
barking trees		5.8	6.2	6.5	6.9	7.3	7.6	8.0	8.4
carrying logs		8.7	9.3	9.9	10.4	11.0	11.5	12.1	12.6
felling trees		6.2	6.6	7.0	7.4	7.8	8.2	8.6	9.0
hoeing		4.2	4.6	4.8	5.1	5.4	5.6	5.9	6.2
planting by hand		5.1	5.5	5.8	6.1	6.4	6.8	7.1	7.4
sawing by hand		5.7	6.1	6.5	6.8	7.2	7.6	7.9	8.3
sawing, power		3.5	3.8	4.0	4.2	4.4	4.7	4.9	5.1
stacking firewood		4.2	4.4	4.7	4.9	5.2	5.5	5.7	6.0
trimming trees		6.1	6.5	6.8	7.2	7.6	8.0	8.4	8.8
weeding		3.4	3.6	3.8	4.0	4.2	4.5	4.7	4.9

71 157	74 163	77 170	80 176	83 183	86 190	89 196	92 203	95 209	98 216
5.9	6.1	6.4	6.6	6.9	7.1	7.4	7.6	7.9	8.1
6.4	6.7	6.9	7.2	7.5	7.7	8.0	8.3	8.6	8.8
5.6	5.9	6.2	6.5	6.8	7.1	7.4	7.7	8.0	8.3
4.2	4.4	4.5	4.7	4.9	5.1	5.3	5.4	5.6	5.8
4.5	4.7	4.9	5.1	5.3	5.5	5.7	5.9	6.1	6.3
7.1	7.4	7.7	8.0	8.3	8.6	8.9	9.2	9.5	9.8
12.0	12.5	13.0	13.5	14.0	14.5	15.0	15.5	16.1	16.6
6.9	7.2	7.5	7.8	8.1	8.4	8.8	9.1	9.4	9.7
7.3	7.6	7.9	8.2	8.5	8.9	9.2	9.5	9.8	10.1
9.6	10.0	10.4	10.8	11.2	11.6	12.0	12.4	12.8	13.2
3.6	3.8	3.9	4.1	4.2	4.4	4.5	4.7	4.8	5.0
7.3	7.6	7.9	8.2	8.5	8.9	9.2	9.5	9.8	10.1
11.9	12.4	12.9	13.4	13.9	14.4	15.0	15.5	16.0	16.5
5.1	5.3	5.6	5.8	6.0	6.2	6.4	6.7	6.9	7.1
10.3	10.7	11.2	11.6	12.0	12.5	12.9	13.3	13.8	14.2
2.6	2.7	2.8	2.9	3.0	3.1	3.2	3.3	3.4	3.5
1.6	1.7	1.8	1.8	1.9	2.0	2.0	2.1	2.2	2.3
4.1	4.3	4.5	4.6	4.8	5.0	5.2	5.3	5.5	5.7
9.6	10.0	10.4	10.8	11.2	11.6	12.0	12.4	12.8	13.2
2.8	3.0	3.1	3.2	3.3	3.4	3.6	3.7	3.8	3.9
2.6	2.7	2.8	3.0	3.1	3.2	3.3	3.4	3.5	3.6
6.0	6.3	6.5	6.8	7.1	7.3	7.6	7.8	8.1	8.3
4.6	4.8	5.0	5.2	5.4	5.6	5.8	6.0	6.2	6.4
9.8	10.2	10.6	11.0	11.5	11.9	12.3	12.7	13.1	13.5
3.8	4.0	4.2	4.3	4.5	4.6	4.8	5.0	5.1	5.3
1.6	1.7	1.8	1.8	1.9	2.0	2.0	2.1	2.2	2.3
6.0	6.3	6.5	6.8	7.1	7.3	7.6	7.8	8.1	8.3
11.2	11.7	12.1	12.6	13.1	13.5	14.0	14.4	14.9	15.5
5.6	5.8	6.1	6.3	6.5	6.8	7.0	7.2	7.4	7.7
9.5	9.9	10.3	10.7	11.1	11.5	11.9	12.3	12.7	13.1
4.4	4.6	4.8	5.0	5.1	5.3	5.5	5.7	5.9	6.1
4.4	4.6	4.8	5.0	5.1	5.3	5.5	5.7	5.9	6.1
9.4	9.8	10.2	10.6	11.0	11.4	11.7	12.1	12.5	12.9
21.1	22.0	22.9	23.8	24.7	25.5	26.4	27.3	28.2	29.1
6.0	6.3	6.5	6.8	7.1	7.3	7.6	7.8	8.1	8.3
8.7	9.1	9.5	9.8	10.2	10.6	10.9	11.3	11.7	12.1
13.2	13.8	14.3	14.9	15.4	16.0	16.6	17.1	17.7	18.2
9.4	9.8	10.2	10.6	11.0	11.4	11.7	12.1	12.5	12.9
6.5	6.7	7.0	7.3	7.6	7.8	8.1	8.4	8.6	8.9
7.7	8.1	8.4	8.7	9.0	9.4	9.7	10.0	10.4	10.7
8.7	9.0	9.4	9.8	10.1	10.5	10.9	11.2	11.6	12.0
5.3	5.6	5.8	6.0	6.2	6.5	6.7	6.9	7.1	7.4
6.2	6.5	6.8	7.0	7.3	7.6	7.8	8.1	8.4	8.6
9.2	9.5	9.9	10.3	10.7	11.1	11.5	11.9	12.3	12.6
5.1	5.3	5.5	5.8	6.0	6.2	6.4	6.6	6.8	7.1

YOUR BODY WEIGHT—continued

Activity	kg lb	47 104	50 110	53 117	56 123	59 130	62 137	65 143	68 150
Frisbee		4.7	5.0	5.3	5.5	5.9	6.2	6.4	6.8
Furriery		3.9	4.2	4.4	4.6	4.9	5.1	5.4	5.6
Gardening									
digging		5.9	6.3	6.7	7.1	7.4	7.8	8.2	8.6
hedging		3.3	3.9	4.1	4.3	4.5	4.8	5.0	5.2
mowing		5.3	5.6	5.9	6.3	6.6	6.9	7.3	7.6
raking		2.5	2.7	2.9	3.0	3.2	3.3	3.5	3.7
Golf		4.0	4.3	4.5	4.8	5.0	5.3	5.5	5.8
Gymnastics		3.0	3.3	3.5	3.7	3.9	4.1	4.3	4.5
Handball		6.9	7.2	7.7	8.1	8.5	9.0	9.4	9.8
Horse-grooming		6.0	6.4	6.8	7.2	7.6	7.9	8.3	8.7
Horseback riding									
galloping		6.4	6.9	7.3	7.7	8.1	8.5	8.9	9.3
trotting		5.2	5.5	5.8	6.2	6.5	6.8	7.2	7.5
walking		1.9	2.1	2.2	2.3	2.4	2.5	2.7	2.8
Horseshoes		3.3	3.4	3.5	3.7	3.9	4.1	4.3	4.5
Housework									
mopping floors		2.8	3.1	3.3	3.5	3.7	3.8	4.0	4.2
dusting		3.0	3.3	3.4	3.6	3.8	4.0	4.2	4.4
laundry		3.1	3.4	3.5	3.7	3.9	4.1	4.3	4.5
washing windows		3.2	3.5	3.6	3.8	4.0	4.2	4.4	4.6
vacuuming		3.0	3.3	3.4	3.6	3.8	4.0	4.2	4.4
Hunting		4.1	4.4	4.7	4.9	5.2	5.5	5.7	6.0
Ice hockey		7.4	7.7	8.2	8.6	9.1	9.6	10.0	10.5
Ironing clothes		1.6	1.7	1.7	1.8	1.9	2.0	2.1	2.2
Judo		9.2	9.8	10.3	10.9	11.5	12.1	12.7	13.3
Jumping rope									
70 per min		7.6	8.1	8.6	9.1	9.6	10.0	10.5	11.0
80 per min		7.7	8.2	8.7	9.2	9.7	10.2	10.7	11.2
125 per min		8.3	8.9	9.4	9.9	10.4	11.0	11.5	12.0
145 per min		9.3	9.9	10.4	11.0	11.6	12.2	12.8	13.4
Karate		9.5	9.8	10.3	10.9	11.5	12.1	12.7	13.3
Kendo		9.3	9.7	10.2	10.8	11.4	12.0	12.6	13.2
Knitting, sewing		1.1	1.1	1.2	1.2	1.3	1.4	1.4	1.5
Lacrosse		7.0	7.4	7.9	8.3	8.7	9.2	9.6	10.1
Locksmith		2.8	2.9	3.0	3.2	3.4	3.5	3.7	3.9
Lying at ease		1.0	1.1	1.2	1.2	1.3	1.4	1.4	1.5
Machine-tooling									
machining		2.3	2.4	2.5	2.7	2.8	3.0	3.1	3.3
operating lathe		2.5	2.6	2.8	2.9	3.1	3.2	3.4	3.5
operating punch press		4.2	4.4	4.7	4.9	5.2	5.5	5.7	6.0
tapping and drilling		3.2	3.3	3.4	3.6	3.8	4.0	4.2	4.4
welding		2.4	2.6	2.8	2.9	3.1	3.2	3.4	3.5
working sheet metal		2.3	2.4	2.5	2.7	2.8	3.0	3.1	3.3
Marching, rapid		6.7	7.1	7.5	8.0	8.4	8.8	9.2	9.7
Mountain climbing		7.4	7.9	8.4	8.9	9.4	9.9	10.3	10.8
Motorcycle riding		6.5	6.9	7.3	7.7	8.1	8.5	8.9	9.3

| 71 | 74 | 77 | 80 | 83 | 86 | 89 | 92 | 95 | 98 |
157	163	170	176	183	190	196	203	209	216
7.1	7.4	7.7	8.0	8.2	8.5	8.8	9.1	9.4	9.7
5.9	6.1	6.4	6.6	6.9	7.1	7.4	7.6	7.9	8.1
8.9	9.3	9.7	10.1	10.5	10.8	11.2	11.6	12.0	12.3
5.5	5.7	5.9	6.2	6.4	6.6	6.9	7.1	7.3	7.5
8.0	8.3	8.6	9.0	9.3	9.6	10.0	10.3	10.6	11.0
3.8	4.0	4.2	4.3	4.5	4.6	4.8	5.0	5.1	5.3
6.0	6.3	6.5	6.8	7.1	7.3	7.6	7.8	8.1	8.3
4.7	4.9	5.1	5.3	5.5	5.7	5.9	6.1	6.3	6.5
10.3	10.7	11.2	11.5	12.0	12.5	12.9	13.3	13.7	14.2
9.1	9.5	9.9	10.2	10.6	11.0	11.4	11.8	12.2	12.5
9.7	10.1	10.6	11.0	11.4	11.8	12.2	12.6	13.0	13.4
7.8	8.1	8.5	8.8	9.1	9.5	9.8	10.1	10.5	10.8
2.9	3.0	3.2	3.3	3.4	3.5	3.6	3.8	3.9	4.0
4.7	4.9	5.1	5.3	5.5	5.7	5.9	6.1	6.3	6.5
4.4	4.6	4.8	5.0	5.2	5.4	5.6	5.8	6.0	6.2
4.6	4.7	4.9	5.1	5.3	5.5	5.7	5.9	6.1	6.3
4.7	4.9	5.1	5.3	5.5	5.7	5.9	6.1	6.3	6.5
4.8	5.0	5.2	5.4	5.6	5.8	6.0	6.2	6.4	6.6
4.6	4.8	5.0	5.2	5.4	5.6	5.8	6.0	6.2	6.4
6.2	6.5	6.7	7.0	7.2	7.5	7.8	8.0	8.2	8.5
11.0	11.5	12.0	12.5	13.1	13.6	14.1	14.6	15.1	15.7
2.3	2.4	2.5	2.6	2.7	2.8	2.9	3.0	3.1	3.2
13.8	14.4	15.0	15.6	16.2	16.8	17.4	17.9	18.5	19.1
11.5	12.0	12.5	13.0	13.4	13.9	14.4	14.9	15.4	15.9
11.6	12.1	12.6	13.1	13.6	14.1	14.6	14.6	15.6	16.1
12.6	13.1	13.6	14.2	14.7	15.2	15.8	16.3	16.8	17.3
14.0	14.6	15.2	15.8	16.4	16.9	17.5	18.1	18.7	19.3
13.8	14.4	15.0	15.6	16.2	16.8	17.4	17.9	18.5	19.1
13.7	14.3	14.9	15.5	16.1	16.7	17.3	17.8	18.4	19.0
1.6	1.6	1.7	1.8	1.8	1.9	2.0	2.0	2.1	2.2
10.4	10.7	11.0	11.2	11.5	11.8	12.1	12.4	12.7	13.0
4.0	4.2	4.4	4.6	4.7	4.9	5.1	5.2	5.4	5.6
1.6	1.6	1.7	1.8	1.8	1.9	2.0	2.0	2.1	2.2
3.4	3.6	3.7	3.8	4.0	4.1	4.3	4.4	4.6	4.7
3.7	3.8	4.0	4.2	4.3	4.5	4.6	4.8	4.9	5.1
6.2	6.5	6.8	7.0	7.3	7.6	7.8	8.1	8.4	8.6
4.6	4.8	5.0	5.2	5.4	5.6	5.8	6.0	6.2	6.4
3.7	3.8	4.0	4.2	4.3	4.5	4.6	4.8	4.9	5.1
3.4	3.6	3.7	3.8	4.0	4.1	4.3	4.4	4.6	4.7
10.1	10.5	10.9	11.4	11.8	12.2	12.6	13.1	13.5	13.9
11.3	11.7	12.2	12.7	13.2	13.7	14.1	14.6	15.0	15.6
9.7	10.1	10.5	10.9	11.3	11.7	12.1	12.5	12.9	13.3

YOUR BODY WEIGHT—*continued*

Activity	kg lb	47 104	50 110	53 117	56 123	59 130	62 137	65 143	68 150
Music playing									
accordion (sitting)		1.5	1.6	1.7	1.8	1.9	2.0	2.1	2.2
cello (sitting)		2.0	2.1	2.2	2.3	2.4	2.5	2.7	2.8
conducting		1.9	2.0	2.1	2.2	2.3	2.4	2.5	2.7
drums (sitting)		3.1	3.3	3.5	3.7	3.9	4.1	4.3	4.5
flute (sitting)		1.7	1.8	1.9	2.0	2.1	2.2	2.3	2.4
horn (sitting)		1.4	1.5	1.5	1.6	1.7	1.8	1.9	2.0
organ (sitting)		2.6	2.7	2.8	3.0	3.1	3.3	3.4	3.6
piano (sitting)		1.9	2.0	2.1	2.2	2.4	2.5	2.6	2.7
trumpet (standing)		1.5	1.6	1.6	1.7	1.8	1.9	2.0	2.1
violin (sitting)		2.2	2.3	2.4	2.5	2.7	2.8	2.9	3.1
woodwind (sitting)		1.5	1.6	1.7	1.8	1.9	2.0	2.1	2.2
Paddleball		8.5	8.9	9.4	10.0	10.5	11.0	11.6	12.1
Paddle tennis		8.4	8.6	9.1	9.6	10.1	10.7	11.1	11.7
Painting									
inside projects		1.6	1.7	1.8	1.9	2.0	2.1	2.2	2.3
outside projects		3.7	3.9	4.1	4.3	4.5	4.8	5.0	5.2
scraping		3.1	3.2	3.3	3.5	3.7	3.9	4.1	4.3
Planting seedings		3.3	3.5	3.7	3.9	4.1	4.3	4.6	4.8
Plastering		3.7	3.9	4.1	4.4	4.6	4.8	5.1	5.3
Printing press work		1.7	1.8	1.9	2.0	2.1	2.2	2.3	2.4
Racquetball		8.4	8.9	9.4	10.0	10.5	11.0	11.6	12.1
Roller skating, leisure		5.3	5.8	6.2	6.5	6.9	7.3	7.3	8.0
Rope jumping									
110 rpm		6.7	7.1	7.5	7.9	8.4	8.8	9.2	9.7
120 rpm		6.4	6.8	7.3	7.7	8.1	8.5	8.9	9.3
130 rpm		6.0	6.4	6.8	7.1	7.5	7.7	8.3	8.7
Rowing									
machine, moderate		5.7	6.0	6.3	6.7	7.0	7.4	7.7	8.1
machine, race pace		8.6	8.9	9.4	10.0	10.5	11.0	11.6	12.1
skull, leisure		4.7	5.0	5.3	5.5	5.9	6.2	6.4	6.8
skull, race pace		8.7	8.9	9.4	10.0	10.5	11.0	11.6	12.1
Running, cross-country		7.8	8.2	8.6	9.1	9.6	10.1	10.6	11.1
Running, on flat surface									
11 min, 30 s per mile		6.3	6.8	7.2	7.6	8.0	8.4	8.8	9.2
9 min per mile		9.1	9.7	10.2	10.8	11.4	12.0	12.5	13.1
8 min per mile		9.8	10.8	11.3	11.9	12.5	13.1	13.6	14.2
7 min per mile		10.7	12.2	12.7	13.3	13.9	14.5	15.0	15.6
6 min per mile		11.8	13.9	14.4	15.0	15.6	16.2	16.7	17.3
5 min, 30 s per mile		13.6	14.5	15.3	16.2	17.1	17.9	18.8	19.7
Sailing, leisure		2.1	2.2	2.3	2.5	2.6	2.7	2.9	3.0
Scrubbing floors		5.1	5.5	5.8	6.1	6.4	6.8	7.1	7.4
Scuba diving		10.9	11.2	11.5	11.8	12.1	12.4	12.7	13.0
Shoe repair, general		2.2	2.3	2.4	2.5	2.7	2.8	2.9	3.1
Sitting quietly		1.0	1.1	1.1	1.2	1.2	1.3	1.4	1.4
Skateboarding		5.6	5.8	6.2	6.5	6.9	7.2	7.5	7.9
Skiing, hard snow									
level, moderate speed		5.6	6.0	6.3	6.7	7.0	7.4	7.7	8.1
level, walking speed		6.7	7.2	7.6	8.0	8.4	8.9	9.3	9.7
uphill, "fast" speed		12.9	13.7	14.5	15.3	16.2	17.0	17.8	18.6

| 71 | 74 | 77 | 80 | 83 | 86 | 89 | 92 | 95 | 98 |
157	163	170	176	183	190	196	203	209	216
2.3	2.4	2.5	2.6	2.7	2.8	2.8	2.9	3.0	3.1
2.9	3.0	3.2	3.3	3.4	3.5	3.6	3.8	3.9	4.0
2.8	2.9	3.0	3.1	3.2	3.4	3.5	3.6	3.7	3.8
4.7	4.9	5.1	5.3	5.5	5.7	5.9	6.1	6.3	6.6
2.5	2.6	2.7	2.8	2.9	3.0	3.1	3.2	3.3	3.4
2.1	2.1	2.2	2.3	2.4	2.5	2.6	2.7	2.8	2.8
3.8	3.9	4.1	4.2	4.4	4.6	4.7	4.9	5.0	5.2
2.8	3.0	3.1	3.2	3.3	3.4	3.6	3.7	3.8	3.9
2.2	2.3	2.4	2.5	2.6	2.7	2.8	2.9	2.9	3.0
3.2	3.3	3.5	3.6	3.7	3.9	4.0	4.1	4.3	4.4
2.3	2.4	2.5	2.6	2.7	2.8	2.8	2.9	3.0	3.1
12.6	13.2	13.7	14.2	14.8	15.3	15.8	16.4	16.9	17.4
12.2	12.7	13.2	13.7	14.2	14.2	15.2	15.8	16.3	16.8
2.4	2.5	2.6	2.7	2.8	2.9	3.0	3.1	3.2	3.3
5.5	5.7	5.9	6.2	6.4	6.6	6.9	7.1	7.3	7.5
4.5	4.7	4.9	5.0	5.2	5.4	5.6	5.8	6.0	6.2
5.0	5.2	5.4	5.6	5.8	6.0	6.2	6.4	6.7	6.9
5.5	5.8	6.0	6.2	6.5	6.7	6.9	7.2	7.4	7.6
2.5	2.6	2.7	2.8	2.9	3.0	3.1	3.2	3.3	3.4
12.6	13.2	13.7	14.2	14.8	15.3	15.8	16.4	16.9	17.4
8.3	8.6	9.0	9.3	9.7	10.1	10.4	10.8	11.1	11.4
10.1	10.5	10.5	11.3	11.8	12.2	12.6	13.1	13.5	13.9
9.8	10.1	10.6	10.9	11.4	11.8	12.2	12.6	13.0	13.4
9.1	9.4	9.8	10.2	10.6	11.0	11.3	11.7	12.1	12.5
8.5	8.9	9.3	9.7	10.1	10.6	11.1	11.6	12.1	12.6
12.6	13.2	13.7	14.2	14.8	15.3	15.8	16.4	16.9	17.4
7.2	7.6	8.0	8.4	8.8	9.2	9.6	10.0	10.4	10.8
12.6	13.2	13.7	14.2	14.8	15.3	15.8	16.4	16.9	17.4
11.6	12.1	12.6	13.0	13.5	14.0	14.5	15.0	15.5	16.0
9.6	10.0	10.5	10.9	11.3	11.7	12.1	12.5	12.9	13.3
13.7	14.3	14.9	15.4	16.0	16.6	17.2	17.8	18.3	18.9
14.8	15.4	16.0	16.5	17.1	17.7	18.3	18.9	19.4	20.0
16.2	16.8	17.4	17.9	18.5	19.1	19.7	20.3	20.8	21.4
17.9	18.5	19.1	19.6	20.2	20.8	21.4	22.0	22.5	23.1
20.5	21.4	22.3	23.1	24.0	24.9	25.7	26.6	27.5	28.3
3.1	3.3	3.4	3.5	3.7	3.8	3.9	4.1	4.2	4.3
7.7	8.1	8.4	8.7	9.0	9.4	9.7	10.0	10.4	10.7
13.3	13.6	13.9	14.2	14.5	14.8	15.1	15.4	15.7	16.0
3.2	3.3	3.5	3.6	3.7	3.9	4.0	4.1	4.3	4.4
1.5	1.6	1.6	1.7	1.7	1.8	1.9	1.9	2.0	2.1
8.3	8.6	8.9	9.3	9.6	10.0	10.3	10.7	11.0	11.4
8.4	8.8	9.2	9.5	9.9	10.2	10.6	10.9	11.3	11.7
10.2	10.6	11.0	11.4	11.9	12.3	12.7	13.2	13.6	14.0
19.5	20.3	21.1	21.9	22.7	23.6	24.4	25.2	26.0	26.9

YOUR BODY WEIGHT—*continued*

Activity	kg / lb	47 / 104	50 / 110	53 / 117	56 / 123	59 / 130	62 / 137	65 / 143	68 / 150
Skiing, soft snow									
leisure (F)		4.6	4.9	5.2	5.5	5.8	6.1	6.4	6.7
leisure (M)		5.2	5.6	5.9	6.2	6.5	6.9	7.2	7.5
Skindiving									
considerable motion		13.0	13.8	14.6	15.5	16.3	17.1	17.9	18.8
moderate motion		9.7	10.3	10.9	11.5	12.2	12.8	13.4	14.0
Snorkeling		4.3	4.6	4.9	5.2	5.5	5.8	6.0	6.3
Snowshoeing, soft snow		7.8	8.3	8.8	9.3	9.8	10.3	10.8	11.3
Snowmobiling		3.4	3.7	4.0	4.2	4.4	4.7	4.9	5.1
Soccer		6.5	6.8	7.3	7.7	8.1	8.5	8.9	9.3
Softball		3.3	3.5	3.7	3.9	4.1	4.3	4.5	4.7
Squash		10.0	10.6	11.2	11.9	12.5	13.1	13.8	14.4
Standing quietly (M)		1.3	1.4	1.4	1.5	1.6	1.7	1.8	1.8
Steel mill, working in									
fettling		4.3	4.5	4.7	5.0	5.3	5.5	5.8	6.1
forging		4.7	5.0	5.3	5.6	5.9	6.2	6.5	6.8
hand rolling		6.4	6.9	7.3	7.7	8.1	8.5	8.9	9.3
merchant mill rolling		6.8	7.3	7.7	8.1	8.6	9.0	9.4	9.9
removing slag		8.4	8.9	9.4	10.0	10.5	11.0	11.6	12.1
tending furnace		5.9	6.3	6.7	7.1	7.4	7.8	8.2	8.6
tipping molds		4.3	4.6	4.9	5.2	5.4	5.7	6.0	6.3
Surfing		3.9	4.1	4.3	4.5	4.8	5.0	5.3	5.5
Stock clerking		2.5	2.7	2.9	3.0	3.2	3.3	3.5	3.7
Swimming, fitness swims									
back stroke		7.9	8.5	9.0	9.5	10.0	10.5	11.0	11.5
breast stroke		7.6	8.1	8.6	9.1	9.6	10.0	10.5	11.0
butterfly			8.6	9.1	9.6	10.1	10.7	11.1	11.7
crawl, fast		7.3	7.8	8.3	8.7	9.2	9.7	10.1	10.6
crawl, slow		6.0	6.4	6.8	7.2	7.6	7.9	8.3	8.7
side stroke		5.7	6.1	6.5	6.8	7.2	7.6	7.9	8.3
treading, fast		8.0	8.5	9.0	9.5	10.0	10.5	11.1	11.6
treading, normal		2.9	3.1	3.3	3.5	3.7	3.8	4.0	4.2
Table tennis (ping pong)		3.2	3.4	3.6	3.8	4.0	4.2	4.4	4.6
Tailoring									
cutting		2.0	2.1	2.2	2.3	2.4	2.5	2.7	2.8
hand-sewing		1.5	1.6	1.7	1.8	1.9	2.0	2.1	2.2
machine-sewing		2.2	2.3	2.4	2.5	2.7	2.8	2.9	3.1
pressing		2.9	3.1	3.3	3.5	3.7	3.8	4.0	4.2
Tennis									
competition		6.9	7.3	7.8	8.2	8.7	9.1	9.5	9.9
recreational		5.1	5.5	5.8	6.1	6.4	6.8	7.1	7.4
Typing									
electric (computer)		1.3	1.4	1.4	1.5	1.6	1.7	1.8	1.8
manual		1.5	1.6	1.6	1.7	1.8	1.9	2.0	2.1
Volleyball									
competition		5.9	7.3	7.8	8.2	8.7	9.1	9.5	10.0
recreational		2.4	2.5	2.7	2.8	3.0	3.1	3.3	3.4
Walking, leisure outdoors									
asphalt road		3.8	4.0	4.2	4.5	4.7	5.0	5.2	5.4
fields and hillsides		3.9	4.1	4.3	4.6	4.8	5.1	5.3	5.6
grass track		3.8	4.1	4.3	4.5	4.8	5.0	5.3	5.5
plowed field		3.6	3.9	4.1	4.3	4.5	4.8	5.0	5.2

| 71 | 74 | 77 | 80 | 83 | 86 | 89 | 92 | 95 | 98 |
157	163	170	176	183	190	196	203	209	216
7.0	7.3	7.5	7.8	8.1	8.4	8.7	9.0	9.3	9.6
7.9	8.2	8.5	8.9	9.2	9.5	9.9	10.2	10.5	10.9
19.6	20.4	21.3	22.1	22.9	23.7	24.6	25.4	26.2	27.0
14.6	15.2	15.9	16.5	17.1	17.7	18.3	19.0	19.6	20.2
6.6	6.8	7.1	7.4	7.7	8.0	8.2	8.5	8.8	9.1
11.8	12.3	12.8	13.3	13.8	14.3	14.8	15.3	15.8	16.3
5.3	5.5	5.8	6.0	6.2	6.5	6.7	6.9	7.1	7.3
9.8	10.1	10.6	10.9	11.4	11.8	12.2	12.6	13.0	13.4
4.9	5.1	5.3	5.5	5.7	5.9	6.1	6.3	6.5	6.7
15.1	15.7	16.3	17.0	17.6	18.2	18.9	19.5	20.1	20.8
1.9	2.0	2.1	2.2	2.2	2.3	2.4	2.5	2.6	2.6
6.3	6.6	6.9	7.1	7.4	7.7	7.9	8.2	8.5	8.7
7.1	7.4	7.7	8.0	8.3	8.6	8.9	9.2	9.5	9.8
9.7	10.1	10.6	11.0	11.4	11.8	12.2	12.6	13.0	13.4
10.3	10.7	11.2	11.6	12.0	12.5	12.9	13.3	13.8	14.2
12.6	13.2	13.7	14.2	14.8	15.3	15.8	16.4	16.9	17.4
8.9	9.3	9.7	10.1	10.5	10.8	11.2	11.6	12.0	12.3
6.5	6.8	7.1	7.4	7.6	7.9	8.2	8.5	8.7	9.0
5.7	6.0	6.3	6.5	6.8	7.0	7.2	7.4	7.6	7.9
3.8	4.0	4.2	4.3	4.5	4.6	4.8	5.0	5.1	5.3
12.0	12.5	13.0	13.5	14.0	14.5	15.0	15.5	16.1	16.6
11.5	12.0	12.5	13.0	13.4	13.9	14.4	14.9	15.4	15.9
12.2	12.7	13.2	13.7	14.2	14.2	15.2	15.8	16.3	16.8
11.1	11.5	12.0	12.5	12.9	13.4	13.9	14.4	14.8	15.3
9.1	9.5	9.9	10.2	10.6	11.0	11.4	11.8	12.2	12.5
8.7	9.0	9.4	9.8	10.1	10.5	10.9	11.2	11.6	12.0
12.1	12.6	13.1	13.6	14.1	14.6	15.1	15.6	16.2	16.7
4.4	4.6	4.8	5.0	5.1	5.3	5.5	5.7	5.9	6.1
4.8	5.0	5.2	5.4	5.6	5.8	6.1	6.3	6.5	6.7
2.9	3.0	3.2	3.3	3.4	3.5	3.6	3.8	3.9	4.0
2.3	2.4	2.5	2.6	2.7	2.8	2.8	2.9	3.0	3.1
3.2	3.3	3.5	3.6	3.7	3.9	4.0	4.1	4.3	4.4
4.4	4.6	4.8	5.0	5.1	5.3	5.5	5.7	5.9	6.1
10.2	10.6	11.1	11.5	11.9	12.4	12.8	13.2	13.7	14.1
7.7	8.1	8.4	8.7	9.0	9.4	9.7	10.0	10.4	10.7
1.9	2.0	2.1	2.2	2.2	2.3	2.4	2.5	2.6	2.6
2.2	2.3	2.4	2.5	2.6	2.7	2.8	2.9	2.9	3.0
3.6	3.7	3.9	4.0	4.2	4.3	4.5	4.6	4.8	4.9
10.5	10.9	11.4	11.8	12.3	12.7	13.1	13.6	14.0	14.5
5.7	5.9	6.2	6.4	6.6	6.9	7.1	7.4	7.6	7.8
5.8	6.1	6.3	6.6	6.8	7.1	7.3	7.5	7.8	8.0
5.8	6.0	6.2	6.5	6.7	7.0	7.2	7.5	7.7	7.9
5.5	5.7	5.9	6.2	6.4	6.6	6.9	7.1	7.3	7.5

YOUR BODY WEIGHT—*continued*

Activity	kg lb	47 104	50 110	53 117	56 123	59 130	62 137	65 143	68 150
Walking, treadmill level									
2.0 mph		2.4	2.6	2.8	3.0	3.1	3.3	3.4	3.6
2.5 mph		3.0	3.2	3.4	3.6	3.8	4.0	4.2	4.4
3.0 mph		3.6	3.8	4.0	4.2	4.4	4.6	4.8	5.0
3.5 mph		4.0	4.3	4.6	4.8	5.1	5.3	5.6	6.1
4.0 mph		4.6	4.9	5.2	5.4	5.7	6.0	6.3	6.6
Wallpapering		2.3	2.4	2.5	2.7	2.8	3.0	3.1	3.3
Water polo, recreation		7.0	7.4	7.7	8.1	8.5	8.9	9.3	9.7
Water polo, competition		9.4	9.9	10.4	11.0	11.5	12.0	12.5	13.1
Water-skiing		5.6	6.0	6.4	6.7	7.1	7.5	7.8	8.2
Watch repairing		1.2	1.3	1.3	1.4	1.5	1.6	1.6	1.7
Whitewater rafting, recreational		4.1	4.4	4.6	4.9	5.2	5.4	5.7	6.0
Window cleaning		2.9	3.0	3.1	3.3	3.5	3.7	3.8	4.0
Wind surfing		3.3	3.5	3.7	3.9	4.1	4.3	4.6	4.8
Wrestling, competition		9.1	9.7	10.3	10.8	11.4	12.0	12.6	13.2
Writing (sitting)		1.4	1.5	1.5	1.6	1.7	1.8	1.9	2.0
Yoga		2.9	3.1	3.3	3.5	3.7	3.8	4.0	4.2

71 157	74 163	77 170	80 176	83 183	86 190	89 196	92 203	95 209	98 216
3.7	3.9	4.1	4.2	4.4	4.5	4.7	4.9	5.0	5.2
4.5	4.7	4.9	5.1	5.3	5.5	5.7	5.9	6.1	6.3
5.3	5.5	5.7	5.9	6.2	6.5	6.7	6.9	7.1	7.3
6.1	6.4	6.6	6.9	7.1	7.4	7.7	7.9	8.2	8.4
6.9	7.2	7.5	7.8	8.1	8.4	8.7	8.9	9.2	9.5
3.4	3.6	3.7	3.8	4.0	4.1	4.3	4.4	4.6	4.7
10.1	10.5	10.9	11.3	11.7	12.1	12.5	12.9	13.3	13.7
13.6	14.1	14.7	15.2	15.7	16.3	16.8	17.3	17.9	18.4
8.7	9.1	9.4	9.8	10.1	10.5	10.9	11.2	11.6	12.0
1.8	1.9	1.9	2.0	2.1	2.2	2.2	2.3	2.4	2.5
6.2	6.5	6.7	7.0	7.3	7.5	7.8	8.1	8.3	8.6
4.2	4.4	4.5	4.7	4.9	5.1	5.3	5.4	5.6	5.8
5.0	5.2	5.4	5.6	5.8	6.0	6.2	6.4	6.7	6.9
13.8	14.3	14.9	15.5	16.1	16.7	17.2	17.8	18.4	19.0
2.1	2.1	2.2	2.3	2.4	2.5	2.6	2.7	2.8	2.8
4.4	4.6	4.8	5.0	5.1	5.3	5.5	5.7	5.9	6.1

Nutritive Values for Common Foods, Alcoholic and Nonalcoholic Beverages, and Specialty and Fast-Food Items

THIS APPENDIX HAS three parts. Part 1 lists nutritive values for common foods, Part 2 lists nutritive values for alcoholic and nonalcoholic beverages, and Part 3 presents nutritive values for specialty and fast-food items. The nutritive values of foods and alcoholic and nonalcoholic beverages are expressed in 1-ounce (28.4 g) portions so comparisons can readily be made between the different food categories. Thus, for example, the protein content of 1.55 g for 1 ounce of banana nut bread can be compared directly to the protein content of 6.28 g for 1 ounce of processed American cheese.

PART 1

NUTRITIVE VALUES FOR COMMON FOODS[a]

The foods are grouped into categories and are listed in alphabetical order within each category. The categories include breads, cakes and pies, cookies, candy bars, chocolate, desserts, cereals, cheese, fish, fruits, meats, eggs, dairy products, vegetables, and typical salad bar entries. An additional section labeled Variety consists of food items such as soups, sandwiches, salad dressings, oils, some condiments, and other "goodies." The nutritive value for each food is expressed per ounce or 28.4 g of that food item. The specific values for each food include the caloric content (kcal) for 1 ounce and the protein, total fat, carbohydrate, calcium, iron, vitamin B_1, vitamin B_2, fiber, and cholesterol content.

---

[a] The information about the nutritive value of the foods was taken from a variety of sources. This includes primarily data from Watt, B.K., and Merrill, A.L.: *Composition of Foods—Raw, Processed and Prepared.* U.S. Department of Agriculture, Washington, DC, 1963; Adams, C., and Richardson, M.: *Nutritive Value of Foods.* Home and Garden Bulletin No. 72, rev, Washington, DC, U.S. Government Printing Office, 1981; and Pennington, J.A.T., and Church, H.N.: *Food Values of Portions Commonly Used,* 14th ed. New York, Harper & Row, 1985. Other sources include a comprehensive database on the Cyber mainframe computer at the University of Massachusetts, the consumer relations departments of manufacturers, and journal articles that evaluated specific foods items. *NA indicates data not available.*

BREADS

	kcal	Protein (g)	Fat (g)	CHO (g)	Ca (mg)	Fe (mg)	B₁ (mg)	B₂ (mg)	Fiber (g)	Cholesterol (mg)
Breads										
Banana nut	91	1.55	4.00	12.7	10.0	0.470	0.054	0.046	0.66	18.3
Boston brown—canned	60	1.26	0.39	13.2	25.8	0.567	0.038	0.025	1.34	1.9
Cornmeal muffin—recipe	91	1.89	3.15	13.2	41.6	0.567	0.069	0.069	1.00	14.5
Croutons—dry	105	3.69	1.04	20.5	35.0	1.020	0.099	0.099	0.09	0
Cracked wheat	74	2.63	0.99	14.2	18.1	0.755	0.108	0.108	1.50	0
Cracked wheat—toast	88	3.00	1.17	16.9	21.6	0.899	0.100	0.128	1.82	0
French—chunk	81	2.67	1.10	14.3	31.6	0.875	0.130	0.097	0.57	0
Italian	78	2.55	0.25	16.0	4.7	0.756	0.116	0.066	0.47	0
Mixed grain	74	2.27	1.05	13.6	30.6	0.907	0.113	0.113	1.78	0
Mixed grain—toast	80	2.47	1.15	14.8	33.3	0.986	0.099	0.123	1.97	0
Oatmeal	74	2.37	1.25	13.6	17.0	0.794	0.130	0.075	1.10	0
Oatmeal—toast	80	2.47	1.36	14.8	18.5	0.863	0.110	0.081	1.20	0
Pita pocket	78	2.94	0.42	15.6	23.2	0.685	0.129	0.061	0.45	0
Pumpernickel	71	2.60	0.98	13.6	20.4	0.777	0.097	0.147	1.67	0
Pumpernickel—toast	78	2.86	1.08	15.0	22.5	0.857	0.088	0.162	1.87	0
Raisin—	77	2.15	1.12	15.0	28.4	0.879	0.093	0.176	0.68	0
Raisin—toasted	92	2.57	1.34	17.6	33.8	1.080	0.081	0.209	0.81	0
Rye—light	74	2.40	1.04	13.6	22.7	0.771	0.116	0.090	1.87	0
Rye—light—toast	84	2.73	1.18	15.5	25.8	0.876	0.107	0.103	2.15	0
Vienna	79	2.72	1.10	14.4	31.2	0.873	0.130	0.100	0.91	0
White	76	2.35	1.10	13.8	35.7	0.806	0.133	0.088	0.54	0
White—toast	84	2.67	1.26	15.7	40.6	0.915	0.121	0.103	0.64	0
Whole wheat	69	2.84	1.22	12.9	20.2	0.964	0.100	0.059	2.10	0
Whole wheat—toasted	79	3.42	1.47	14.4	22.5	1.090	0.090	0.066	2.74	0
Bread crumbs—dry grated	111	3.69	1.42	20.7	34.6	1.160	0.099	0.099	1.15	1.4
Bread crumbs—soft	76	2.35	1.10	13.9	35.9	0.806	0.134	0.088	0.54	0
Bread sticks wo/salt	109	3.40	0.82	21.3	7.9	0.255	0.017	0.020	0.43	0
Bread sticks w/salt	86	2.67	0.89	16.4	13.0	0.243	0.016	0.024	0.41	0

CAKES AND PIES

	kcal	Protein (g)	Fat (g)	CHO (g)	Ca (mg)	Fe (mg)	B₁ (mg)	B₂ (mg)	Fiber (g)	Cholesterol (mg)
Cakes										
Angel food cake	67	1.71	0.09	15.2	23.5	0.123	0.014	0.057	0	0
Boston cream pie	61	0.59	1.89	10.4	6.1	0.142	0.002	0.043	0	4.7
Carrot cake	103	1.05	5.32	13.2	6.9	0.304	0.030	0.035	0	14.6
Cheesecake	86	1.54	5.45	8.1	15.9	0.136	0.009	0.037	0	52.4
Choc cupcake/choc frosting	97	1.24	3.29	16.5	16.9	0.575	0.029	0.041	0	15.2
Coffee cake	91	1.78	2.70	14.8	17.3	0.480	0.054	0.059	0	18.5
Dark fruitcake	109	1.32	4.62	16.5	27.0	0.791	0.053	0.053	0	13.2
Gingerbread cake	91	1.15	2.86	15.2	12.2	0.706	0.042	0.038	0	7.8
Pound cake	113	1.89	4.72	14.2	18.9	0.472	0.047	0.057	0	30.2
Sheet cake—plain	104	1.32	3.96	15.8	18.1	0.429	0.046	0.049	0	20.1
Sheet cake—white frosting	104	0.94	3.28	18.0	14.3	0.281	0.030	0.037	0	16.4
Sponge cake	83	2.01	1.27	16.0	10.8	0.524	0.043	0.046	0	58.8
White cake/coconut	109	1.30	4.05	17.0	13.7	0.454	0.041	0.053	0	1.2

CAKES AND PIES—*continued*

	kcal	Protein (g)	Fat (g)	CHO (g)	Ca (mg)	Fe (mg)	B_1 (mg)	B_2 (mg)	Fiber (g)	Cholesterol (mg)
Cakes—cont'd										
White cake/white frosting	104	1.20	3.59	16.8	13.2	0.399	0.080	0.052	0	1.2
Yellow cake/chocolate frosting	101	1.03	4.48	15.9	9.5	0.509	0.020	0.058	0	15.6
Pies										
Apple pie	73	0.66	3.14	10.7	5.0	0.300	0.031	0.023	0	0
Apple pie—fried	85	0.73	4.67	10.7	4.0	0.312	0.030	0.020	0	4.7
Banana cream pie	46	0.90	1.85	6.7	21.0	0.156	0.022	0.042	0	2.2
Blueberry pie	68	0.72	3.05	9.9	4.7	0.377	0.031	0.025	0	0
Boston cream pie	61	0.59	1.89	10.4	6.1	0.142	0.002	0.043	0	4.7
Cherry pie	74	0.77	3.19	10.9	6.6	0.569	0.034	0.025	0	0
Cherry pie—fried	83	0.68	4.74	10.7	3.7	0.233	0.020	0.020	0	4.3
Chocolate cream pie	50	1.20	2.04	6.9	25.9	0.175	0.024	0.049	0	2.4
Coconut cream pie	57	1.03	2.79	7.2	24.0	0.198	0.021	0.042	0	2.5
Coconut custard pie	66	1.69	3.85	6.3	25.0	0.304	0.029	0.055	0	31.4
Cream pie	85	0.56	4.29	11.0	8.6	0.205	0.011	0.028	0	1.5
Custard pie	55	1.43	2.65	6.3	23.1	0.269	0.026	0.050	0	27.6
Lemon meringue pie	72	0.95	2.90	10.7	5.1	0.283	0.020	0.028	0	27.7
Mincemeat pie	70	0.65	2.13	12.8	6.9	0.360	0.028	0.024	0	0
Peach pie	73	0.63	3.14	10.9	4.8	0.340	0.031	0.028	0	0
Pecan pie	120	1.30	4.87	18.9	7.2	0.380	0.045	0.034	0	28.1
Pumpkin pie	52	1.28	2.23	7.3	30.0	0.373	0.019	0.042	0	15.5
Strawberry chiffon pie	65	0.85	3.46	8.0	7.7	0.254	0.022	0.023	0	7.1

COOKIES

	kcal	Protein (g)	Fat (g)	CHO (g)	Ca (mg)	Fe (mg)	B_1 (mg)	B_2 (mg)	Fiber (g)	Cholesterol (mg)
Animal cookies	120	1.90	2.89	22.0	3.0	0.918	0.080	0.130	0	0.1
Brownies w/nuts	135	1.84	8.93	15.6	12.8	0.567	0.070	0.070	0	25.5
Butter cookies	130	1.76	4.82	20.2	36.3	0.170	0.011	0.017	0	4.1
Fig bars	106	1.02	1.93	21.4	20.2	0.689	0.039	0.037	0	13.7
Lady fingers	102	2.19	2.19	18.3	11.6	0.515	0.019	0.039	0	101.0
Oatmeal raisin cookies	134	1.64	5.45	19.6	9.8	0.600	0.049	0.044	0	1.1
Peanut butter cookies	145	2.36	8.27	16.5	12.4	0.650	0.041	0.041	0	13.0
Sandwich type cookies	138	1.42	5.67	20.6	8.5	0.992	0.064	0.050	0	0
Shortbread cookies	137	1.77	7.09	17.7	11.5	0.709	0.089	0.080	0	23.9
Sugar cookies	139	1.18	7.09	18.3	29.5	0.532	0.053	0.035	0	17.1
Vanilla wafers	131	1.42	4.96	20.6	11.3	0.567	0.050	0.070	0	17.7

CANDY BARS

	kcal	Protein (g)	Fat (g)	CHO (g)	Ca (mg)	Fe (mg)	B_1 (mg)	B_2 (mg)	Fiber (g)	Cholesterol (mg)
Almond Joy	151	1.69	7.82	18.5	2.0	0.778	0	0	0	0
Sugar-coated almonds	146	3.10	9.12	14.6	39.6	0.775	0.042	0.156	0	0

CANDY BARS—continued

	kcal	Protein (g)	Fat (g)	CHO (g)	Ca (mg)	Fe (mg)	B₁ (mg)	B₂ (mg)	Fiber (g)	Cholesterol (mg)
Bittersweet chocolate	141	1.90	9.73	15.7	13.0	1.040	0.015	0.050	0	0
Caramel—plain or chocolate	115	1.00	2.99	22.0	41.9	0.399	0.010	0.050	0	1.0
Chocolate candy kisses	154	2.10	8.98	15.9	52.9	0.499	0.020	0.080	0	0
Chocolate-coated almonds	161	3.92	12.70	8.0	47.8	1.090	0.052	0.186	0	0
Chocolate-covered coconut	133	0.91	7.10	17.5	8.4	0.614	0.008	0.016	0	0
Chocolate-covered mints	116	0.50	2.99	23.0	16.0	0.299	0.010	0.020	0	0
Chocolate-covered peanuts	159	5.00	11.70	9.8	32.9	0.689	0.086	0.043	0	0
Chocolate-covered raisins	111	1.06	2.71	20.6	12.2	0.663	0.034	0.025	0	0
Chocolate fudge	115	0.56	2.78	21.0	22.0	0.299	0.010	0.030	0	1.0
Chocolate fudge with nuts	114	1.06	4.99	18.8	22.0	0.299	0.016	0.030	0	7.4
English toffee	195	0.89	16.90	9.8	0	0.177	0.470	0.044	0	0
Gum drops	98	0	0.20	24.8	2.0	0.100	0	0	0	0
Hard candy	109	0	0	27.6	6.0	0.100	0	0	0	0
Jelly beans	104	0	0.10	26.4	1.0	0.299	0	0	0	0
Kit Kat	138	1.98	7.25	16.5	42.9	0.369	0.020	0.073	0	0
Krackle	149	2.00	8.09	16.9	50.0	0.400	0.017	0.075	0	0
Malted milk balls	135	2.30	6.99	17.8	62.9	0	0	0	0	0
M&M's plain chocolate	140	1.95	6.08	19.5	46.7	0.449	0.015	0.073	0	0
M&M's peanut chocolate	144	3.23	7.25	16.5	35.4	0.402	0.016	0.056	0	0
Mars bar	136	2.27	6.24	17.0	48.2	0.312	0.014	0.093	0	0
Milk chocolate—plain	145	2.00	8.98	16.0	49.9	0.399	0.020	0.100	0	6.0
Milk chocolate w/almonds	150	2.90	10.40	15.0	60.9	0.559	0.030	0.130	0	4.5
Milk chocolate w/peanuts	155	4.89	11.70	10.0	31.9	0.679	0.112	0.065	0	3.0
Milk chocolate + rice cereal	140	2.00	6.99	18.0	47.9	0.200	0.010	0.080	0	6.0
Milky Way	123	1.53	4.25	20.3	40.6	0.232	0.013	0.070	0	6.6
Mr. Goodbar	151	3.62	9.05	13.9	39.2	0.567	0.030	0.072	0	4.2
Reese's peanut butter cup	151	3.65	9.07	13.9	21.7	0.430	0.020	0.032	0	1.6
Snickers	134	3.08	6.62	17.0	32.4	0.227	0.013	0.050	0	0
Vanilla fudge	118	0.70	3.15	22.0	29.9	0.030	0.006	0.025	0	10.0
Vanilla fudge with nuts	122	1.00	5.01	18.3	25.0	0.159	0.017	0.026	0	8.5

CHOCOLATE

	kcal	Protein (g)	Fat (g)	CHO (g)	Ca (mg)	Fe (mg)	B₁ (mg)	B₂ (mg)	Fiber (g)	Cholesterol (mg)
Baking chocolate	145	3.49	15.00	7.5	22.0	1.900	0.015	0.099	0	0
Bittersweet chocolate	141	1.90	9.73	15.7	13.0	1.040	0.015	0.050	0	0
Milk chocolate—plain	145	2.00	8.98	16.0	49.9	0.399	0.020	0.100	0	6.0
Semi-sweet chocolate chips	143	1.17	10.20	16.2	8.5	0.967	0.017	0.023	0	0
Dark chocolate—sweet	150	1.00	9.98	16.0	7.0	0.599	0.010	0.040	0	0
Chocolate cupcake/ chocolate frosting	97	1.24	3.29	16.5	16.9	0.575	0.029	0.041	0	15.2
Chocolate candy kisses	154	2.10	8.98	15.9	52.9	0.499	0.020	0.080	0	0
Chocolate chip cookies	122	1.54	5.94	18.9	11.0	0.540	0.068	0.155	0	3.4

CHOCOLATE—continued

	kcal	Protein (g)	Fat (g)	CHO (g)	Ca (mg)	Fe (mg)	B_1 (mg)	B_2 (mg)	Fiber (g)	Cholesterol (mg)
Chocolate coated almonds	161	3.92	12.70	8.0	47.8	1.090	0.052	0.186	0	0
Chocolate coated peanuts	159	5.00	11.70	9.8	32.9	0.689	0.086	0.043	0	0
Chocolate covered mints	116	0.50	2.99	23.0	16.0	0.299	0.010	0.020	0	0
Chocolate covered raisins	111	1.06	2.71	20.6	12.2	0.663	0.034	0.025	0	0
Chocolate cream pie	50	1.20	2.04	6.9	25.9	0.175	0.024	0.049	0	2.4
Chocolate fudge	115	0.56	2.78	21.0	22.0	0.299	0.010	0.030	0	1.0
Chocolate fudge with nuts	114	1.06	4.99	18.8	22.0	0.299	0.016	0.030	0	7.4
Cake flour-baked value	103	2.08	0.28	22.4	4.5	1.250	0.154	0.096	0	0
Reese's peanut butter cup	151	3.65	9.07	13.9	21.7	0.430	0.020	0.032	0	1.6
Chocolate pudding/recipe	42	0.88	1.25	7.3	27.3	0.142	0.005	0.039	0	4.3
Chocolate pudding instant	34	0.85	0.818	5.9	28.4	0.065	0.009	0.039	0	3.1

DESSERTS AND BREAKFAST PASTRIES

	kcal	Protein (g)	Fat (g)	CHO (g)	Ca (mg)	Fe (mg)	B_1 (mg)	B_2 (mg)	Fiber (g)	Cholesterol (mg)
Apple brown betty	43	0.30	1.60	7.40	5.4	0.130	0.016	0.012	0	3.8
Apple cobbler	55	0.53	1.74	9.57	8.8	0.206	0.023	0.019	0	0.3
Apple crisp	53	0.33	1.93	9.09	7.4	0.278	0.018	0.013	0	0
Apple dumpling	55	0.32	2.37	8.64	7.1	0.253	0.012	0.013	0	0
Banana nut bread	91	1.60	4.00	12.70	10.0	0.470	0.054	0.046	0	18.3
Bread + raisin pudding	60	1.20	2.47	8.54	27.7	0.304	0.030	0.048	0	24.4
Cheesecake	86	1.50	5.45	8.10	15.9	0.136	0.009	0.037	0	52.4
Cherry cobbler	44	0.53	1.37	7.52	8.5	0.391	0.019	0.021	0	0.3
Cherry & cream cheese torte	79	1.28	3.96	10.00	28.5	0.266	0.015	0.052	0	11.2
Vanilla milkshake	32	0.98	0.841	5.09	34.5	0.026	0.013	0.052	0	3.2
Cream puff w/custard fill	72	1.24	4.54	6.83	16.4	0.276	0.015	0.040	0	58.8
Chocolate eclair w/custard fill	79	1.20	4.43	8.96	18.6	0.258	0.019	0.041	0	50.4
Gelatin salad	17	0.43	0	3.99	0.5	0.024	0.002	0.002	0	0
Peach cobbler	28	0.50	1.35	7.96	7.6	0.197	0.018	0.017	0	0.3
Peach crisp	34	0.31	1.06	6.18	4.8	0.203	0.010	0.010	0	0
Crepe, unfilled	49	2.06	1.32	7.07	25.0	0.475	0.045	0.070	0.21	43.0
Pancakes—plain	63	2.10	2.10	9.45	28.4	0.525	0.063	0.074	0.42	16.8
Croissant	117	2.32	6.02	13.40	10.0	1.040	0.085	0.065	0.54	6.5
Danish pastry—plain	109	1.99	5.97	12.90	29.8	0.547	0.080	0.085	0	24.4
Danish pastry w/fruit	102	1.74	5.67	12.20	7.41	0.567	0.070	0.061	0	24.4
Doughnut—cake type	119	1.33	6.75	13.90	13.0	0.454	0.068	0.068	0	11.3
Doughnut—jelly filled	99	1.48	3.84	13.00	12.2	0.349	0.052	0.044	0	0
Doughnut—yeast-raised	111	1.89	6.28	12.30	8.0	0.661	0.132	0.057	0	9.9
Chocolate pudding	42	0.88	1.25	7.28	27.3	0.142	0.005	0.039	0	4.3
Tapioca pudding	38	1.43	1.44	4.85	29.7	0.120	0.012	0.052	0	27.3
Vanilla pudding	32	0.99	1.10	4.50	33.1	0.089	0.009	0.046	0	4.1
Chocolate pudding—instant	34	0.85	0.82	5.89	28.4	0.065	0.009	0.039	0	3.1
Rice pudding	33	0.86	0.86	5.80	28.6	0.107	0.021	0.039	0	3.2
Butterscotch pudding pop	47	1.19	1.29	7.80	37.8	0.020	0.015	0.055	0	0.5
Chocolate pudding pop	49	1.34	1.34	8.20	42.8	0.179	0.015	0.055	0	0.5
Vanilla pudding pop	46	1.19	1.29	7.80	37.8	0.020	0.015	0.055	0	0.5

CEREALS (WITHOUT MILK)

	kcal	Protein (g)	Fat (g)	CHO (g)	Ca (mg)	Fe (mg)	B₁ (mg)	B₂ (mg)	Fiber (g)	Cholesterol (mg)
All-Bran	70	3.99	0.50	21.0	23.00	4.49	0.369	0.429	8.490	0
Alpha Bits	111	2.20	0.60	24.6	7.99	1.80	0.399	0.399	0.650	0
Apple Jacks	110	1.50	0.10	25.7	2.99	4.49	0.399	0.399	0.200	0
Bran Buds	73	3.95	0.68	21.6	18.90	4.52	0.371	0.439	7.860	0
Bran Chex	90	2.95	0.81	22.6	16.80	4.51	0.347	0.150	5.200	0
Buc Wheats	110	2.00	1.00	24.0	59.90	8.09	0.674	0.764	2.000	0
C.W. Post—plain	126	2.54	4.44	20.3	13.70	4.50	0.380	0.438	0.643	0
C.W. Post w/raisins	123	2.45	4.05	20.3	14.00	4.51	0.358	0.413	0.660	0
Cap'n Crunch	120	1.46	2.60	22.9	4.60	7.53	0.506	0.544	0.709	0
Cap'n Crunchberries	118	1.46	2.35	23.0	8.91	7.32	0.478	0.543	0.324	0
Cap'n Crunch—peanut butter	125	2.03	3.64	21.5	5.67	7.37	0.486	0.567	0.324	0
Cheerios	110	4.24	1.77	19.4	47.30	4.44	0.394	0.394	3.000	0
Cocoa Krispies	109	1.50	0.39	25.2	4.73	1.81	0.394	0.394	0.354	0
Cocoa Pebbles	117	1.35	1.49	24.7	5.40	1.75	0.405	0.405	0.312	0
Corn Bran	98	1.97	1.02	23.9	32.30	9.60	0.299	0.551	5.390	0
Corn Chex	111	2.00	0.10	24.9	2.99	1.80	0.399	0.070	0.499	0
Corn flakes—Kellogg's	110	2.30	0.09	24.4	1.00	1.80	0.367	0.424	0.594	0
Corn flakes—Post Toasties	110	2.30	0.09	24.4	1.00	0.70	0.367	0.424	0.594	0
Corn grits—enriched yellow dry	105	2.49	0.33	22.5	0.55	1.10	0.182	0.107	3.270	0
Corn grits—enriched ckd	17	0.41	0.06	3.7	0.12	0.18	0.028	0.018	0.527	0
Cracklin' Oat Bran	108	2.60	4.16	19.4	18.90	1.80	0.378	0.425	4.280	0
Cream of Rice	15	0.24	0.01	3.3	0.93	0.05	0.012	0	0.163	0
Cream of Wheat	16	0.42	0.07	3.4	6.27	1.27	0.028	0.008	0.395	0
Crispy Wheat 'n Raisins	99	2.00	0.46	23.1	46.80	4.48	0.396	0.396	1.320	0
Farina—cooked	14	0.41	0.02	3.0	0.49	0.14	0.023	0.015	0.389	0
Fortified Oat Flakes	105	5.32	0.41	20.5	40.20	8.09	0.354	0.413	0.827	0
40% Bran Flakes—Kellogg's	91	3.60	0.54	22.2	13.80	8.14	0.369	0.430	0.850	0
40% Bran Flakes—Post	92	3.20	0.45	22.3	12.70	4.50	0.374	0.435	3.800	0
Froot Loops	111	1.70	1.00	25.0	2.99	4.49	0.399	0.399	0.299	0
Frosted Mini-Wheats	102	2.93	0.27	23.4	9.15	1.83	0.366	0.457	2.160	0
Frosted Rice Krispies	109	1.30	0.10	25.7	1.00	1.80	0.399	0.399	0.998	0
Fruit & Fiber w/apples	90	2.99	1.00	22.0	9.98	4.49	0.374	0.424	4.190	0
Fruit & Fiber w/dates	90	2.99	1.00	21.0	9.98	4.49	0.374	0.424	4.190	0
Fruitful Bran	92	2.50	0	22.5	8.34	6.75	0.313	0.354	4.170	0
Fruity Pebbles	115	1.10	1.50	24.4	2.99	1.80	0.399	0.399	0.226	0
Golden Grahams	109	1.60	1.09	24.1	17.40	4.50	0.363	0.436	1.670	0
Granola—homemade	138	3.49	7.69	15.6	17.70	1.12	0.170	0.072	2.970	0
Granola—Nature Valley	126	2.89	4.92	18.9	17.80	0.95	0.098	0.048	2.960	0
Grape Nuts	100	3.28	0.11	23.2	10.90	1.22	0.398	0.398	1.840	0
Grape Nuts Flakes	102	2.99	0.30	23.2	11.00	4.49	0.399	0.399	1.900	0
Honey & Nut Corn Flakes	113	1.80	1.50	23.3	2.99	1.80	0.399	0.399	0.299	0
Honey Bran	96	2.51	0.57	23.2	13.00	4.54	0.405	0.405	3.160	0
Honey Comb	111	1.68	0.52	25.3	5.15	1.80	0.387	0.387	0.387	0
Honey Nut Cheerios	107	3.09	0.69	22.8	19.80	4.47	0.344	0.430	0.790	0
King Vitamin	115	1.49	1.62	24.0	NA	17.10	0.124	1.430	0.135	0
Kix	109	2.49	0.70	23.3	34.80	8.06	0.398	0.398	0.398	0
Life	104	5.22	0.52	20.3	99.20	7.47	0.612	0.644	0.902	0
Lucky Charms	111	2.57	1.06	23.1	31.90	4.52	0.354	0.443	0.624	0
Malt-O-Meal	14	0.43	0.03	3.1	0.59	1.13	0.057	0.028	0.354	0
Maypo—cooked	1	0.02	0.01	0.1	0.52	0.04	0.003	0.003	0.012	0

CEREALS (WITHOUT MILK)—*continued*

	kcal	Protein (g)	Fat (g)	CHO (g)	Ca (mg)	Fe (mg)	B_1 (mg)	B_2 (mg)	Fiber (g)	Cholesterol (mg)
Nutri-Grain—barley	106	3.11	0.21	23.4	7.60	1.00	0.346	0.415	1.660	0
Nutri-Grain—corn	108	2.30	0.68	24.0	0.68	0.60	0.338	0.405	1.750	0
Nutri-Grain—rye	102	2.48	0.21	24.0	5.67	0.80	0.354	0.425	2.160	0
Nutri-Grain—wheat	102	2.45	0.32	24.0	7.73	0.80	0.387	0.451	1.800	0
Oatmeal—prepared	18	0.73	0.29	3.1	2.42	0.19	0.032	0.006	0.497	0
Rolled Oats	109	4.55	1.78	19.0	14.70	1.19	0.206	0.038	3.090	0
Instant Oatmeal w/apples	26	0.74	0.30	5.0	30.00	1.15	0.091	0.053	0.552	0
Instant Oatmeal w/bran & raisins	23	0.71	0.28	4.4	25.20	1.10	0.081	0.092	0.480	0
Instant Oatmeal w/maple	30	0.84	0.35	5.8	29.60	1.16	0.097	0.059	0.530	0
Instant Oatmeal w/cinnamon & spice	31	0.85	0.34	6.2	30.30	1.17	0.099	0.60	0.510	0
Instant Oatmeal w/raisins & spice	29	0.77	0.32	5.7	29.60	1.18	0.092	0.065	0.556	0
100% Bran	77	3.57	1.42	20.7	19.80	3.49	0.687	0.773	8.380	0
100% Natural	135	3.02	6.02	18.0	48.90	0.83	0.085	0.150	3.390	0
100% Natural—w/apples	130	2.92	5.32	19.0	42.80	0.79	0.090	0.158	1.300	0
100% Natural—w/raisins & dates	128	2.89	5.23	18.7	41.20	0.80	0.077	0.165	1.080	0
Product 19	108	2.75	0.17	23.5	3.44	18.00	1.460	1.720	0.369	0
Puffed Rice	111	1.79	0.20	25.5	2.03	0.30	0.030	0.028	0.227	0
Puffed Wheat	104	4.25	0.24	22.4	7.09	1.35	0.047	0.070	5.430	0
Quisp	117	1.42	2.08	23.6	8.50	5.96	0.510	0.718	0.378	0
Raisin Bran—Kellogg's	91	3.07	0.46	21.4	14.50	13.90	0.293	0.332	3.410	0
Raisin Bran—Post	86	2.68	0.55	21.4	13.70	4.56	0.373	0.430	3.190	0
Raisins, Rice & Rye	96	1.60	0.06	24.2	6.16	3.45	0.308	0.370	0.308	0
Ralston—cooked	15	0.62	0.09	3.2	1.57	0.18	0.022	0.020	0.370	0
Rice Chex	112	1.49	1.00	25.2	3.88	1.79	0.400	0.298	1.840	0
Rice Krispies	109	1.86	0.20	24.2	3.91	1.76	0.391	0.391	0.312	0
Roman Meal—dry	91	4.07	0.60	20.4	18.40	1.31	0.142	0.069	0.905	0
Roman Meal—cooked	17	0.77	0.11	3.9	3.45	0.25	0.028	0.014	0.877	0
Shredded Wheat	102	3.09	0.71	22.5	11.00	1.20	0.070	0.080	3.100	0
Shredded wheat	97	3.06	0.45	16.4	11.20	0.89	0.082	0.075	2.900	0
Special K	111	5.58	0.10	21.3	7.97	4.48	0.399	0.399	0.266	0
Sugar Corn Pops	108	1.40	0.10	25.6	0.10	1.80	0.399	0.399	0.100	0
Sugar Frosted Flakes	108	1.46	0.08	25.7	0.81	1.78	0.405	0.405	0.446	0
Sugar Smacks	106	2.00	0.50	24.7	2.99	1.80	0.369	0.429	0.319	0
Super Golden Crisp	106	1.80	0.26	25.6	6.01	1.80	0.344	0.430	0.430	0
Team	111	1.82	0.48	24.3	4.05	1.73	0.371	0.425	0.270	0
Total	105	2.84	0.60	22.3	172.00	18.00	1.460	1.720	2.060	0
Trix	108	1.50	0.40	24.9	5.99	4.49	0.399	0.399	0.184	0
Wheat & Raisin Chex	97	2.68	0.21	22.6	NA	4.04	0.263	0.315	1.890	0
Wheat Chex	104	2.77	0.68	23.3	11.00	4.50	0.370	0.105	2.100	0
Wheat germ—toasted	108	8.25	3.09	14.0	12.50	2.19	0.474	0.233	3.910	0
Wheat germ w/brown sugar, honey	107	6.19	2.30	17.2	8.98	1.93	0.349	0.180	3.390	0
Wheatena—cooked	16	0.58	0.13	3.4	1.28	0.16	0.002	0.006	0.385	0
Wheaties	99	2.74	0.51	22.6	43.00	4.50	0.391	0.391	2.540	0
Whole wheat berries	16	0.54	0.11	3.2	1.70	0.17	0.023	0.006	0.680	0
Whole wheat cereal—cooked	18	0.58	0.11	3.9	1.99	0.18	0.020	0.014	0.457	0

CHEESE

	kcal	Protein (g)	Fat (g)	CHO (g)	Ca (mg)	Fe (mg)	B₁ (mg)	B₂ (mg)	Fiber (g)	Cholesterol (mg)
American—processed	106	6.28	8.84	0.45	174	0.110	0.008	0.111	0	27.0
American cheese food—cold pack	94	5.23	6.78	2.36	145	0.240	0.009	0.274	0	18.0
American cheese spread	82	5.16	6.00	2.48	159	0.090	0.014	0.380	0	16.0
Blue	100	6.09	8.14	0.66	150	0.090	0.008	0.395	0	21.0
Brick	105	6.40	8.40	0.79	191	0.130	0.004	0.159	0	27.0
Brie	95	5.87	7.84	0.13	52	0.140	0.020	0.147	0	28.0
Camembert	85	5.60	6.86	0.13	110	0.094	0.008	0.138	0	20.0
Caraway	107	7.13	8.27	0.87	191	0.100	0.009	0.196	0	25.0
Cheddar	114	7.05	9.38	0.36	204	0.197	0.008	0.106	0	29.9
Cheshire	110	6.60	8.66	1.36	182	0.060	0.013	0.198	0	28.9
Colby	112	6.73	9.08	0.73	194	0.216	0.004	0.171	0	27.0
Cottage	29	3.54	1.20	0.76	17	0.040	0.006	0.115	0	4.2
Cottage—lowfat 2%	26	3.90	0.55	1.03	20	0.045	0.007	0.052	0	2.4
Cottage—lowfat 1%	21	3.51	0.29	0.77	18	0.040	0.006	0.115	0	1.3
Cottage—dry curd	24	4.89	0.12	0.52	9	0.065	0.007	0.004	0	2.0
Cottage—w/fruit	35	2.80	0.96	3.78	14	0.031	0.005	0.115	0	3.1
Cream	99	2.10	9.87	0.75	23	0.337	0.005	0.056	0	30.9
Edam	101	7.07	7.79	0.40	207	0.125	0.010	0.274	0	25.0
Feta	75	4.49	6.19	1.16	140	0.180	0.040	0.315	0	25.0
Fontina	110	7.25	8.62	0.44	156	0.060	0.006	NA	0	32.9
Gjetost	132	2.74	8.32	12.00	113	0.130	0.009	0.170	0	25.0
Gorgonzola	111	6.99	8.98	0	149	0.120	0.010	0.512	0	25.0
Gouda	101	7.06	7.72	0.63	198	0.070	0.009	0.232	0	31.9
Gruyere	117	8.44	9.05	0.10	286	0.060	0.017	0.095	0	30.9
Liederkranz	87	4.99	7.99	0	110	0.120	0.010	0.389	0	21.0
Limburger	93	5.67	7.59	0.14	141	0.040	0.023	0.227	0	26.0
Monterey jack	106	6.93	8.56	0.19	212	0.200	0.004	0.119	0	26.0
Mozzarella—skim, low moist	80	7.60	4.67	0.89	207	0.076	0.006	0.150	0	15.0
Mozzarella—whole milk, regular	80	5.50	5.75	0.63	147	0.050	0.004	0.106	0	22.0
Mozzarella—whole milk, moist	90	6.10	7.19	0.43	163	0.060	0.005	0.119	0	25.0
Muenster	104	6.40	8.42	0.32	203	0.125	0.004	0.178	0	27.0
Neufchatel	74	2.82	6.70	0.83	21	0.080	0.004	0.113	0	22.0
Parmesan—hard	111	10.00	7.30	0.91	335	0.230	0.010	0.453	0	19.0
Parmesan—grated	129	11.80	8.50	1.06	389	0.270	0.013	0.527	0	22.0
Pimento processed	106	6.26	8.82	0.49	174	0.120	0.008	0.404	0	27.0
Port du salut	100	6.73	7.99	0.16	84	0.140	0.004	0.151	0	34.9
Provolone	100	7.13	7.54	0.61	214	0.146	0.005	0.248	0	20.0
Ricotta—part skim	39	3.23	2.25	1.45	77	0.126	0.006	0.052	0	8.8
Ricotta—whole milk	49	3.19	3.68	0.86	59	0.108	0.004	0.024	0	14.3
Romano	110	9.00	7.63	1.03	301	0.230	0.010	0.339	0	28.9
Romano—grated	128	10.50	8.86	1.20	350	0.270	0.013	0.394	0	32.9
Roquefort	105	6.10	8.93	0.57	188	0.172	0.010	0.512	0	26.0
Swiss	107	8.03	7.79	0.96	272	0.050	0.006	0.074	0	26.0
Swiss processed	95	7.00	6.97	0.60	219	0.170	0.004	0.078	0	24.0

FISH

	kcal	Protein (g)	Fat (g)	CHO (g)	Ca (mg)	Fe (mg)	B_1 (mg)	B_2 (mg)	Fiber (g)	Cholesterol (mg)
Bass—freshwater raw	32	5.36	1.05	0	22.7	0.422	0.028	0.009	0	19.3
Bluefish—baked/broiled	45	7.43	1.42	0	2.6	0.174	0.022	0.030	0	17.9
Bluefish—fried in crumbs	58	6.44	2.78	1.33	2.3	0.151	0.017	0.023	0	17
Bluefish—raw	35	5.67	1.20	0	2.0	0.136	0.016	0.023	0	16.7
Carp—raw	36	5.05	1.59	0	11.6	0.352	0.013	0.011	0	18.7
Catfish—channel—raw	33	5.16	1.20	0	11.3	0.275	0.013	0.030	0	16.4
Cod—baked w/butter	37	6.46	0.94	0	5.7	0.139	0.025	0.022	0	17.0
Cod—batter-fried	56	5.56	2.92	2.13	22.7	0.142	0.011	0.011	0	15.6
Cod—baked/broiled	30	6.46	0.24	0	4.0	0.139	0.025	0.022	0	15.6
Cod—poached	29	6.24	0.24	0	4.0	0.139	0.025	0.022	0	15.6
Cod—steamed	29	6.24	0.24	0	4.0	0.139	0.025	0.022	0	15.9
Cod—smoked	22	5.19	0.17	0	4.0	0.113	0.023	0.020	0	14.2
Cod—Atlantic—raw	23	5.05	0.19	0	4.5	0.108	0.022	0.018	0	12.2
Cod liver oil	255	0	28.40	0	0	0	0	0	0	162.0
Eel—smoked	94	5.27	7.88	0.23	26.9	0.198	0.040	0.099	0	19.8
Haddock—breaded/fried	58	5.67	3.00	2.33	11.3	0.384	0.020	0.033	0.01	18.3
Haddock—smoked	33	7.14	0.27	0	13.9	0.397	0.013	0.014	0	21.8
Haddock—raw	22	5.36	0.20	0	9.4	0.298	0.010	0.010	0	16.2
Herring—pickled	74	4.03	5.10	2.73	21.8	0.346	0.010	0.039	0	3.7
Herring—smoked/ kippered	62	6.97	3.52	0	23.8	0.428	0.036	0.090	0	22.7
Herring—canned w/liquid	59	5.64	3.86	0	41.7	0.879	0.007	0.051	0	27.5
Mackerel—fried	49	7.00	2.35	0	4.3	0.445	0.045	0.116	0	19.8
Mackerel—Atlantic— baked/broiled	74	6.78	5.05	0	4.3	0.445	0.045	0.117	0	21.3
Mackerel—Atlantic—raw	58	5.27	3.94	0	3.4	0.462	0.050	0.088	0	19.8
Mackerel—Pacific—raw	45	6.12	2.84	0	2.3	0.567	0.043	0.096	0	22.7
Northern pike—raw	25	5.47	0.20	0	16.2	0.156	0.017	0.018	0	11.0
Ocean perch—breaded/ fried	62	5.34	3.67	2.33	30.7	0.400	0.033	0.037	0.03	15.3
Pollock—baked/broiled	28	6.60	0.31	0	19.3	0.149	0.014	0.057	0	19.8
Pollock—poached	36	6.60	0.31	0	17.0	0.149	0.010	0.050	0	19.8
Salmon—broiled/baked	61	7.74	3.10	0	2.0	0.157	0.061	0.048	0	24.7
Coho salmon—steamed/ poached	52	7.77	2.14	0	8.22	0.252	0.057	0.031	0	13.9
Smoked salmon— Chinook	33	5.17	1.22	0	03.0	0.240	0.007	0.029	0	6.7
Atlantic salmon— small can	36	5.05	1.62	0	3.1	0.204	0.057	0.097	0	17.0
Pink salmon—raw	33	5.64	0.98	0	11.3	0.218	0.040	0.057	0	14.7
Sardines	59	7.00	3.24	0	108.0	0.826	0.023	0.064	0	40.4
Sea trout steelhead—raw	30	4.73	1.02	0	4.8	0.077	0.023	0.057	0	23.5
Sea trout steelhead— cooked	37	6.07	1.42	0	5.7	0.088	0.024	0.064	0	32.3
Shad—baked with bacon	57	6.58	3.20	0	6.8	0.170	0.037	0.074	0	17.0
Smelt—rainbow—raw	28	4.99	0.69	0	17.0	0.255	0.016	0.034	0	19.8
Snapper—baked or broiled	36	7.46	0.49	0	11.3	0.068	0.015	0.021	0	13.3
Snapper—raw	28	5.81	0.38	0	9.1	0.051	0.013	0.017	0	10.5
Sole/flounder—baked w/butter	40	5.34	2.00	0	5.3	0.093	0.023	0.032	0	22.7
Sole/flounder—baked/ broiled	33	6.84	0.43	0	5.3	0.093	0.023	0.032	0	19.3

FISH—continued

	kcal	Protein (g)	Fat (g)	CHO (g)	Ca (mg)	Fe (mg)	B₁ (mg)	B₂ (mg)	Fiber (g)	Cholesterol (mg)
Sole/flounder—batter-fried	83	4.47	5.10	4.07	16.7	0.239	0.057	0.042	0.01	15.0
Sole/flounder—breaded/fried	53	4.96	2.55	2.54	11.3	0.128	0.037	0.034	0	15.0
Sole/flounder—steamed	26	5.67	0.33	0	4.5	0.079	0.017	0.027	0	14.7
Sole/flounder—raw	26	5.33	0.34	0	5.1	0.102	0.025	0.022	0	13.6
Lemon sole—raw	23	4.85	0.21	0	4.8	0.088	0.026	0.023	0	17.0
Lemon sole—fried w/crumbs	56	4.56	3.12	2.64	26.9	0.176	0.020	0.023	0	18.4
Lemon sole—steamed	26	5.84	0.26	0	6.0	0.147	0.026	0.026	0	17.0
Swordfish—raw	34	5.61	1.14	0	1.1	0.230	0.010	0.027	0	11.0
Swordfish—broiled/baked	44	7.20	1.46	0	1.7	0.295	0.012	0.033	0	14.2
Trout—baked/broiled	43	7.47	1.22	0	24.3	0.690	0.024	0.064	0	20.7
Tuna—oil pack	56	8.26	2.34	0	3.8	0.395	0.010	0.030	0	5.0
Tuna—water pack	37	8.38	0.14	0	3.4	0.409	0.010	0.033	0	16.0
Tuna—raw	31	6.63	0.27	0	4.5	0.207	0.123	0.013	0	12.8
Whiting—flour/bread-fried	54	5.13	1.56	1.98	11.3	0.198	0.023	0.020	0	18.4

FRUITS

	kcal	Protein (g)	Fat (g)	CHO (g)	Ca (mg)	Fe (mg)	B₁ (mg)	B₂ (mg)	Fiber (g)	Cholesterol (mg)
Apple w/peel	16	0.055	0.100	4.31	2.05	0.051	0.005	0.004	0.709	0
Apple slices w/peel—fresh	17	0.054	0.100	4.33	2.06	0.052	0.005	0.004	0.709	0
Apple juice—canned/bottled	13	0.017	0.032	3.32	1.94	0.105	0.006	0.005	0.034	0
Apple juice—frozen concentrate	47	0.144	0.105	11.60	5.78	0.258	0.003	0.015	0.089	0
Applesauce—sweetened	22	0.052	0.052	5.67	1.11	0.111	0.003	0.008	0.397	0
Apricot—fresh halves	14	0.397	0.110	3.15	4.02	0.154	0.009	0.011	0.538	0
Apricot halves—light syrup	18	0.150	0.013	4.67	3.34	0.110	0.005	0.006	0.319	0
Apricot nectar—canned	16	0.104	0.025	4.08	2.03	0.108	0.003	0.004	0.170	0
Avocado—average	46	0.563	0.340	2.10	3.07	0.284	0.030	0.035	2.720	0
Banana—fresh slices	26	0.293	0.136	6.63	1.74	0.088	0.013	0.028	0.578	0
Blackberries—canned	26	0.370	0.040	6.54	5.98	0.184	0.008	0.011	1.011	0
Blackberries—fresh	15	0.205	0.110	3.62	9.06	0.158	0.008	0.011	1.910	0
Blackberries—frozen	18	0.334	0.122	4.45	8.26	0.173	0.008	0.013	1.460	0
Blueberries—fresh	16	0.190	0.108	4.00	1.76	0.047	0.014	0.014	0.763	0
Blueberries-frozen unsweetened	14	0.119	0.181	3.46	2.19	0.051	0.009	0.010	0.658	0
Boysenberries—frozen	14	0.314	0.075	3.46	7.73	0.240	0.015	0.010	1.100	0
Sour cherries—frozen	13	0.260	0.124	3.13	3.66	0.150	0.012	0.010	0.384	0
Sweet cherries—fresh	20	0.340	0.272	4.69	4.10	0.110	0.014	0.017	0.430	0
Sweet cherries—frozen	25	0.325	0.037	6.34	3.39	0.099	0.008	0.013	0.224	0
Cranberries—whole—raw	14	0.110	0.057	3.58	2.09	0.057	0.009	0.006	1.190	0
Cranberry/apple juice	19	0.015	0.090	4.82	2.02	0.017	0.001	0.006	0.070	0
Cranberry juice cocktail	16	0.009	0.015	4.03	0.90	0.043	0.002	0.002	0.085	0
Date—whole—each	78	0.557	0.127	20.80	9.22	0.342	0.026	0.028	2.300	0

FRUITS—continued

	kcal	Protein (g)	Fat (g)	CHO (g)	Ca (mg)	Fe (mg)	B_1 (mg)	B_2 (mg)	Fiber (g)	Cholesterol (mg)
Figs—medium—fresh	21	0.215	0.085	5.44	10.20	0.102	0.017	0.014	1.050	0
Fig—dried—each	72	0.864	0.330	18.50	40.80	0.634	0.020	0.025	3.140	0
Fruit cocktail—heavy syrup	21	0.111	0.020	5.36	1.78	0.081	0.005	0.005	0.280	0
Fruit cocktail—light syrup	16	0.114	0.020	4.23	1.80	0.082	0.005	0.005	0.284	0
Grapefruit half—pink/red	9	0.157	0.028	2.18	3.00	0.034	0.010	0.006	0.369	0
Grapefruit half—white	10	0.195	0.029	2.38	3.36	0.017	0.010	0.006	0.368	0
Grapefuit sections/fresh	9	0.179	0.028	2.29	3.33	0.025	0.010	0.006	0.370	0
Grapefruit sections—canned	17	0.160	0.028	4.38	4.02	0.114	0.010	0.006	0.313	0
Grapefruit juice—fresh	11	0.142	0.029	2.60	2.53	0.056	0.011	0.006	0.113	0
Grapefruit juice—sweetened	13	0.164	0.026	3.15	2.27	0.102	0.011	0.007	0.076	0
Grapefruit juice—unsweetened	11	0.148	0.028	2.54	1.95	0.057	0.012	0.006	0.077	0
Grapefruit juice—frozen concentrate	41	0.548	0.137	9.86	7.67	0.140	0.041	0.022	0.383	0
Grapes—Thompson	20	0.188	0.163	5.03	3.01	0.073	0.026	0.016	0.333	0
Grape juice—bottled/canned	17	0.158	0.021	4.25	2.47	0.068	0.007	0.010	0.141	0
Grape juice—frozen concentrate	51	0.184	0.088	12.60	3.68	0.102	0.015	0.026	0.492	0
Grape juice—prep frozen	15	0.053	0.026	3.62	1.13	0.029	0.004	0.007	0.142	0
Kiwi fruit	17	0.280	0.127	4.22	7.46	0.112	0.007	0.015	0.962	0
Lemon—fresh wo/peel	8	0.313	0.083	2.64	7.33	0.171	0.011	0.006	0.582	0
Lemon juice—fresh	7	0.107	0.081	2.45	2.09	0.009	0.008	0.003	0.099	0
Lemon juice—bottled	6	0.114	0.081	1.84	3.02	0.036	0.012	0.003	0.085	0
Lime—fresh	9	0.199	0.055	2.99	9.30	0.169	0.008	0.006	0.228	0
Lime juice—fresh	8	0.124	0.029	2.56	2.54	0.009	0.006	0.003	0.113	0
Lime juice—bottled	6	0.115	0.115	1.84	3.46	0.069	0.009	0.001	0.099	0
Loganberries—fresh	20	0.430	0.088	3.69	8.50	0.181	0.014	0.010	1.760	0
Loganberries—frozen	16	0.430	0.089	3.68	7.33	0.181	0.014	0.010	1.760	0
Mango—fresh—slices	19	0.146	0.077	4.83	2.92	0.360	0.016	0.016	0.997	0
Mango—fresh—whole	19	0.145	0.078	4.82	2.88	0.356	0.016	0.016	1.010	0
Cantaloupe—cubes	10	0.250	0.079	2.37	3.19	0.060	0.006	0.006	0.284	0
Casaba melon—cubes	8	0.255	0.028	1.75	1.50	0.113	0.017	0.006	0.284	0
Honeydew melon—cubes	10	0.128	0.028	2.60	1.67	0.020	0.022	0.005	0.307	0
Melon balls—mixed—frozen	9	0.239	0.023	2.25	2.79	0.008	0.005	0.006	0.295	0
Mixed fruit—dried	69	0.697	0.139	18.20	10.60	0.767	0.012	0.045	1.220	0
Mixed fruit—frozen—thawed	28	0.397	0.052	6.87	2.04	0.079	0.005	0.010	0.386	0
Nectarine	14	0.267	0.129	3.34	1.25	0.044	0.005	0.012	0.554	0
Orange	13	0.266	0.035	3.33	11.30	0.029	0.025	0.011	0.680	0
Orange sections—fresh	13	0.266	0.035	3.34	11.30	0.029	0.025	0.011	0.680	0
Mandarin oranges—canned	17	0.113	0.011	4.61	2.03	0.101	0.015	0.012	0.478	0
Orange juice—fresh	13	0.199	0.057	2.95	3.09	0.057	0.025	0.008	0.113	0
Oranged juice—frozen concentrate	45	0.679	0.059	10.80	9.05	0.099	0.079	0.018	0.313	0

FRUITS—continued

	kcal	Protein (g)	Fat (g)	CHO (g)	Ca (mg)	Fe (mg)	B₁ (mg)	B₂ (mg)	Fiber (g)	Cholesterol (mg)
Orange juice—frozen	13	0.191	0.016	3.05	2.50	0.031	0.023	0.005	0.057	0
Papaya—whole fresh	11	0.173	0.040	2.78	6.71	0.028	0.008	0.009	0.482	0
Papaya—slices fresh	12	0.174	0.040	2.77	6.68	0.060	0.008	0.009	0.482	0
Papaya nectar—canned	16	0.049	0.043	4.12	2.72	0.098	0.002	0.001	0.170	0
Peaches—fresh	12	0.199	0.026	3.14	1.30	0.031	0.005	0.012	0.489	0
Peach slices—frozen/thawed	27	0.177	0.037	6.80	0.91	0.105	0.004	0.010	0.467	0
Peach halves—heavy syrup	21	0.130	0.028	5.67	1.05	0.077	0.003	0.007	0.315	0
Peach halves—light syrup	15	0.126	0.010	4.13	1.05	0.101	0.002	0.007	0.402	0
Peach halves—dried	68	0.020	0.216	17.40	8.07	1.150	0	0.060	2.330	0
Peach nectar—canned	15	0.076	0.006	3.95	1.48	0.054	0	0.004	0.170	0
Pears—Bartlett	17	0.111	0.113	4.29	3.24	0.070	0.006	0.011	0.779	0
Pear halves—heavy syrup	21	0.057	0.036	5.42	1.44	0.061	0.004	0.006	0.395	0
Pear halves—light syrup	16	0.054	0.007	4.30	1.44	0.082	0.003	0.005	0.395	0
Pear nectar—canned	17	0.030	0.003	4.47	1.25	0.073	0	0.004	0.204	0
Pineapple slices—heavy syrup	22	0.098	0.034	5.72	3.91	0.108	0.025	0.007	0.270	0
Pineapple slices—light syrup	15	0.103	0.034	3.81	3.91	0.110	0.026	0.007	0.268	0
Pineapple—frozen sweetened	24	0.113	0.029	6.29	2.55	0.113	0.028	0.009	0.496	0
Pineapple juice—frozen concentrate	51	0.369	0.029	12.60	11.00	0.255	0.065	0.017	0.255	0
Plums	16	0.223	0.176	3.69	1.29	0.030	0.012	0.027	0.550	0
Plums—canned—heavy syrup	25	0.102	0.028	6.59	2.53	0.238	0.005	0.010	0.434	0
Plums—canned—light syrup	18	0.105	0.029	4.61	2.70	0.243	0.005	0.011	0.444	0
Prunes—dried	68	0.739	0.145	17.80	14.50	0.702	0.023	0.046	2.700	0
Prune juice—bottled	20	0.172	0.009	4.95	3.43	0.334	0.005	0.020	0.310	0
Raisins—seedless	85	0.914	0.130	22.50	13.90	0.594	0.044	0.025	1.670	0
Raspberries—fresh	14	0.256	0.157	3.27	6.22	0.162	0.009	0.026	1.770	0
Raspberries—canned w/liquid	26	0.235	0.034	6.62	2.99	0.120	0.006	0.009	1.200	0
Raspberries—frozen	29	0.197	0.044	7.42	4.30	0.184	0.005	0.013	1.300	0
Rhubarb—raw—diced	6	0.253	0.056	1.29	39.50	0.062	0.006	0.009	0.737	0
Rhubarb—cooked w/sugar	33	0.111	0.013	8.85	41.10	0.060	0.005	0.006	0.624	0
Strawberries—fresh	9	0.173	0.105	2.00	4.00	0.108	0.006	0.019	0.736	0
Strawberries—frozen	10	0.120	0.030	2.59	4.38	0.213	0.006	0.010	0.736	0
Tangerine—fresh	13	0.179	0.054	3.17	4.05	0.028	0.030	0.006	0.574	0
Tangerines—canned—light syrup	17	0.127	0.028	4.61	2.03	0.105	0.015	0.012	0.453	0
Watermelon	9	0.175	0.121	2.04	2.24	0.048	0.023	0.006	0.114	0

MEATS

	kcal	Protein (g)	Fat (g)	CHO (g)	Ca (mg)	Fe (mg)	B_1 (mg)	B_2 (mg)	Fiber (g)	Cholesterol (mg)
Beef chuck—pot roasted	108	7.20	8.64	0	3.67	0.840	0.020	0.065	0	29.0
Beef chuck—pot roasted lean	77	8.80	4.34	0	3.67	1.040	0.024	0.080	0	30.0
Beef round—pot roasted lean & fat	74	8.44	4.20	0	1.67	0.920	0.020	0.069	0	27.0
Beef round—pot roasted lean	63	8.97	2.74	0	1.33	0.980	0.021	0.074	0	27.0
Ground beef—lean	77	7.00	5.34	0	3.00	0.600	0.013	0.060	0	24.7
Ground beef—regular	82	6.67	5.94	0	3.00	0.700	0.010	0.053	0	25.3
Sirloin steak—lean	57	8.10	2.53	0	2.33	0.700	0.026	0.056	0	21.7
T-bone steak—lean & fat	92	6.80	6.97	0	2.67	0.720	0.026	0.059	0	23.7
Beef lunchmeat—thin-sliced	50	7.96	1.09	1.62	2.99	0.759	0.023	0.054	0	12.0
Beef lunchmeat—loaf/roll	87	4.06	7.42	0.82	2.99	0.659	0.030	0.062	0	18.0
Beef rib—oven roasted—lean	68	7.70	3.90	0	3.34	0.740	0.023	0.060	0	22.7
Beef round—oven roasted—lean	54	8.14	2.12	0	1.67	0.834	0.028	0.076	0	23.0
Beef rump roast—lean only	51	8.40	1.89	0	1.13	0.567	0.026	0.049	0	19.6
Beef brains—pan-fried	56	3.57	4.50	0	2.67	0.630	0.037	0.074	0	566.0
Beef heart	47	8.17	1.59	0.12	1.67	2.130	0.040	0.436	0	54.7
Beef kidney	41	7.23	0.97	0.27	5.00	2.070	0.054	1.150	0	110.0
Beef liver—fried	61	7.57	2.27	2.23	3.00	1.780	0.060	1.170	0	137.0
Beef tongue—cooked	80	6.27	5.87	0.09	2.00	0.960	0.009	0.009	0	30.4
Beef tripe—raw	28	4.14	1.12	0	36.00	0.553	0.002	0.047	0	26.9
Beef tripe—pickled	17	3.29	0.40	0	25.00	0.389	0	0.028	0	15.0
Corned beef—canned	71	7.67	4.24	0	5.67	0.590	0.006	0.042	0	24.3
Corned beef hash—canned	49	2.35	1.29	2.82	3.74	0.567	0.016	0.052	0.153	17.0
Beef—dried/cured	47	8.24	1.10	0.44	2.00	1.280	0.050	0.230	0	45.9
Beef & vegetable stew	26	1.85	1.27	1.74	3.36	0.336	0.017	0.020	0.393	8.2
Beef stew—canned	22	1.64	0.88	2.06	2.66	0.368	0.008	0.014	0.150	1.7
Burrito—beef & bean	63	3.40	2.84	6.48	26.70	0.437	0.042	0.047	0.810	8.4
Tostada w/beans & beef	49	2.72	3.06	2.98	27.50	0.319	0.012	0.036	0.583	9.1
Beef + macaroni + tomato	24	1.25	0.73	3.16	3.81	0.300	0.024	0.021	0.291	2.8
Beef enchilada	69	3.09	3.26	3.69	60.20	0.418	0.017	0.039	0.465	8.9
Frankfurter—beef	92	3.20	8.36	0.68	3.48	0.378	0.014	0.029	0	13.4
Frankfurter—beef & pork	91	3.20	8.26	0.73	2.98	0.328	0.056	0.034	0	14.4
Beef pot pie—frozen	52	1.99	2.73	4.77	2.42	0.436	0.022	0.018	0.109	5.0
Beef pie—recipe	70	2.84	4.05	5.27	3.92	0.513	0.039	0.039	0.155	5.7
Beef taco	75	4.94	4.80	3.67	30.90	0.469	0.010	0.049	0.407	16.2
Chicken meat—all-fried	62	8.67	2.59	0.48	4.86	0.383	0.024	0.056	0.002	26.5
Chicken meat—all-roasted	54	8.20	2.10	0	4.25	0.342	0.020	0.050	0	25.3
Chicken meat—all-stewed	50	7.74	1.90	0	4.05	0.330	0.014	0.046	0	23.5
Boned chicken w/broth	47	6.17	2.26	0	3.99	0.439	0.004	0.037	0	17.6
Chicken—dark meat—fried	68	8.22	3.30	0.74	5.06	0.423	0.026	0.070	0.002	27.3
Chicken—dark meat—roasted	58	7.76	2.75	0	4.25	0.377	0.020	0.064	0	26.3
Chicken—dark meat—stewed	55	7.37	2.55	0	4.05	0.385	0.016	0.057	0	24.9

MEATS—continued

	kcal	Protein (g)	Fat (g)	CHO (g)	Ca (mg)	Fe (mg)	B_1 (mg)	B_2 (mg)	Fiber (g)	Cholesterol (mg)
Chicken—light meat—fried	54	9.31	1.57	0.12	4.45	0.322	0.020	0.036	0	25.3
Chicken—light meat—roasted	49	8.77	1.28	0	4.25	0.302	0.018	0.033	0	23.9
Chicken—light meat—stewed	45	8.18	1.17	0	3.64	0.265	0.012	0.033	0	21.7
Chicken breast—no skin	47	8.80	0.99	0	4.29	0.295	0.020	0.032	0	24.0
Chicken breast meat—stewed	43	8.20	0.86	0	3.58	0.250	0.012	0.034	0	21.8
Chicken drumstick—batter fried	76	6.22	4.45	2.36	4.73	0.382	0.032	0.061	0.008	24.4
Chicken drumstick—roasted	61	7.69	3.16	0	3.27	0.376	0.020	0.061	0	26.2
Chicken wing—batter-fried	92	5.64	6.19	3.10	5.79	0.365	0.030	0.043	0.012	22.6
Chicken wing—flour-fried	91	7.40	6.28	0.67	4.43	0.354	0.017	0.039	0.009	23.0
Chicken wing—roasted	83	7.48	5.53	0	4.17	0.359	0.012	0.037	0	24.2
Chicken gizzards—simmered	44	7.73	1.04	0.32	2.58	1.180	0.008	0.070	0	54.9
Chicken hearts—simmered	52	7.49	2.23	0.03	5.27	2.560	0.017	0.206	0	68.7
Chicken livers—simmered	44	6.90	1.55	0.25	4.05	2.400	0.043	0.496	0	179.0
Chicken roll—light meat	45	5.52	2.08	0..69	11.90	0.274	0.018	0.037	0	13.9
Chicken frankfurter	73	3.67	5.52	1.93	27.00	0.567	0.019	0.033	0	28.4
Chicken a la king	54	3.12	3.93	1.93	14.70	0.289	0.012	0.049	0.154	25.6
Chicken + noodles	43	2.60	2.13	3.07	3.07	0.278	0.006	0.020	0.142	12.2
Chicken chow mein	29	2.60	1.25	1.13	6.58	0.284	0.009	0.026	0.466	8.5
Chicken curry	26	2.21	1.53	0.64	2.52	0.170	0.009	0.019	0.033	5.3
Chicken frankfurter	72	3.67	5.52	1.93	27.00	0.567	0.019	0.033	0	28.4
Chicken pot pie—frozen	53	1.84	2.84	5.08	3.70	0.382	0.020	0.020	0.210	4.9
Chicken roll—light meat	45	5.52	2.08	0.69	11.90	0.274	0.018	0.037	0	13.9
Chicken salad w/celery	97	3.82	8.90	0.47	5.92	0.239	0.012	0.028	0.109	17.3
Chicken patty sandwich	79	4.48	4.06	6.10	7.95	0.338	0.052	0.047	0.244	12.3
Chicken broth—from dry	2	0.16	0.13	0.17	1.74	0.009	0	0.004	0.001	0.1
Chicken broth—from cube	2	0.11	0.04	0.18	0.04	0.014	0.001	0.003	0	0.1
Chicken noodle soup	9	0.48	0.29	1.10	2.00	0.092	0.006	0.007	0.085	0.8
Tostada w/beans/chicken	45	3.50	2.06	3.38	29.30	0.305	0.013	0.034	0.668	9.6
Chicken taco	63	5.60	3.03	3.67	31.60	0.237	0.014	0.043	0.407	16.5
Chicken enchilada	64	3.38	2.48	3.69	60.50	0.359	0.018	0.036	0.465	9.1
Turkey dark meat—roasted	53	8.10	2.05	0	9.11	0.662	0.018	0.070	0	24.0
Turkey white meat—roasted	44	8.48	0.91	0	5.47	0.380	0.017	0.037	0	19.6
Turkey breast—barbecued	40	6.39	1.40	0	2.00	0.120	0.010	0.030	0	16.0
Turkey gizzards	46	8.34	1.10	0.17	4.32	1.540	0.009	0.093	0	65.6
Turkey hearts	50	7.58	1.73	0.58	3.72	1.950	0.019	0.250	0	64.0
Turkey livers	48	6.80	1.69	0.97	3.02	2.210	0.015	0.404	0	177.0
Turkey loaf	31	6.38	0.45	0	2.00	0.113	0.011	0.030	0	11.6
Turkey roll	41	5.27	2.03	0.15	11.40	0.358	0.025	0.064	0	11.9
Turkey bologna	56	3.86	4.27	0.27	23.40	0.432	0.015	0.047	0	28.0
Turkey frankfurter	64	4.05	5.22	0.42	36.50	0.485	0.023	0.050	0	24.6
Turkey ham	36	5.37	1.49	0.42	2.49	0.776	0.020	0.075	0	15.9
Turkey pastrami	37	5.22	1.75	0.43	2.49	0.403	0.022	0.075	0	14.9
Turkey salami	55	4.62	3.89	0.15	5.47	0.463	0.029	0.075	0	22.9
Turkey pot pie—frozen	51	1.80	2.75	4.65	7.79	0.256	0.020	0.020	0.110	2.4

EGGS

	kcal	Protein (g)	Fat (g)	CHO (g)	Ca (mg)	Fe (mg)	B_1 (mg)	B_2 (mg)	Fiber (g)	Cholesterol (mg)
Egg white, cooked	13	2.68	0	0.33	3.20	0.008	0.002	0.072	0	0
Egg yolk, cooked	108	4.76	8.73	0.07	44.40	1.620	0.044	0.121	0	355.0
Egg, fried in butter	56	3.54	3.45	0.38	15.70	0.536	0.018	0.148	0	129.0
Egg, hard cooked	40	3.52	2.79	0.34	13.80	0.474	0.014	0.132	0	113.0
Egg, poached	40	3.50	2.79	0.34	13.80	0.474	0.014	0.132	0	113.0
Egg, scrambled milk + butter	40	2.88	2.57	0.61	23.90	0.412	0.013	0.106	0	93.9
Egg raw—large	40	3.52	2.79	0.34	13.80	0.474	0.017	0.139	0	113.0
Egg white—raw	13	2.68	0	0.33	3.20	0.008	0.002	0.075	0	0
Egg yolk, raw	108	4.76	8.73	0.07	44.40	1.620	0.051	0.126	0	355.0
Egg substitute, frozen	45	3.20	3.15	0.91	20.80	0.562	0.034	0.110	0	0.5
Egg substitute, powder	125	15.60	3.66	6.12	90.70	0.879	0.062	0.493	0	162.0

DAIRY PRODUCTS

	kcal	Protein (g)	Fat (g)	CHO (g)	Ca (mg)	Fe (mg)	B_1 (mg)	B_2 (mg)	Fiber (g)	Cholesterol (mg)
Milk—1% lowfat	12	0.93	0.30	1.36	34.9	0.014	0.011	0.047	0	1.16
Milk—2% lowfat	14	0.94	0.56	1.36	34.5	0.012	0.011	0.047	0	2.56
Milk—skim	10	0.97	0.05	1.38	34.9	0.012	0.010	0.040	0	0.46
Milk—whole	17	0.93	0.95	1.32	33.8	0.014	0.010	0.046	0	3.83
Buttermilk	12	0.94	0.25	1.35	33.0	0.014	0.010	0.044	0	1.04
Milk—instant nonfat dry	102	9.96	0.21	14.80	349.0	0.088	0.117	0.496	0	5.00
Canned skim milk— evaporated	22	2.11	0.06	3.22	82.0	0.078	0.013	0.088	0	1.11
Canned whole milk— evaporated	38	1.91	2.20	2.81	73.9	0.054	0.014	0.090	0	8.33
Carob flavor mix—powder	106	0.47	0.05	26.50	0	1.300	0.002	0	4.020	0
Chocolate milk—1%	18	0.92	0.28	2.96	32.5	0.068	0.010	0.047	0.425	0.79
Chocolate milk—2%	20	0.91	0.57	2.95	32.2	0.068	0.010	0.046	0.425	1.93
Chocolate milk—whole	24	0.90	0.96	2.94	31.8	0.068	0.010	0.046	0.425	3.52
Hot cocoa—with whole milk	25	1.03	1.03	2.93	33.8	0.088	0.012	0.049	0.340	3.74
Instant breakfast w/2% milk	25	1.52	0.47	3.50	31.0	0.807	0.040	0.048	0	1.82
Instant breakfast w/1% milk	23	1.51	0.25	3.50	31.3	0.807	0.040	0.048	0	1.00
Instant breakfast w/skim milk	22	1.55	0.04	3.50	31.4	0.804	0.039	0.041	0	0.40
Instant breakfast w/whole milk	28	1.51	0.82	3.47	30.4	0.807	0.040	0.047	0	3.33
Egg nog	38	1.08	2.12	3.84	36.8	0.057	0.010	0.054	0	16.60
Kefir	20	1.13	0.55	1.07	42.6	0.060	0.055	0.054	0	1.22
Malt powder—chocolate flavored	107	1.49	1.08	24.80	17.6	0.648	0.049	0.057	0.540	1.35
Malted milk powder	117	3.12	2.30	21.50	85.0	0.209	0.143	0.260	0.405	5.40
Malted milk drink— chocolate	25	1.00	0.95	3.19	32.5	0.064	0.014	0.047	0.043	3.64

DAIRY PRODUCTS—*continued*

	kcal	Protein (g)	Fat (g)	CHO (g)	Ca (mg)	Fe (mg)	B₁ (mg)	B₂ (mg)	Fiber (g)	Cholesterol (mg)
Chocolate milkshake	36	0.96	1.05	5.80	32.0	0.088	0.016	0.069	0.035	3.70
Strawberry milkshake	32	0.95	0.80	5.35	32.0	0.030	0.013	0.055	0.024	3.10
Vanilla milkshake	32	0.98	0.84	5.09	34.5	0.026	0.013	0.052	0.019	3.20
Ovaltine powder— chocolate flavored	102	2.00	0.85	23.70	134.0	6.190	0.719	0.772	0.013	0
Ovaltine powder—malt flavored	104	2.53	0.24	23.60	106.0	5.820	0.772	1.010	0.040	0
Ovaltine drink—chocolate flavored	24	1.02	0.94	3.12	41.9	0.510	0.067	0.104	0.001	3.53
Ovaltine drink—malt flavored	24	1.06	0.89	3.10	39.7	0.480	0.072	0.124	0.003	3.53
Milk—goat	20	1.00	1.17	1.27	37.9	0.014	0.014	0.039	0	3.25
Milk—sheep	31	1.70	1.99	1.52	54.8	0.028	0.018	0.100	0	0
Milk—soybean	9	0.78	0.54	0.51	1.2	0.163	0.046	0.020	0	0
Ice cream—regular-vanilla	57	1.02	3.05	6.76	37.5	0.026	0.011	0.070	0	12.60
Ice cream—rich-vanilla	67	0.79	4.54	6.13	28.9	0.019	0.008	0.054	0	16.90
Ice cream—soft-serve	62	1.15	3.69	6.28	38.7	0.070	0.013	0.073	0	25.00
Creamsicle ice cream bar	44	0.52	1.33	7.56	19.8	0	0.009	0.034	0	0
Drumstick ice cream bar	88	1.23	4.68	10.20	31.7	0.047	0.009	0.043	0	0
Fudgesicle ice cream bar	35	1.48	0.08	7.22	50.0	0.039	0.012	0.070	0	0
Ice milk	40	1.12	1.22	6.28	38.0	0.039	0.016	0.075	0	3.90
Ice milk—soft serve— 3% fat	36	1.30	0.75	6.22	44.4	0.045	0.019	0.088	0	2.10
Yogurt—coffee-vanilla	24	1.40	0.35	3.90	48.5	0.020	0.012	0.057	0	1.42
Yogurt—lowfat with fruit	29	1.24	0.31	5.37	43.0	0.020	0.010	0.050	0	1.25
Yogurt—lowfat-plain	18	1.49	0.43	2.00	51.8	0.022	0.012	0.060	0	1.75
Yogurt—nonfat milk	16	1.62	0.05	2.17	56.5	0.025	0.014	0.066	0	0.50
Yogurt—whole milk	17	0.98	0.92	1.32	34.3	0.014	0.008	0.040	0	3.68

VEGETABLES

	kcal	Protein (g)	Fat (g)	CHO (g)	Ca (mg)	Fe (mg)	B₁ (mg)	B₂ (mg)	Fiber (g)	Cholesterol (mg)
Alfalfa sprouts	9	1.13	0.200	1.07	9.5	0.272	0.021	0.036	1.030	0
Artichoke hearts— marinated	28	0.680	0.250	2.18	6.5	0.270	0.010	0.029	1.780	0
Asparagus—raw spears	6	0.865	0.063	1.05	6.4	0.193	0.032	0.035	0.395	0
Asparagus—canned spears	5	0.606	0.184	0.70	3.9	0.177	0.017	0.025	0.454	0
Bamboo shoots—sliced— raw	8	0.738	0.088	1.47	3.8	0.143	0.043	0.020	0.738	0
Bamboo shoots—sliced, canned	5	0.489	0.113	0.91	2.2	0.090	0.007	0.007	0.706	0
Bean sprouts—fresh raw	9	0.861	0.050	1.68	3.8	0.258	0.024	0.035	0.736	0
Bean sprouts—boiled	6	0.576	0.025	1.19	3.4	0.185	0.014	0.029	0.572	0
Bean sprouts—stir fried	14	1.220	0.059	3.00	3.7	0.549	0.040	0.050	0.777	0
Black beans—cooked	37	2.500	0.152	6.72	7.8	0.593	0.069	0.017	2.540	0

VEGETABLES—continued

	kcal	Protein (g)	Fat (g)	CHO (g)	Ca (mg)	Fe (mg)	B_1 (mg)	B_2 (mg)	Fiber (g)	Cholesterol (mg)
Green beans—raw uncooked	9	0.515	0.034	2.02	10.6	0.363	0.024	0.030	0.644	0
Green beans—fresh— cooked	10	0.535	0.082	2.24	13.2	0.363	0.021	0.027	0.737	0
Green beans—frozen— cooked	8	0.386	0.038	1.73	12.8	0.233	0.014	0.021	0.880	0
Green beans—canned/ drained	6	0.326	0.028	1.28	7.6	0.256	0.004	0.016	0.378	0
Red kidney beans—dry	94	6.690	0.234	16.90	40.5	2.330	0.150	0.062	6.160	0
Lima beans—dry large	96	6.080	0.194	18.00	22.9	2.130	0.144	0.057	8.600	0
Lima beans—fresh— cooked	35	1.930	0.090	6.70	9.0	0.695	0.040	0.027	2.670	0
Lima beans—dry small	98	5.790	0.397	18.20	18.4	2.270	0.136	0.048	8.500	0
Lima beans—canned/ drained	27	1.530	0.100	5.20	8.0	0.487	0.010	0.013	2.420	0
Beans/w/franks—canned	40	1.900	1.860	4.37	13.6	0.490	0.016	0.016	1.950	1.7
Pork & beans—canned	32	1.500	0.413	5.95	17.4	0.470	0.013	0.017	1.560	1.9
Navy beans—dry, cooked	40	2.460	0.162	7.77	19.9	0.703	0.057	0.017	2.490	0
Pinto beans—dry, cooked	39	2.320	0.148	7.28	13.6	0.741	0.053	0.026	3.230	0
Refried beans—canned	30	1.770	0.303	5.24	13.2	0.500	0.014	0.016	2.470	0
Soybeans—dry	118	10.400	5.650	8.55	78.5	4.450	0.248	0.247	1.570	0
White beans—dry	95	5.990	0.334	17.70	36.0	2.190	0.210	0.059	0.766	0
White beans—dry, cooked	40	2.550	0.182	7.32	20.7	0.808	0.067	0.017	2.230	0
Yellow wax beans—raw	9	0.515	0.034	2.02	10.6	0.294	0.024	0.030	0.644	0
Yellow wax beans—raw	10	0.535	0.082	2.24	13.2	0.363	0.021	0.027	0.726	0
Yellow wax beans—frozen	8	0.386	0.038	1.73	12.8	0.233	0.014	0.021	0.880	0
Beets—cooked	9	0.300	0.014	1.90	3.1	0.176	0.009	0.004	0.539	0
Beets—pickled slices	18	0.227	0.028	4.63	3.1	0.116	0.006	0.014	0.587	0
Broccoli—raw chopped	8	0.844	0.097	1.49	13.5	0.251	0.019	0.034	0.934	0
Broccoli—raw spears	8	0.845	0.098	1.49	13.5	0.250	0.018	0.034	0.935	0
Broccoli—frozen cooked spears	8	0.879	0.034	1.51	14.5	0.173	0.015	0.023	0.826	0
Brussels sprouts—raw	12	0.960	0.084	2.54	11.6	0.396	0.039	0.026	1.260	0
Brussels sprouts—cooked	11	1.090	0.145	2.45	10.2	0.342	0.030	0.023	1.220	0
Brussels sprouts—frozen cooked	12	1.030	0.112	2.36	7.0	0.210	0.029	0.032	1.230	0
Cabbage—raw, shredded	7	0.340	0.049	1.52	13.0	0.162	0.015	0.009	0.680	0
Cabbage—cooked	6	0.272	0.070	1.35	9.5	0.110	0.016	0.016	0.661	0
Bok choy—raw, shredded	4	0.425	0.057	0.62	30.0	0.227	0.011	0.020	0.486	0
Bok choy—cooked	3	0.442	0.045	0.51	26.3	0.295	0.009	0.018	0.454	0
Red cabbage—raw	8	0.393	0.073	1.74	14.6	0.142	0.018	0.009	0.648	0
Red cabbage—cooked	6	0.299	0.057	1.32	10.6	0.102	0.010	0.006	1.567	0
Carrot—whole, raw	12	0.291	0.055	2.87	7.5	0.142	0.028	0.017	1.906	0
Carrot—grated, raw	12	0.289	0.052	2.88	7.7	0.142	0.027	0.016	0.907	0
Carrots—sliced, cooked	13	0.309	0.050	2.97	8.7	0.176	0.010	0.016	0.992	0
Carrots—frozen, cooked	10	0.338	0.031	2.34	8.2	0.136	0.008	0.010	1.050	0
Carrots—canned, drained	7	0.183	0.054	1.57	7.4	0.181	0.005	0.009	0.435	0
Carrot juice	11	0.267	0.041	2.63	6.7	0.130	0.026	0.015	0.385	0
Cauliflower—raw	7	0.561	0.051	1.39	7.9	0.164	0.022	0.016	0.720	0
Cauliflower—cooked	7	0.530	0.050	1.31	7.8	0.119	0.018	0.018	0.622	0

VEGETABLES—continued

	kcal	Protein (g)	Fat (g)	CHO (g)	Ca (mg)	Fe (mg)	B_1 (mg)	B_2 (mg)	Fiber (g)	Cholesterol (mg)
Cauliflower—frozen, cooked	5	0.457	0.061	1.06	4.9	0.116	0.010	0.015	0.535	0
Celery—raw—chopped	5	0.189	0.033	1.03	10.4	0.137	0.009	0.009	0.472	0
Swiss chard—raw	5	0.510	0.057	1.06	14.5	0.510	0.011	0.025	0.512	0
Swiss chard—cooked	6	0.533	0.023	1.17	16.5	0.642	0.010	0.024	0.616	0
Collards—fresh	5	0.445	0.062	1.07	33.0	0.299	0.009	0.018	0.590	0
Collards—fresh, cooked	4	0.313	0.043	0.75	22.0	0.116	0.005	0.012	0.798	0
Collards—frozen, cooked	10	0.840	0.115	2.02	59.5	0.317	0.013	0.033	0.794	0
Corn—kernels raw	24	0.913	0.335	5.38	0.6	0.147	0.057	0.017	1.220	0
Corn on the cob—cooked	31	0.943	0.363	7.14	0.6	0.173	0.061	0.020	1.190	0
Corn—cooked from frozen	23	0.857	0.020	5.80	0.6	0.085	0.020	0.020	1.190	0
Corn—canned, drained	23	0.743	0.283	5.26	1.4	0.142	0.009	0.014	0.398	0
Corn—canned cream style	21	0.494	0.119	5.14	0.9	0.108	0.007	0.015	0.354	0
Cucumber slices w/peel	4	0.153	0.037	0.82	4.0	0.079	0.009	0.006	0.329	0
Eggplant—cooked	8	0.236	0.066	1.88	1.7	0.099	0.022	0.006	1.060	0
Escarole/curly endive—chopped	5	0.354	0.057	0.95	14.7	0.235	0.023	0.022	0.369	0
Garbanzo/chickpeas—dry	103	5.470	1.720	17.20	29.9	1.770	0.135	0.060	5.390	0
Garbanzo/chickpeas—cooked	47	2.500	0.735	7.78	13.8	0.819	0.033	0.018	1.920	0
Jerusalem artichoke—raw	22	0.567	0.004	4.95	4.0	0.964	0.057	0.017	0.369	0
Kale—fresh, chopped	14	0.935	0.198	2.84	38.0	0.482	0.031	0.037	1.650	0
Kohlrabi—raw slices	8	0.482	0.028	1.76	6.9	0.113	0.014	0.006	0.405	0
Kohlrabi—cooked	8	0.510	0.030	1.96	7.0	0.113	0.011	0.006	0.395	0
Leeks—chopped raw	17	0.425	0.085	4.00	16.7	0.594	0.017	0.008	0.668	0
Leeks—cooked, chopped	9	0.230	0.057	2.16	8.5	0.310	0.007	0.006	0.927	0
Lentils—dry	96	7.960	0.273	16.20	14.6	2.550	0.135	0.069	3.400	0
Lentils—cooked from dry	33	2.560	0.106	5.73	5.3	0.944	0.048	0.020	1.430	0
Lentils—sprouted, raw	30	2.540	0.156	6.30	7.0	0.909	0.065	0.036	1.150	0
Lettuce—butterhead	4	0.367	0.062	0.66	9.5	0.085	0.017	0.017	0.397	0
Lettuce—iceberg	4	0.286	0.054	0.59	5.4	0.142	0.013	0.009	0.347	0
Lettuce—Romaine	5	0.459	0.057	0.67	10.2	0.312	0.028	0.028	0.482	0
Mushrooms—raw sliced	7	0.593	0.119	1.32	1.4	0.352	0.029	0.127	0.508	0
Mushrooms—cooked	8	0.614	0.134	1.46	1.7	0.494	0.020	0.085	0.625	0
Mushrooms—canned, drained	7	0.530	0.082	1.40	3.1	0.224	0.017	0.063	0.596	0
Mustard greens—fresh	7	0.764	0.057	1.39	29.4	0.414	0.023	0.031	0.764	0
Mustard greens—cooked	4	0.640	0.068	0.60	21.0	0.316	0.012	0.018	0.587	0
Okra pods—cooked	9	0.530	0.048	2.04	17.9	0.128	0.037	0.016	0.624	0
Okra slices—cooked	11	0.589	0.085	2.32	27.1	0.190	0.028	0.035	0.709	0
Onions—chopped, raw	10	0.335	0.074	2.07	7.1	0.105	0.017	0.003	0.454	0
Onion slices—raw	10	0.335	0.074	2.08	7.2	0.105	0.017	0.003	0.454	0
Onion—dehydrated flakes	91	2.530	0.122	23.70	72.9	0.446	0.022	0.018	2.510	0
Onion rings—frozen, heated	115	1.520	7.570	10.80	8.8	0.482	0.079	0.040	0.240	0
Parsley—freeze dried	81	8.910	1.420	11.90	40.5	15.200	0.304	0.648	22.000	0
Parsley—fresh chopped	9	0.624	0.085	1.96	36.9	1.760	0.023	0.031	1.550	0
Parsnips—sliced raw	21	0.341	0.085	5.09	10.0	0.167	0.026	0.014	1.280	0
Fresh peas—uncooked	23	1.530	0.113	4.10	7.0	0.416	0.075	0.037	1.380	0
Peas—cooked	24	1.520	0.060	4.43	7.8	0.438	0.073	0.042	1.360	0
Peas—frozen, cooked	22	1.460	0.078	4.04	6.7	0.443	0.080	0.050	1.280	0
Peas—edible pods—fresh	12	0.794	0.057	2.15	12.1	0.589	0.043	0.023	0.794	0
Split peas—dry	97	6.970	0.328	17.10	15.5	1.250	0.206	0.061	4.030	0

VEGETABLES—continued

	kcal	Protein (g)	Fat (g)	CHO (g)	Ca (mg)	Fe (mg)	B₁ (mg)	B₂ (mg)	Fiber (g)	Cholesterol (mg)
Peas + carrots—frozen, cooked	14	0.875	0.120	2.87	6.4	0.266	0.064	0.020	1.170	0
Green chili pepper—raw	11	0.557	0.057	2.68	5.0	0.340	0.026	0.026	0.504	0
Red chili peppers—raw/ chopped	11	0.567	0.057	2.68	4.9	0.340	0.026	0.026	0.454	0
Jalapeno peppers—canned chopped	7	0.225	0.170	1.39	7.5	0.792	0.008	0.014	0.850	0
Baked potato with skin	31	0.653	0.028	7.16	2.8	0.386	0.030	0.009	0.660	0
Baked potato—flesh only	26	0.556	0.029	6.10	1.5	0.100	0.030	0.006	0.436	0
Potato skin—oven baked	56	1.220	0.029	13.20	9.8	1.080	0.035	0.034	1.130	0
Potato + peel— microwaved	30	0.692	0.028	6.83	3.1	0.350	0.034	0.009	0.660	0
Peeled potato—boiled	24	0.485	0.029	5.67	2.1	0.088	0.028	0.005	0.426	0
French fries—oven heated	63	0.980	2.480	9.64	2.3	0.380	0.035	0.009	0.567	0
French fries—frozen— vegetable oil	90	1.140	4.690	11.20	5.7	0.215	0.050	0.008	0.567	0
Cottage-fried potatoes	62	0.975	2.320	9.64	2.8	0.425	0.034	0.009	0.567	0
Hash-brown potatoes	30	0.343	1.980	3.02	1.1	0.115	0.010	0.003	0.567	0
Mashed potatoes prep/ milk	22	0.548	0.166	4.98	7.4	0.077	0.025	0.011	0.405	0.5
Mashed potatoes—milk & margarine	30	0.533	1.200	4.74	7.3	0.074	0.024	0.014	0.405	0.5
Potato pancakes	88	1.730	4.700	9.85	7.8	0.451	0.039	0.035	0.563	34.7
Potatoes au gratin mix	26	0.653	1.170	3.65	23.5	0.090	0.006	0.023	0.487	1.4
Scalloped potatoes— recipe	24	0.813	1.040	3.05	16.2	0.163	0.020	0.026	0.289	3.4
Potato chips	148	1.590	10.000	14.70	7.0	0.339	0.040	0.006	1.360	0
Potato flour	100	2.260	0.226	22.60	9.3	4.880	0.119	0.040	0.317	0
Pumpkin—canned	10	0.311	0.080	2.28	7.4	0.394	0.007	0.015	0.519	0
Red radishes	4	0.170	0.151	1.01	5.7	0.082	0.001	0.013	0.624	0
Rutabaga—cooked cubes	10	0.314	0.053	2.19	12.0	0.133	0.020	0.010	0.434	0
Sauerkraut—canned liquid	5	0.258	0.040	1.21	8.7	0.417	0.006	0.006	0.529	0
Soybeans—mature, raw	37	3.700	1.900	3.17	19.4	0.599	0.096	0.033	0.656	0
Spinach—cooked from fresh	7	0.843	0.074	1.06	38.4	1.010	0.027	0.067	0.702	0
Summer squash—raw slices	6	0.334	0.061	1.23	5.7	0.130	0.018	0.010	0.425	0
Zucchini squash—cooked	5	0.181	0.014	1.11	3.6	0.099	0.012	0.012	0.567	0
Acorn squash—boiled/ mashed	10	0.190	0.023	2.49	7.5	0.159	0.028	0.002	0.680	0
Butternut squash/baked— cube	12	0.256	0.026	2.97	11.6	0.170	0.020	0.005	0.794	0
Spaghetti squash—baked/ boiled	8	0.187	0.073	1.83	6.0	0.095	0.010	0.006	0.794	0
Winter squash—boiled	10	0.319	0.050	2.40	5.2	0.136	0.018	0.006	0.794	0
Sweet potato—baked in skin	29	0.487	0.032	6.89	8.0	0.129	0.020	0.036	0.850	0
Candied sweet potatoes	39	0.246	0.920	7.91	7.3	0.324	0.005	0.012	0.545	0
Tofu (soybean curd)	22	2.290	1.360	0.53	29.7	1.520	0.023	0.015	0.343	0
Tomato—fresh whole	6	0.251	0.060	1.23	2.1	0.136	0.017	0.014	0.415	0
Tomatoes—whole canned	6	0.265	0.070	1.22	7.4	0.171	0.013	0.009	0.298	0

VEGETABLES—continued

	kcal	Protein (g)	Fat (g)	CHO (g)	Ca (mg)	Fe (mg)	B₁ (mg)	B₂ (mg)	Fiber (g)	Cholesterol (mg)
Tomato sauce—canned	9	0.376	0.047	2.04	3.9	0.218	0.019	0.016	0.425	0
Tomato paste—canned	24	1.070	0.249	5.33	9.9	0.848	0.044	0.054	1.210	0
Tomato juice—canned	5	0.215	0.017	1.20	2.6	0.164	0.013	0.009	0.220	0
Turnip cubes—raw	8	0.255	0.028	1.76	8.5	0.085	0.011	0.009	0.587	0
Mixed vegetables—frozen, cooked	17	0.812	0.043	3.70	7.2	0.232	0.020	0.034	1.120	0
Vegetable juice cocktail	6	0.178	0.026	1.29	3.1	0.119	0.012	0.008	0.178	0
Water chestnuts—raw	30	0.398	0.027	6.77	3.2	0.170	0.040	0.057	0.869	0
Watercress—fresh	3	0.650	0.033	0.37	33.4	0.050	0.025	0.033	0.719	0
White yams—raw	34	0.438	0.049	7.90	8.7	0.153	0.032	0.009	0.822	0

SALAD BAR

	kcal	Protein (g)	Fat (g)	CHO (g)	Ca (mg)	Fe (mg)	B₁ (mg)	B₂ (mg)	Fiber (g)	Cholesterol (mg)
Alfalfa sprouts	9	1.130	0.196	1.07	9.5	0.272	0.021	0.036	1.030	0
Artichoke hearts, marinated	28	0.680	2.250	2.18	6.5	0.270	0.010	0.029	1.780	0
Asparagus	6	0.867	0.062	1.05	6.4	0.193	0.032	0.035	0.432	0
Avocado	46	0.563	4.340	2.10	3.1	0.284	0.030	0.035	2.720	0
Bacon, regular	163	8.640	14.000	0.16	3.0	0.482	0.195	0.080	0	23.9
Bean sprouts	9	0.861	0.050	1.68	3.8	0.258	0.024	0.035	0.7365	0
Beets	9	0.300	0.013	1.90	3.0	0.176	0.009	0.004	0.567	0
Beets, canned, diced	9	0.260	0.040	2.04	4.3	0.517	0.003	0.012	0.590	0
Broccoli, raw	8	0.844	0.097	1.49	13.5	0.251	0.019	0.034	0.934	0
Cabbage	6	0.340	0.049	1.52	13.0	0.162	0.015	0.009	0.680	0
Cabbage, red	8	0.393	0.073	1.74	14.6	0.142	0.018	0.009	0.648	0
Carrots, grated	12	0.289	0.052	2.88	7.7	0.142	0.027	0.016	0.907	0
Cauliflower	7	0.561	0.051	1.39	7.9	0.164	0.022	0.016	0.720	0
Celery	5	0.189	0.030	1.03	10.4	0.137	0.009	0.009	0.472	0
Chicken salad	97	3.820	8.900	0.47	5.9	0.239	0.012	0.028	0.109	17.3
Crab, cooked	24	5.050	0.561	0.14	12.9	0.104	0.012	0.044	0	18.0
Croutons, dry bread cubes	105	3.690	1.040	20.50	35.0	1.020	0.099	0.099	0.085	0
Cucumber slices	4	0.153	0.037	0.82	4.0	0.079	0.009	0.006	0.329	0
Egg, chopped	40	3.520	2.790	0.34	13.8	0.475	0.014	0.133	0	113
Escarole/curly endive	5	0.354	0.057	0.95	14.7	0.235	0.023	0.022	0.369	0
Garbanzo/chickpeas, cooked	47	2.500	0.735	7.78	13.8	0.819	0.033	0.018	1.920	0
Green pepper, sweet	7	0.244	0.130	1.50	1.7	0.357	0.024	0.014	0.454	0
Ham salad	52	5.000	3.000	0.88	2.0	0.280	0.244	0.072	0	16
Ham, minced	74	4.620	5.860	0.53	2.7	0.216	0.203	0.054	0	20.2
Leeks	17	0.425	0.085	4.00	16.7	0.594	0.017	0.008	0.688	0
Lettuce, butterhead	4	0.366	0.062	0.66	9.5	0.085	0.017	0.017	0.370	0
Lettuce, iceberg	4	0.287	0.054	0.59	5.4	0.142	0.013	0.009	0.370	0
Lettuce, loose leaf	5	0.369	0.085	0.99	19.2	0.397	0.014	0.023	0.391	0
Lettuce, Romaine	5	0.459	0.057	0.67	10.2	0.312	0.028	0.028	0.482	0
Lobster meat	28	5.800	0.168	0.36	17.2	0.111	0.020	0.019	0	20.3

SALAD BAR—continued

	kcal	Protein (g)	Fat (g)	CHO (g)	Ca (mg)	Fe (mg)	B_1 (mg)	B_2 (mg)	Fiber (g)	Cholesterol (mg)
Mushrooms, raw	7	0.593	0.119	1.32	1.4	0.352	0.029	0.127	0.508	0
Onions	16	0.335	0.074	2.07	7.1	0.105	0.017	0.003	0.454	0
Parmesan cheese, grated	129	11.800	8.500	1.06	389	0.270	0.013	0.109	0	22.0
Peas, cooked	22	1.460	0.078	4.04	6.7	0.443	0.080	0.050	1.280	0
Sesame seed kernels, dried	167	7.480	15.500	2.66	37.2	2.210	0.204	0.024	1.950	0
Shrimp, boiled	28	5.930	0.306	0	11.0	0.876	0.009	0.009	0	55.3
Spinach, fresh	6	0.810	0.099	0.99	28.0	0.770	0.022	0.054	0.947	0
Sunflower seeds, dry	162	6.460	14.000	5.32	32.9	1.920	0.650	0.070	1.970	0
Tomatoes	6	0.252	0.061	1.23	1.9	0.135	0.017	0.014	0.416	0
Tuna salad	53	4.550	2.630	2.67	4.8	0.282	0.009	0.019	0.340	3.73
Turkey meat	41	5.270	2.030	0.15	11.4	0.358	0.025	0.064	0	11.9

VARIETY

	kcal	Protein (g)	Fat (g)	CHO (g)	Ca (mg)	Fe (mg)	B_1 (mg)	B_2 (mg)	Fiber (g)	Cholesterol (mg)
Chips & crackers										
Doritos—nacho flavor	139	2.20	6.79	18.00	17.0	0.399	0.040	0.030	1.10	0
Doritos—taco flavor	140	2.60	6.59	17.60	44.9	0.699	0.080	0.090	1.10	0
Potato chips—sour cream & onion	153	2.40	9.48	14.60	21.0	0.474	0.040	0.055	1.35	1.0
Wheat cracker—thin	124	3.19	4.96	17.70	10.6	1.060	0.142	0.106	1.84	0
Whole wheat crackers	124	3.19	5.32	17.70	10.6	1.850	0.070	0.106	2.94	0
Condiments										
Catsup	30	0.52	0.11	7.17	6.2	0.228	0.026	0.020	0.45	0
Mustard	21	1.34	1.25	1.81	23.8	0.567	0.024	0.057	0.11	0
Soy sauce	14	1.46	0.02	2.40	4.7	0.567	0.014	0.036	0	0
Deli meats										
Bologna—beef	89	3.32	8.04	0.56	3.7	0.394	0.016	0.036	0	16.0
Bratwurst	92	4.05	7.90	0.84	13.8	0.292	0.070	0.064	0	17.8
Keilbasa sausage	88	3.76	7.70	0.61	12.0	0.414	0.064	0.061	0	18.5
Knockwurst sausage	87	3.37	7.88	0.05	2.9	0.258	0.097	0.040	0	16.3
Liverwurst	93	4.00	8.10	0.63	7.9	1.810	0.077	0.291	0	44.1
Pepperoni sausage	140	5.94	12.50	0.80	2.8	0.397	0.09	0.07		9.79
Polish sausage	92	3.99	8.13	0.46	3.0	0.409	0.142	0.042	0	20.0
Salami—beef	72	4.17	5.69	0.70	2.47	0.567	0.036	0.073	0	17.3
Salami—pork & beef	72	3.94	5.70	0.64	3.68	0.755	0.068	0.106	0	18.5
Salami—turkey	55	4.62	3.89	0.15	5.47	0.463	0.029	0.075	0	22.9
Salami—dry—beef & pork	120	6.49	9.75	0.74	2.84	0.425	0.170	0.082	0	22.7
Turkey pastrami	37	5.22	1.75	0.43	2.49	0.403	0.022	0.075	0	14.9
Mexican foods										
Beef taco	75.2	4.94	4.80	3.67	30.9	0.469	0.01	0.049	0.407	16.2
Beef enchilada	69.0	3.09	3.26	3.69	60.2	0.418	0.017	0.039	0.465	8.93
Cheese enchilada	78.0	3.12	4.2	3.78	108.0	0.324	0.015	0.050	0.465	10.2
Chicken enchilada	63.6	3.38	2.48	3.69	60.5	0.359	0.018	0.036	0.465	9.10
Corn tortilla, enriched, regular	61.4	1.89	0.964	12.30	39.7	0.567	0.047	0.028	2.27	0

VARIETY—continued

	kcal	Protein (g)	Fat (g)	CHO (g)	Ca (mg)	Fe (mg)	B_1 (mg)	B_2 (mg)	Fiber (g)	Cholesterol (mg)
Mexican Foods—continued										
Corn tortilla, enriched, thin	61.0	1.64	0.95	12.30	39.8	0.567	0.046	0.028	2.26	0
Corn tortilla, fried	82.2	2.08	2.84	12.30	39.7	0.567	0.047	0.028	2.27	0
Enchirito	60.4	3.15	2.75	3.31	51.5	0.410	0.015	0.037	0.748	9.18
Flour tortilla	84	2.07	2.15	15.50	17.0	0.440	0.102	0.062	0.800	0
Refried beans, canned	30.3	1.77	0.303	5.24	13.2	0.500	0.014	0.016	2.47	0
Nuts & seeds										
Almonds—dried, chopped	167	5.65	14.80	5.78	75.5	1.040	0.060	0.220	3.36	0
Almonds—whole toasted	167	5.77	14.40	6.48	80.0	1.400	0.037	0.170	3.99	0
Sunflower seeds—dry	162	6.46	14.00	5.32	32.9	1.920	0.650	0.070	1.97	0
Oils & shortening										
Cocoa butter oil	251	0	28.40	0	0	0	0	0	0	0
Corn oil	251	0	28.40	0	0	0.001	0	0	0	0
Cottonseed oil	251	0	28.40	0	0	0	0	0	0	0
Olive oil	251	0	28.40	0	0.1	0.109	0	0	0	0
Palm oil	251	0	28.40	0	0.1	0.003	0	0	0	0
Palm kernel oil	251	0	28.40	0	0	0	0	0	0	0
Peanut oil	251	0	28.40	0	0	0.008	0	0	0	0
Safflower oil	251	0	28.40	0	0	0	0	0	0	0
Sesame oil	250	0	28.40	0	0	0	0	0	0	0
Soybean oil	251	0	28.40	0	0	0.007	0	0	0	0
Sunflower oil	251	0	28.40	0	0	0	0	0	0	0
Walnut oil	251	0	28.40	0	0	0	0	0	0	0
Wheat germ oil	250	0	28.40	0	0	0	0	0	0	0
Vegetable shortening	251	0	28.40	0	0	0	0	0	0	0
Pasta & noodles										
Spaghetti, cooked firm, hot	41	1.42	0.142	8.53	3.1	0.454	0.051	0.028	0.482	0
Spaghetti, cooked tender, hot	31	1.01	0.111	6.48	3.0	0.405	0.04	0.022	0.425	0
Whole wheat spaghetti, cooked	35	1.53	0.113	7.49	4.3	0.244	0.048	0.020	1.040	0
Spaghetti + sauce + cheese, canned	22	0.68	0.227	4.42	4.5	0.318	0.040	0.032	0.284	0.3
Spaghetti + sauce + cheese, homemade	30	1.02	1.02	4.20	9.07	0.260	0.028	0.020	0.284	0.9
Spaghetti + sauce + meat, canned	30	1.36	1.13	4.42	6.01	0.374	0.017	0.020	0.312	2.6
Spaghetti + sauce + meat, homemade	38	2.17	1.37	4.46	14.20	0.423	0.029	0.034	0.314	10.2
Spaghetti sauce, homemade	23	0.77	1.25	2.95	6.70	0.380	0.026	0.017	0.343	0
Spaghetti sauce, canned	31	0.52	1.35	4.52	7.97	0.184	0.016	0.017	0.343	0
Spaghetti meat sauce,	30	1.03	1.30	3.72	4.95	0.385	0.028	0.022	0.193	2.3
Spaghetti sauce, dry, packet	79	1.70	0.28	18.20	48.20	0.765	NA	0.162	0.057	0
Spaghetti sauce + mushrooms, packet	85	2.84	2.55	13.90	113.00	0.510	NA	0.136	0.085	0
Egg noodles, cooked	35	1.17	0.35	6.60	3.19	0.400	0.039	0.023	0.624	8.9

VARIETY—continued

	kcal	Protein (g)	Fat (g)	CHO (g)	Ca (mg)	Fe (mg)	B_1 (mg)	B_2 (mg)	Fiber (g)	Cholesterol (mg)
Pasta & noodles—continued										
Chow mein noodles, dry	139	3.72	6.93	16.40	8.82	0.252	0.032	0.019	1.100	3.2
Spinach noodles, dry	108	3.97	1.08	20.20	11.60	1.290	0.278	0.133	1.930	0
Spinach noodles, cooked	32	1.13	0.36	5.97	3.37	0.429	0.043	0.027	0.569	0
Chicken + noodles, recipe	43	2.60	2.13	3.07	3.07	0.278	0.006	0.020	0.142	12.2
Chicken + noodles, frozen	32	2.17	1.30	2.49	15.70	0.393	0.009	0.018	0.022	8.0
Noodles-ramen-beef, cooked	28	0.76	0.94	4.17	NA	NA	NA	NA	0.500	NA
Noodles, ramen, chicken, cooked	25	0.76	0.85	3.63	NA	NA	NA	NA	0.512	NA
Noodles, ramen, oriental	26	0.74	1.07	3.83	NA	NA	NA	NA	0.512	NA
Lasagna, frozen entree	38	2.32	1.71	2.61	34.00	0.343	0.026	0.045	0.194	12.4
Pizza										
Pizza—cheese	69	3.54	2.13	9.21	52.00	0.378	0.080	0.069	0.510	13.2
Pizza—mozzarella	80	7.60	4.67	0.89	207.00	0.076	0.006	0.097	0	15.0
Pizza—Canadian bacon	52	6.82	2.36	0.38	3.00	0.229	0.231	0.055	0	16.3
Pizza—pepperoni	140	5.94	12.50	0.81	2.80	0.397	0.090	0.070	0	9.8
Pizza—onion	10	0.34	0.07	2.07	7.10	1.105	0.017	0.003	0.450	0
Popcorn										
Popcorn—plain, air popped	106	3.50	1.42	21.30	3.50	0.709	0.106	0.035	4.600	0
Popcorn—cooked in oil/salted	142	2.32	7.99	15.50	7.70	0.696	0.026	0.052	3.090	0
Popcorn—syrup-coated	109	1.60	0.81	24.30	1.60	0.405	0.106	0.016	0.810	0
Rice										
Brown—dry	102	2.13	0.54	21.90	9.04	0.510	0.096	0.014	0.965	0
Brown—cooked	34	0.709	0.17	7.23	3.40	0.170	0.026	0.006	0.483	0
White—regular, dry	103	1.90	0.11	22.80	6.74	0.828	0.125	0.009	0.340	0
White—regular, cooked	31	0.567	0.03	6.86	2.84	0.397	0.03	0.003	0.102	0
White—converted, dry	105	2.10	0.15	23.00	17.00	0.828	0.124	0.010	0.624	0
White—converted, cooked	30	0.599	0.02	6.60	5.35	0.227	0.03	0.003	0.180	0
White—instant, dry	106	2.13	0.06	23.40	1.42	1.300	0.125	0.008	0.737	0
White—instant, prepared	31	0.624	0.03	6.86	0.85	0.227	0.037	0.003	0.216	0
Wild—cooked	26	1.02	0.06	5.39	1.42	0.312	0.031	0.045	0.709	0
Rice bran	78	3.77	5.44	14.40	21.50	5.500	0.64	0.070	6.150	0
Rice polish	75	3.43	3.62	16.40	19.40	4.560	0.521	0.051	0.680	0
Salad dressings										
Blue cheese salad dressing	143	1.37	14.80	2.09	22.90	0.057	0.003	0.028	0.020	7.6
Caesar's salad dressing	126	2.66	12.70	0.67	44.40	0.239	0.007	0.025	0.050	33.9
French dressing	150	0.16	16.00	1.81	3.55	0.113	0	0	0.220	0
Italian dressing—low calorie	15	0.02	1.18	1.37	0.59	0.059	0	0	0.080	1.7

VARIETY—continued

	kcal	Protein (g)	Fat (g)	CHO (g)	Ca (mg)	Fe (mg)	B₁ (mg)	B₂ (mg)	Fiber (g)	Cholesterol (mg)
Salad dressings—continued										
Mayonnaise	203	0.31	22.60	0.77	5.67	0.168	0.005	0.012	0	16.8
Imitation mayonnaise	66	0	5.67	3.78	0	0	0	0	0	7.6
Ranch salad dressing	104	0.86	10.70	1.31	28.40	0.075	0.010	0.040	0	11.1
Russian salad dressing	140	0.45	14.50	3.00	5.44	0.174	0.014	0.014	0.080	18.4
1000 island dressing	107	0.26	10.10	4.30	3.52	0.170	0.006	0.009	0.060	7.3
1000 island dressing—low calorie	45	0.22	3.00	4.58	3.12	1.174	0.006	0.008	0.340	3.4
Vinegar & oil dressing	124	0	14.20	0	0	0	0	0	0	0
Salads, prepared										
Chicken salad w/celery	97	3.82	8.90	0.47	5.92	0.239	0.012	0.028	0.110	17.3
Cole slaw	20	0.36	0.74	3.52	12.80	0.166	0.019	0.017	0.570	2.3
Egg salad	68	2.91	6.01	0.45	14.50	0.525	0.019	0.070	0	97.4
Ham salad spread	62	2.46	4.39	3.01	2.24	0.168	0.123	0.034	0.030	10.4
Macaroni salad—no cheese	75	0.54	6.66	3.52	5.50	0.229	0.020	0.014	0.270	4.9
Potato salad w/mayo + eggs	41	0.76	2.32	3.16	5.44	0.185	0.022	0.017	0.420	19.3
Tuna salad	53	4.55	2.53	2.67	4.84	0.282	0.009	0.019	0.340	3.7
Waldorf salad	85	0.72	8.33	2.62	8.82	0.196	0.020	0.013	0.720	4.3
Sandwiches										
Avocado & cheese—white	64	2.02	4.00	5.39	43.1	0.418	0.057	0.059	0.98	4.4
Avocado & cheese—whole wheat	62	2.14	3.97	5.24	37.8	0.477	0.047	0.05	1.76	4.3
BLT —whole wheat	68	2.49	3.77	6.45	11.4	0.570	0.077	0.043	1.55	4.1
BLT—white	70	2.30	3.77	6.70	18.2	0.489	0.092	0.055	0.43	4.2
Grilled cheese—wheat	91	4.22	5.37	7.10	87.4	0.565	0.057	0.076	1.59	11.8
Grilled cheese—part WW	95	4.39	5.82	6.59	103.0	0.526	0.067	0.093	0.61	13.3
Grilled cheese—white	97	4.22	5.79	6.88	103.0	0.441	0.068	0.092	0.30	13.3
Chicken salad—wheat	80	3.00	4.25	8.13	14.7	0.679	0.066	0.046	1.88	6.2
Chicken salad—white	85	2.83	4.63	8.05	22.7	0.552	0.080	0.060	0.39	7.1
Corn dog	84	2.55	5.10	6.97	8.7	0.495	0.072	0.043	0.03	9.5
Corned beef & swiss on rye	83	5.26	4.59	4.90	63.8	0.768	0.044	0.078	0.97	16.4
English muffin (egg/cheese/bacon)	74	3.70	3.70	6.37	40.5	0.637	0.095	0.103	0.32	43.8
Egg salad—wheat	79	2.60	4.56	7.44	17.0	0.744	0.063	0.059	1.67	48.8
Egg salad—soft white	83	2.41	4.90	7.25	24.5	0.636	0.075	0.074	0.30	41.6
Ham—rye bread	59	3.84	2.09	6.10	12.0	0.474	0.182	0.073	1.24	7.1
Ham—whole wheat	59	3.79	2.04	6.84	12.4	0.617	0.164	0.060	1.54	6.1
Ham—soft white	61	3.74	2.08	6.60	18.6	0.504	0.186	0.073	0.29	6.7
Ham & swiss—rye	68	4.65	3.23	5.08	63.5	0.389	0.147	0.079	0.99	10.8
Ham & cheese—wheat	67	4.20	3.23	5.72	40.5	0.527	0.136	0.066	1.27	9.7
Ham & cheese—soft white	69	4.20	3.36	5.43	48.0	0.428	0.152	0.078	0.23	10.6
Ham salad—wheat	75	2.45	4.02	7.83	11.5	0.569	0.104	0.045	1.52	5.6
Ham salad—white	78	2.25	4.26	7.71	17.5	0.454	0.119	0.057	0.28	6.2
Hotdog/frankfurter & bun	87	2.80	5.10	7.04	19.6	0.570	0.095	0.062	0.40	7.6

VARIETY—continued

	kcal	Protein (g)	Fat (g)	CHO (g)	Ca (mg)	Fe (mg)	B_1 (mg)	B_2 (mg)	Fiber (g)	Cholesterol (mg)
Sandwiches—continued										
Patty melt—gound beef/rye	91	5.09	6.07	3.96	36.5	0.533	0.040	0.072	0.81	17.1
Peanut butter & jam—whole wheat	92	3.40	3.85	12.30	15.4	0.751	0.070	0.045	2.29	0
Peanut butter & jam—white	98	3.29	4.14	12.80	23.4	0.632	0.085	0.059	0.85	0
Reuben grilled	58	3.43	3.38	3.53	43.6	0.633	0.030	0.052	0.80	10.4
Roast beef—whole wheat	64	4.00	2.52	6.71	12.3	0.760	0.061	0.054	1.53	6.2
Roast beef—white	67	3.97	2.63	6.46	18.5	0.665	0.072	0.066	0.27	6.9
Tuna salad—wheat	72	3.29	3.29	8.03	13.0	0.667	0.057	0.040	1.74	5.5
Tuna salad—white	76	3.18	3.47	7.92	19.6	0.555	0.068	0.052	0.44	6.2
Turkey—whole wheat	62	4.09	2.33	6.67	11.6	0.554	0.056	0.044	1.53	6.0
Turkey—white	64	4.07	2.42	6.41	17.8	0.435	0.066	0.055	0.27	6.7
Turkey & ham—rye	58	3.74	2.12	6.18	12.3	0.743	0.060	0.079	1.23	8.4
Turkey & ham—whole wheat	59	3.71	2.07	6.90	12.6	0.846	0.060	0.064	1.54	7.2
Turkey & ham—white	60	3.65	2.10	6.67	18.8	0.762	0.071	0.078	0.28	8.0
Turkey & ham & cheese on rye	68	4.22	3.46	5.04	44.2	0.616	0.050	0.083	0.99	12.1
Turkey & ham & cheese—wheat	67	4.14	3.25	5.77	40.5	0.716	0.051	0.070	1.27	10.6
Turkey & ham & cheese—white	69	4.13	3.38	5.48	48.3	0.636	0.059	0.082	0.23	11.6
Sauces										
Bordelaise sauce	24	0.33	1.46	1.10	3.80	0.179	0.008	0.010	0.01	3.8
Hot chili sauce, red pepper	5	0.25	0.17	1.10	2.51	0.137	0.003	0.026	2.29	0
Teriyaki sauce	24	1.69	0.09	4.52	6.30	0.488	0.008	0.020	0	0
Seafood										
Anchovy—raw	37	5.78	1.37	0	41.7	0.921	0.016	0.073	0	19.6
Frog legs—raw meat	21	4.65	0.085	0	5.1	0.539	0.040	0.070	0	14.2
Lobster meat—cooked	28	5.80	0.17	0.36	17.2	0.111	0.020	0.019	0	20.3
Scampi—fried in crumbs	69	6.07	3.49	3.26	19.0	0.357	0.037	0.039	0.04	50.2
Shrimp—boiled	28	5.93	0.31	0	11.0	0.876	0.009	0.009	0	55.3
Squid (calamari)—fried in flour	50	5.10	2.12	2.20	11.0	0.287	0.016	0.130	0	73.7
Soups										
Cream of celery	20	0.38	1.27	2.00	9.04	0.141	0.007	0.011	0.09	3.2
Chicken, chunky	20	1.43	0.75	1.95	2.71	0.195	0.010	0.020	0.03	3.4
Chicken + dumpling	23	1.30	1.28	1.39	3.34	0.144	0.004	0.017	0.10	7.6
Chicken gumbo	13	0.60	0.32	1.89	5.53	0.201	0.006	0.009	0.05	0.9
Chicken-noodle—chunky	14	1.50	0.70	0.24	2.84	0.170	0.009	0.020	0.09	2.1
Chili with beans	32	1.62	1.56	3.38	13.20	0.973	0.014	0.030	0.91	4.8
Clam chowder—New England	19	1.08	0.75	1.90	21.40	0.169	0.008	0.027	0.11	2.5
Minestrone—chunky	15	0.60	0.33	2.45	7.20	0.209	0.006	0.014	0.12	0.6
Cream of mushroom	29	0.46	2.15	2.10	7.23	0.119	0.007	0.019	0.06	0.4
Mushroom—barley	14	0.43	0.51	1.69	2.82	0.113	0.006	0.020	0.17	0

VARIETY—continued

	kcal	Protein (g)	Fat (g)	CHO (g)	Ca (mg)	Fe (mg)	B₁ (mg)	B₂ (mg)	Fiber (g)	Cholesterol (mg)
Soups—continued										
Onion—canned	13	0.87	0.40	1.89	6.10	0.156	0.008	0.006	0.11	0
Oyster stew	14	0.49	0.89	0.94	4.96	0.227	0.005	0.008	0	3.1
Pea—prepared w/milk	27	1.40	0.79	3.59	19.30	0.224	0.017	0.030	0.07	2.0
Cream of potato	17	0.39	0.53	2.59	4.52	0.107	0.008	0.008	0.10	1.5
Split pea + ham	22	1.31	0.47	3.17	3.90	0.253	0.014	0.011	0.19	0.8
Tomato—canned	19	0.47	0.43	3.75	3.05	0.396	0.020	0.011	0.11	0
Tomato-beef-noodle	32	1.00	0.97	4.78	3.95	0.252	0.019	0.020	0.03	0.9
Tomato bisque prepared w/milk	22	0.71	0.75	3.32	21.00	0.099	0.013	0.030	0.01`	2.5
Turkey—chunky	16	1.23	0.53	1.69	6.00	0.229	0.010	0.029	0.12	1.1
Turkey noodle	16	0.88	0.45	1.95	2.60	0.212	0.017	0.014	0.03	1.1
Cream vegetable—dry mix	126	2.27	6.84	14.80	1.42	0.539	1.470	0.127	0.22	1.2
Vegetable	16	0.49	0.45	2.77	4.96	0.249	0.012	0.010	0.37	0
Miscellanous										
Garlic cloves	42	1.80	0.14	9.38	51.30	0.482	0.057	0.030	0.47	0
Gelatin salad/dessert	17	0.43	0	3.99	0.50	0.024	0.002	0.002	0.02	0
Quiche lorraine	97	2.09	7.73	4.67	34.00	0.226	0.018	0.052	0.09	45.9
Spinach souffle	45	2.29	3.84	0.59	47.90	0.279	0.019	0.064	0.79	38.4

PART 2

NUTRITIVE VALUES FOR ALCOHOLIC AND NONALCOHOLIC BEVERAGES

The nutritive values for alcoholic and nonalcoholic beverages are expressed in 1-ounce (28.4-g) portions. We have also included the nutritive values for the minerals calcium, iron, magnesium, phosphorus, and potassium and the vitamins B₁ (thiamine), B₂ (riboflavin), niacin, and B₁₂ (cobalamin). The alcoholic beverages contain no cholesterol or fat.

ALCOHOLIC BEVERAGES (1 OUNCE)

	kcal	Protein (g)	CHO (g)	Minerals					Vitamins			
				Ca (mg)	Fe (mg)	Mg (mg)	P (mg)	K (mg)	B₁ (mg)	B₂ (mg)	Niacin (mg)	B₁₂ (mg)
Beer, regular	12	0.072	1.1	1.4	0.009	1.83	3.50	7.09	0.002	0.007	0.128	0.005
Beer, light	8	0.057	0.4	1.4	0.011	1.42	3.44	5.13	0.003	0.008	0.111	0.002
Brandy	69	0	10.6	2.5	0.012		1.01	1.01	0.002	0.002	0.004	0
Champagne	22	0.043	0.6	1.6	0.093	2.40	1.90	22.60	0	0.003	0.019	0
Dessert wine, dry	36	0.057	1.2	2.3	0.068	2.55	2.55	26.20	0.005	0.005	0.060	0
Dessert wine, sweet	44	0.057	3.3	2.3	0.057	2.55	2.64	26.20	0.005	0.005	0.060	0
Gin, rum, vodka, scotch, whiskey, 80 proof	64	0	0	0	0.010	0	0	1.01	0	0	0	0
Gin, rum, vodka, scotch, whiskey, 86 proof	71	0	0	0	0.012	0	1.16	0.55	0.002	0.002	0.004	0

ALCOHOLIC BEVERAGES (1 OUNCE)—continued

	kcal	Protein (g)	CHO (g)	Minerals					Vitamins			
				Ca (mg)	Fe (mg)	Mg (mg)	P (mg)	K (mg)	B_1 (mg)	B_2 (mg)	Niacin (mg)	B_{12} (mg)
Gin, rum, vodka, scotch, whiskey, 90 proof	74	0	0	0	0.010	0	0	0.86	0	0	0	0
Sherry, dry	28	0.024	0.3	2.1	0.052	1.96	2.60	17.80	0.002	0.002	0.024	0
Sherry, medium	40	0.066	2.3	2.3	0.071	2.27	1.89	23.60	0.002	0.008	0.035	0
Vermouth, dry	34	0.028	1.6	2.0	0.096	1.42	1.89	11.30	NA	NA	0.011	0
Vermouth, sweet	44	0.014	4.5	1.7	0.099	1.13	1.65	8.50	NA	NA	0.011	0
Wine, dry white	19	0.029	0.2	2.6	0.093	2.62	1.67	17.40	0	0.001	0.019	0
Wine, medium white	19	0.028	0.2	2.5	0.085	3.03	3.84	22.60	0.001	0.001	0.019	0
Wine, red	20	0.055	0.5	2.2	0.122	3.60	3.84	31.50	0.001	0.008	0.023	0.004
Wine, rosé	20	0.055	0.4	2.4	0.108	2.74	4.08	28.10	0.001	0.004	0.020	0.002
Creme de menthe	105	0	11.8	0	0.023	0	0	0	0	0	0.001	0
Bloody Mary	22	0.153	0.9	1.9	0.105	2.10	4.02	41.40	0.010	0.006	0.123	0
Bourbon and soda	26	0	0	1.0	0.244	0.24	0.48	0.48	0	0	0.005	0
Daiquiri	52	0	1.9	0.9	0.043	0.47	1.89	6.14	0.004	0.	0.012	0
Manhattan	64	0	0.9	0.5	0.025	0.01	1.99	7.46	0.003	0.001	0.026	0
Martini	63	0	0.1	0.4	0.024	0.40	0.81	5.26	0	0	0.004	0
Pina colada	53	0.120	8.0	2.2	0.062		2.01	20.10	0.008	0.004	0.033	0
Screwdriver	23	0.160	2.5	2.1	0.023	2.26	3.86	43.30	0.018	0.004	0.046	0
Tequila	31	0.099	2.4	1.7	0.077	1.98	2.80	29.30	0.010	0.005	0.054	0
Tom collins	16	0.013	0.4	1.3	NA	0.38	0.12	2.30	0	0	0.004	0
Whiskey sour	42	0	3.7	0.3	0.021	0.26	1.60	5.08	0.003	0.002	0.006	0
Coffee + cream liqueur	93	0.784	5.9	4.2	0.036	0.60	13.90	9.05	0	0.016	0.022	0
Coffee liqueur	95	0	13.3	0.5	0.016	0.54	1.64	8.18	0.001	0.003	0.040	0

NONALCOHOLIC BEVERAGES (1 OUNCE)

	kcal	Protein (g)	CHO (g)	Minerals					Vitamins			
				Ca (mg)	Fe (mg)	Mg (mg)	P (mg)	K (mg)	B_1 (mg)	B_2 (mg)	Niacin (mg)	B_{12} (mg)
Hot cocoa with whole milk	25	1.030	2.9	33.8	0.088	6.350	30.60	54.400	0.012	0.049	0.041	0.099
Cocoa mix + water— diet	7	0.561	1.3	13.3	0.110	4.870	19.80	59.800	0.006	0.030	0.024	0
Coffee—brewed	0.2	0.016	0.1	0.5	0.113	1.590	0.32	15.400	0	0.002	0.063	0
Coffee—instant dry powder	1.4	0.016	0.3	0.8	0.019	1.100	2.05	67.70	0	0	0.061	0
Coffee—cappuchino	9.2	0.059	1.6	1.0	0.022	1.330	3.84	17.600	0	0	0.048	0
Coffee—Swiss mocha	7.7	0.078	1.3	1.1	0.036	1.360	4.37	17.900	0	0	0.039	0
Coffee whitener— nondairy,	38.5	0.284	3.2	2.6	0.009	0.060	18.20	54.1	0	0	0	0
liquid powder	155	1.360	15.6	6.3	0.326	1.200	120.00	230.0	0	0.047	0	0
Cola beverage, regular	12	0	3.0	0.7	0.009	0.230	3.52	0.306	0	0	0	0
Diet cola— w/aspartame	0	0	0	1.0	0.009	0.319	2.40	0	0.001	0.007	0	0
Club soda	0	0	0	1.4	0.012	0.319	0	0.479	0	0	0	0

NONALCOHOLIC BEVERAGES (1 OUNCE)—*continued*

	kcal	Protein (g)	CHO (g)	Minerals Ca (mg)	Fe (mg)	Mg (mg)	P (mg)	K (mg)	Vitamins B_1 (mg)	B_2 (mg)	Niacin (mg)	B_{12} (mg)
Cream soda	15	0	3.8	1.5	0.015	0.229	0	0.306	0	0	0	0
Diet soda-avg assorted	0	0	0.0	1.1	0.011	0.200	3.03	0.559	0	0	0	0
Egg nog—commercial	38	1.080	3.8	36.8	0.057	5.250	31.00	46.900	0.010	0.054	0.030	0.127
Five Alive citrus	13	0.135	3.1	1.7	0.021	1.950	2.70	34.000	0.015	0.003	0.060	0
Fruit flavored soda pop	13	0	3.2	1.1	0.020	0.305	0.15	1.520	0	0	0.002	0
Fruit punch drink—canned	13	0.015	3.4	2.1	0.058	0.610	0.31	7.160	0.006	0.006	0.006	0
Gatorade	5	0	1.3	2.8	NA	NA	0	2.840	NA	NA	NA	0
Ginger ale	10	0.008	2.5	0.9	0.051	0.232	0.08	0.387	0	0	0	0
Grape soda carbonated	12	0	3.2	0.9	0.024	0.305	0	0.229	0	0	0	0
Kool-Aid w/ NutraSweet	0	0	0	0	0	0.028	0	0	0	0	0	0
Kool-Aid w/sugar added	12	0	3.0	0	0	0	0	0	0	0	0	0
Lemon-lime soda	12	0	3.0	0.7	0.019	0.154	0.08	0.308	0	0	0.004	0
Lemonade drink from dry	11	0	2.9	7.6	0.016	0.322	3.65	3.540	0	0	0.004	0
Lemonade frozen conc	51	0.078	13.3	1.9	0.205	1.420	2.46	19.200	0.007	0.027	0.020	0
Limeade frozen conc	53	0.052	14.0	1.4	0.029	7.800	1.69	16.800	0.003	0.003	0.028	0
Chocolate milkshake	36	0.962	5.8	32.0	0.088	4.700	28.90	56.800	0.016	0.069	0.046	0.097
Strawberry milkshake	32	0.952	5.4	32.0	0.030	3.600	28.40	51.700	0.013	0.055	0.050	0.088
Vanilla milkshake	32	0.982	5.1	34.5	0.026	3.500	29.00	49.300	0.013	0.052	0.052	0.101
Orange drink/ carbonated	14	0	3.5	1.5	0.018	0.305	0.31	0.686	0	0	0	0
Pepper-type soda	12	0	2.9	0.9	0.010	0.077	3.16	0.154	0	0	0	0
Root beer	12	0.008	3.0	1.5	0.014	0.306	0.15	0.230	0	0	0	0
Pineapple grapefruit drink	13	0.068	3.3	2.0	0.087	1.700	1.59	17.500	0.009	0.005	0.076	0
Pineapple orange drink	14	0.352	3.3	1.5	0.076	1.590	1.13	13.200	0.009	0.005	0.059	0
Tang orange juice crystals	13	0.170	0.06	3.1	4.57	0.002	0.02	0.008	0	0	0	0
Tonic water/Quinine water	10	0	2.5	0.4	0.019	0.077	0	0.077	0	0	0	0
Tea-brewed	0	0.001	0.1	0	0.006	0.796	0.16	10.500	0	0.004	0.012	0
Herbal tea, brewed	0	0	0	0.6	0.022	0.319	0	2.390	0.003	0.001	0	0
Perrier water	0	0	0	3.8	0	0.148	0	0	0	0	0	0
Poland Springs bottled water	0	0	0	0.4	0.001	0.239	0	0	0	0	0	0

Note: Alcoholic beverages contain no fat or cholesterol; light beer contains 0.5 g fiber and regular beer contains 1.2 g fiber per 8 oz. serving. All of the other nonmixed alcoholic beverages have no fiber.

Note: Other nonalcoholic beverages are listed in the sections on fruits and vegetables.

PART 3

NUTRITIVE VALUES FOR SPECIALTY AND FAST-FOOD ITEMS

Nutrient information was kindly provided by the manufacturer or its representative, and is reproduced as presented in their literature. Unlike Parts 1 and 2, nutritive values are not given for 1-ounce portions but for the actual amounts of the foods as sold commercially. To make a direct comparison of the kcal values and the various nutrients, we recommend that the weight of the food and its nutrients be expressed relative to 1-ounce (28.4-g) portions.

ARBY'S

Food Item	Serving Size (g)	kcal	Protein (g)	Fat (g)	CHO (g)
Bacon Cheddar Deluxe	225	561	28	34	78
Baked Potato Plain	312	291	8	1	0
Beef 'n Cheddar	190	490	24	21	51
Chicken Breast Sandwich	210	592	28	27	57
Chocolate Shake	300	384	9	11	32
French Fries	71	211	2	8	6
Hot Ham 'n Cheese Sandwich	161	353	26	13	50
Jamocha Shake	305	424	8	10	31
Junior Roast Beef	86	218	12	8	22
King Roast Beef	192	467	27	19	49
Potato Cakes	85	201	2	14	13
Regular Roast Beef	147	353	22	15	32
Super Roast Beef	234	501	25	22	40
Superstuffed Potato Broccoli and Cheddar	340	541	13	22	24
Superstuffed Potato Deluxe	312	648	18	38	72
Superstuffed Potato Mushroom and Cheese	300	506	16	22	21
Superstuffed Potato Taco	425	619	23	27	145
Turkey Deluxe	197	375	24	17	39
Vanilla Shake	250	295	8	10	30

Source: Arby's Inc. Nutritional information provided by Consumer Affairs, Arby's Inc., Atlanta, GA, 1986.

BURGER KING

Food Item	Serving Size (g)	kcal	Protein (g)	Total Carbo-hydrate (g)	Total Fat (g)	Choles-terol (mg)	Sodium (mg)	Dietary Fiber (g)	Percentage of U.S. RDA*			
									Vit A	Vit C	Ca	Fe
Burgers												
Whopper sandwich	270	640	27	45	39	90	870	3	10	15	8	25
Whopper with cheese sandwich	294	730	33	46	46	115	1300	3	15	15	25	25
Double Whopper sandwich	351	870	46	45	56	170	940	3	10	15	8	40
Double Whopper with cheese sandwich	375	960	52	46	63	195	1360	3	15	15	25	40
Whopper Jr. sandwich	168	420	21	29	24	60	570	2	4	8	6	20
Whopper Jr. with cheese sandwich	180	460	23	29	28	75	780	2	8	8	15	20
Hamburger	129	330	20	28	15	55	570	1	2	0	4	15
Cheeseburger	142	380	23	28	19	65	780	1	6	0	15	15
Double cheese-burger	213	600	41	29	36	135	1040	1	8	0	20	25
Double cheese-burger with bacon	221	640	44	29	39	145	1220	1	8	0	20	25
Sandwich/Side Orders												
BK Big Fish sandwich	255	720	25	59	43	60	1090	2	2	2	6	20
BK Broiler Chicken sandwich	248	540	30	41	29	80	480	2	4	10	4	30
Chicken sandwich	229	700	26	54	43	60	1400	2	°	°	10	20
Chicken Tenders (6 piece)	88	250	16	14	12	35	530	2	°	°	°	4
Broiled Chicken salad†	302	200	21	7	10	60	110	3	100	25	15	20
Garden salad†	215	90	6	7	5	15	110	3	110	50	15	6
Side salad†	133	50	3	4	3	5	55	2	50	20	6	2
French fries (medium, salted)	116	400	5	43	20	0	240	3	°	4	°	6
Onion rings	124	310	4	41	14	0	810	5	°	°	°	°
Dutch apple pie	113	310	3	39	15	0	230	2	°	10	°	8
Drinks												
Vanilla shake (medium)	284	310	9	53	7	20	230	1	6	6	30	°
Chocolate shake (medium)	284	310	9	54	7	20	230	3	6	°	20	10
Chocolate shake (medium, syrup added)	341	460	11	87	7	20	300	1	6	6	30	°
Strawberry shake (medium, syrup added)	341	430	9	83	7	20	260	1	6	6	30	°

BURGER KING—*continued*

Food Item	Serving Size (g)	kcal	Protein (g)	Total Carbohydrate (g)	Total Fat (g)	Cholesterol (mg)	Sodium (mg)	Dietary Fiber (g)	Percentage of U.S. RDA*			
									Vit A	Vit C	Ca	Fe
Drinks—continued												
Coca-Cola Classic (medium)	22 (fl oz)	260	0	70	0	0	@	0	°	°	°	°
Diet Coke (medium)	22 (fl oz)	1	0	<1	0	0	@	0	°	°	°	°
Sprite (medium)	22 (fl oz)	260	0	66	0	0	@	0	°	°	°	°
Tropicana orange juice	311	140	2	33	0	0	0	0	0	100	0	0
Coffee	355	5	0	1	0	0	5	0	°	°	°	°
Milk—2% low fat	244	120	8	12	5	20	120	0	10	4	30	°
Breakfast												
Croissan'wich with bacon, egg and cheese	118	350	15	18	24	225	790	<1	8	°	15	10
Croissan'wich with sausage, egg and cheese	159	530	20	21	41	255	1000	<1	8	°	15	15
Croissan'wich with ham, egg and cheese	144	350	18	19	22	230	1390	<1	8	°	15	10
French toast sticks	141	500	4	60	27	0	490	1	°	°	6	15
Hash browns	71	220	2	25	12	0	320	2	10	8	°	2
A.M. Express grape jam	12	30	0	7	0	0	0	0	0	0	0	0
A.M. Express strawberry jam	12	30	0	8	0	0	5	0	0	0	0	0
Condiments/ Toppings												
Processed American cheese	25	90	6	0	8	25	420	0	6	°	15	°
Lettuce	21	0	0	0	0	0	0	0	°	°	°	°
Tomato	28	5	0	1	0	0	0	0	2	8	°	°
Onion	14	5	0	1	0	0	0	0	°	°	°	°
Pickles	14	0	0	0	0	0	140	0	0	0	0	0
Ketchup	14	15	0	4	0	0	180	0	4	°	°	°
Mustard	3	0	0	0	0	0	40	0	0	0	0	0
Mayonnaise	28	210	0	<1	23	20	160	0	°	°	°	°
Tartar sauce	28	180	0	0	19	15	220	0	°	°	°	°
Land O' Lakes whipped classic blend	10	65	0	0	7	0	75	0	8	°	°	°
Bull's Eye barbecue sauce	14	20	0	5	0	0	140	0	°	°	°	2
Bacon bits	3	15	1	0	1	5	0	0	°	°	°	°
Croutons	7	30	<1	4	1	0	75	0	°	°	°	°

BURGER KING—*continued*

Food Item	Serving Size (g)	kcal	Protein (g)	Total Carbohydrate (g)	Total Fat (g)	Cholesterol (mg)	Sodium (mg)	Dietary Fiber (g)	Vit A	Vit C	Ca	Fe
Burger King												
Salad Dressings												
Thousand Island dressing	30	140	0	7	12	15	190	<1	30	°	°	°
French dressing	30	140	0	11	10	0	190	0	15	°	°	°
Ranch dressing	30	180	<1	2	19	10	170	<1	°	°	°	°
Bleu cheese dressing	30	160	2	1	16	30	260	<1	°	°	°	°
Reduced calorie light Italian dressing#	30	15	0	3	0.5	0	50	0	°	°	°	°
Dipping Sauces												
A.M. Express dip	28	80	0	21	0	0	20	0	°	°	°	°
Honey dipping sauce	28	90	0	23	0	0	10	0	°	°	°	°
Ranch dipping sauce	28	170	0	2	17	0	200	0	°	°	°	°
Barbecue dipping sauce	28	35	0	9	0	0	400	0	2	2	°	°
Sweet & sour dipping sauce	28	45	0	11	0	0	50	0	°	°	°	°

Source: From Burger King Corporation, Miami, FL, 1996. For additional information, call 1-800-937-1800.
† = Without dressing   @ = Depends on the water supply   ° = Less than 2% of the U.S. RDA
★ = Values for vitamins A and C and minerals calcium and iron represent percent daily values based on a 2,000 calorie diet   # = Regular Italian dressing—150 calories—16 grams (g) Fat.
— = Negligible.

DAIRY QUEEN

Food Item	Serving Size (g)	Description	kcal	Protein (g)	Fat (g)	CHO (g)	Ca (mg)	Fe (mg)	Vitamin A (IU)	Vitamin C (mg)	Vitamin B₁ (mg)	Vitamin B₂ (mg)
Banana Split	383		540	9	11	103	—	—	—	—	—	—
Big Brazier	213	deluxe	470	28	24	36	111	5.2	—	<2.5	0.34	0.37
Big Brazier	184	regular	184	27	23	37	113	5.2	—	<2.0	0.37	0.39
Big Brazier	213	w/cheese	553	32	30	38	268	5.2	495	<2.3	0.34	0.53
Blizzard Banana Split	—	regular	763	—	—	—	—	—	—	—	—	—
Blizzard Banana Split	—	large	1333	—	—	—	—	—	—	—	—	—
Blizzard chocolate sandwich cookies	—	regular	600	—	—	—	—	—	—	—	—	—
Blizzard chocolate sandwich cookies	—	large	1050	—	—	—	—	—	—	—	—	—

DAIRY QUEEN—*continued*

Food Item	Serving Size (g)	Description	kcal	Protein (g)	Fat (g)	CHO (g)	Ca (mg)	Fe (mg)	Vitamin A (IU)	Vitamin C (mg)	Vitamin B₁ (mg)	Vitamin B₂ (mg)
Blizzard German chocolate	—	regular	794	—	—	—	—	—	—	—	—	—
Blizzard German chocolate	—	large	1460	—	—	—	—	—	—	—	—	—
Blizzard, Heath	—	regular	824	—	—	—	—	—	—	—	—	—
Blizzard, Heath	—	large	1212	—	—	—	—	—	—	—	—	—
Blizzard, M&M	—	regular	766	—	—	—	—	—	—	—	—	—
Blizzard, M&M	—	large	1154	—	—	—	—	—	—	—	—	—
Brazier cheese dog	113		330	15	19	24	168	1.6	—	—	—	0.18
Brazier chili dog	128		330	13	20	25	86	2.0	—	11.0	0.15	0.23
Brazier dog	99		273	11	15	23	75	1.5	—	11.0	0.12	0.15
Brazier french fries	71	regular	200	2	10	25	tr	0.4	tr	3.6	0.06	tr
Brazier french fries	113	large	320	3	16	40	tr	0.4	tr	4.8	0.09	0.03
Brazier onion rings	85		300	6	17	33	20	0.4	tr	2.4	0.09	tr
Brazier regular	106		260	13	9	28	70	3.5	—	<1.0	0.28	0.26
Brazier w/cheese	121		318	18	14	30	163	3.5	—	<1.2	0.29	0.29
Buster Bar	149		460	10	29	41	—	—	—	—	—	—
Chicken sandwich	220		670	29	41	46	—	—	—	—	—	—
Cone	213	large	340	9	10	57	—	—	—	—	—	—
Cone	142	regular	240	6	7	38	—	—	—	—	—	—
Cone	85	small	140	3	4	22	—	—	—	—	—	—
Dairy Queen Parfait	284		460	10	11	81	300	1.8	400	tr	0.12	0.43
Dilly Bar	85		240	4	15	22	100	0.4	100	tr	0.06	0.17
Dilly Bar	85		210	3	13	21	—	—	—	—	—	—
Dipped, cone	234	large	510	9	24	64	—	—	—	—	—	—
Dipped, cone	156	regular	340	6	16	42	—	—	—	—	—	—
Dipped, cone	92	small	190	3	9	25	—	—	—	—	—	—
Double Delight	255		490	9	20	69	—	—	—	—	—	—
Double hamburger	210		530	36	28	33	—	—	—	—	—	—
Double w/cheese	239		650	43	37	34	—	—	—	—	—	—
Chocolate dipped cone	234	large	450	10	20	58	300	0.4	400	tr	0.12	0.51
Chocolate dipped cone	156	medium	300	7	13	40	200	0.4	300	tr	0.09	0.34
Chocolate dipped cone	78	small	150	3	7	20	100	tr	100	tr	0.03	0.17
Chocolate malt	588	large	840	22	28	125	600	5.4	750	6.0	0.15	0.85
Chocolate malt	418	medium	600	15	20	89	500	3.6	750	3.6	0.12	0.60
Chocolate malt	241	small	340	10	11	51	300	1.8	400	2.4	0.06	0.34
Chocolate sundae	248	large	400	9	9	71	300	1.8	400	tr	0.09	0.43
Chocolate sundae	184	medium	300	6	7	53	200	1.1	300	tr	0.06	0.26

DAIRY QUEEN—*continued*

Food Item	Serving Size (g)	Description	kcal	Protein (g)	Fat (g)	CHO (g)	Ca (mg)	Fe (mg)	Vitamin A (IU)	Vitamin C (mg)	Vitamin B₁ (mg)	Vitamin B₂ (mg)
Chocolate sundae	106	small	170	4	4	30	100	0.7	100	tr	0.03	0.17
Cone	213	large	340	10	10	52	300	tr	400	tr	0.15	0.43
Cone	142	medium	230	6	7	35	200	tr	300	tr	0.09	0.26
Cone	71	small	110	3	3	18	100	tr	100	tr	0.03	0.14
Float	397		330	6	8	59	200	tr	100	tr	0.12	0.17
Freeze	397		520	11	13	89	300	tr	200	tr	0.15	0.34
Sandwich	60		140	3	4	24	60	0.4	100	tr	0.03	0.14
Fiesta sundae	269		570	9	22	84	200	tr	200	tr	0.23	0.26
Fish sandwich	170		400	20	17	41	60	1.1	tr	tr	0.15	0.26
Fish sandwich w/cheese	177		440	24	21	39	150	0.4	100	tr	0.15	0.26
Float	397		410	5	7	82	—	—	—	—	—	—
Freeze	397		500	9	12	89	—	—	—	—	—	—
French fries	71	regular	200	2	10	25	—	—	—	—	—	—
French fries	113	large	320	3	16	40	—	—	—	—	—	—
Frozen dessert	113		180	4	6	27	—	—	—	—	—	—
Hot dog	100		280	11	16	21	—	—	—	—	—	—
Hot dog w/cheese	114		330	15	21	21	—	—	—	—	—	—
Hot dog w/chili	128		320	13	20	23	—	—	—	—	—	—
Hot Fudge brownie delight	266		600	9	25	85	—	—	—	—	—	—
Malt	588	large	1060	20	25	187	—	—	—	—	—	—
Malt	418	regular	760	14	18	134	—	—	—	—	—	—
Malt	291	small	520	10	13	91	—	—	—	—	—	—
Mr. Misty	439	large	340	0	0	84	—	—	—	—	—	—
Mr. Misty	330	regular	250	0	0	63	—	—	—	—	—	—
Mr. Misty	248	small	190	0	0	48	—	—	—	—	—	—
Mr. Misty float	404		440	6	8	85	200	tr	120	tr	0.12	0.17
Mr. Misty float	411		390	5	7	74	—	—	—	—	—	—
Mr. Misty freeze	411		500	9	12	91	—	—	—	—	—	—
Mr. Misty Kiss	89		70	0	0	17	—	—	—	—	—	—
Onion rings	85		280	4	16	31	—	—	—	—	—	—
Parfait	283		430	8	8	76	—	—	—	—	—	—
Peanut Buster Parfait	305		740	16	34	94	—	—	—	—	—	—
Shake	588	large	990	19	26	168	—	—	100	—	—	—
Shake	418	regular	710	14	19	120	—	—	—	—	—	—
Shake	291	small	490	10	13	82	—	—	—	—	—	—
Single hamburger	148		360	21	16	33	—	tr	—	—	—	—
Single w/cheese	162		410	24	20	33	—	—	—	—	—	—
Strawberry shortcake	312		540	10	11	100	—	—	—	—	—	—
Sundae	248	large	440	8	10	78	—	—	—	—	—	—
Sundae	177	regular	310	5	8	56	—	—	—	—	—	—
Sundae	106	small	190	3	4	33	—	—	—	—	—	—
Super Brazier	298		783	53	48	35	282	7.3	—	<3.2	0.39	0.69
Super Brazier chili dog	210		555	23	33	42	158	4.0	—	18.0	0.42	0.48

DAIRY QUEEN—*continued*

Food Item	Serving Size (g)	Description	kcal	Protein (g)	Fat (g)	CHO (g)	Ca (mg)	Fe (mg)	Vitamin A (IU)	Vitamin C (mg)	Vitamin B₁ (mg)	Vitamin B₂ (mg)
Super Brazier dog	182		518	20	30	41	158	4.3	tr	14.0	0.42	0.44
Super Brazier dog w/cheese	203		593	26	36	43	297	4.4	—	14.0	0.43	0.48
Super hot dog	175		520	17	27	44	—	—	—	—	—	—
Super hot dog w/cheese	196		580	22	34	45	—	—	—	—	—	—
Super hot dog w/chili	218		570	21	32	47	—	—	—	—	—	—
Triple hamburger	272		710	51	45	33	—	—	—	—	—	—
Triple w/cheese	301		820	58	50	34	—	—	—	—	—	—

Source: International Dairy Queen, Inc., Minneapolis, MN, 1982. Nutritional information reviewed and edited by Dr. David J. Aulik in cooperation with Raltech Scientific Services.

JACK IN THE BOX

Menu Item	Serving Size (g)	Calories (per serving)	Protein (g)	Fat (g)	Carbo-hydrates (g)	Calcium	Iron	Vitamin A	Vitamin C
Sandwiches									
Beef Gyro	260	620	27	32	55	8	30	4	15
Chicken Fajita Pita	189	290	24	8	29	25	15	10	10
Chicken sandwich	160	400	20	18	38	15	10	4	0
Chicken supreme	245	620	25	36	48	20	15	10	4
Country fried steak sandwich	153	450	14	25	42	6	15	2	8
Fish supreme	245	590	22	32	51	20	20	10	8
Grilled chicken fillet	211	430	29	19	36	15	35	6	10
Smoked chicken cheddar & bacon	223	540	30	30	37	30	15	10	15
Sourdough ranch chicken sandwich	225	490	29	21	45	—	10	—	0
Spicy crispy chicken sandwich	224	560	24	27	55	10	15	4	8
Hamburgers									
Hamburger	97	280	13	11	31	10	15	2	2
Cheeseburger	110	330	16	15	32	20	15	6	2
Double cheeseburger	152	450	24	24	35	25	20	10	0
Jumbo Jack	229	560	26	32	41	10	25	4	10
Jumbo Jack with cheese	242	610	29	36	41	20	30	6	10
Bacon bacon cheeseburger	242	710	35	45	41	25	30	8	15
Grilled sourdough burger	223	670	32	43	39	20	25	15	10
Ultimate cheeseburger	280	830	47	57	33	30	35	15	0
¼ lb. burger	172	510	26	27	39	15	20	6	0
The Colossus burger	272	940	52	60	48	30	35	10	6
Teriyaki Bowls									
Chicken Teriyaki bowl	440	580	28	1.5	115	10	10	110	15
Beef Teriyaki bowl	440	580	28	3	124	15	25	100	10
Soy sauce	9	5	°°	0	°°	0	0	0	0

JACK IN THE BOX—*continued*

Menu Item	Serving Size (g)	Calories (per serving)	Protein (g)	Fat (g)	Carbo-hydrates (g)	Calcium	Iron	Vitamin A	Vitamin C
Breakfast									
Breakfast Jack	121	300	18	12	30	20	15	8	15
Pancake platter	231	610	15	22	87	10	10	8	10
Sausage crescent	156	580	22	43	28	15	15	10	0
Scrambled egg platter	213	560	18	32	50	15	25	15	15
Scrambled egg pocket	183	430	29	21	31	20	20	20	0
Sourdough breakfast sandwich	147	380	21	20	31	25	20	15	15
Supreme crescent	153	530	23	33	34	15	20	15	20
Hash browns	57	160	1	11	14	0	2	0	10
Country Crock Spread	5	25	0	3	0	0	2	4	0
Grape jelly	14	40	0	0	9	0	0	0	0
Pancake syrup	42	120	0	0	30	0	0	0	0
Salads									
Chef salad	324	320	19	30	9	35	15	90	35
Taco salad	397	470	23	34	30	40	25	30	15
Side salad	111	50	3	7	°°	6	0	60	15
Bleu cheese dressing	70	260	22	°°	14	0	0	0	0
Buttermilk house dressing	70	360	36	°°	8	0	0	0	0
Low calorie Italian dressing	70	25	2	°°	2	0	0	0	0
Thousand Island dressing	70	310	30	°°	12	0	0	0	0
Mexican Food									
Taco	78	190	11	7	15	10	6	0	0
Super taco	126	280	17	12	22	15	10	0	4
Guacamole	25	50	4	°°	3	°	°	2	70
Salsa	28	10	0	0	2	°	°	2	°
Sides & Desserts									
Seasoned curly fries	109	360	5	20	39	2	8	0	8
Small french fries	68	220	3	11	28	0	4	0	30
Regular french fries	109	350	4	17	45	0	6	0	40
Jumbo fries	123	400	5	19	51	0	8	0	45
Onion rings	103	380	5	23	38	2	10	0	4
Sesame breadsticks	16	70	2	2	12	0	0	0	0
Tortilla chips	28	140	2	6	18	0	0	0	0
Hot apple turnover	110	350	3	19	48	0	10	0	15
Cheesecake	99	310	8	18	29	10	2	0	0
Chocolate chip cookie dough cheesecake	102	360	7	18	44	15	6	6	0
Cinnamon Churritos	75	330	3	21	34	2	30	0	0
Finger Foods									
Egg rolls-3 piece	165	440	3	24	54	8	15	0	6
Egg rolls-5 piece	285	750	5	41	92	15	20	0	10
Chicken strips (breaded)-4 piece	112	290	25	13	18	0	4	0	0
Chicken strips (breaded)-6 piece	177	450	39	20	28	0	6	0	0
Chicken Taquitos-5 piece	136	350	19	15	34	15	10	4	2
Chicken Taquitos-8 piece	218	560	30	25	54	20	15	8	4
Barbeque sauce	28	45	1	0	11	0	0	0	0
Buttermilk house sauce	25	130	°°	13	3	0	°	0	2
Hot sauce	13	5	°°	0	1	0	0	0	0
Sweet & sour sauce	28	40	°°	0	11	0	0	0	0

JACK IN THE BOX—*continued*

Menu Item	Serving Size (g)	Calories (per serving)	Protein (g)	Fat (g)	Carbo-hydrates (g)	Calcium	Iron	Vitamin A	Vitamin C
Drinks									
Orange juice	183	80	1	0	20	2	2	8	160
Lowfat milk (2%)	244	120	8	5	12	30	0	10	4
Vanilla milk shake (regular)	304	350	9	7	62	30	0	0	0
Chocolate milk shake (regular)	322	330	11	7	59	35	4	0	0
Strawberry milk shake (regular)	298	330	9	7	60	30	0	0	0
Iced tea (small)	16	0	0	0	0	0	0	0	0
Coffee (small)	8	5	0	0	1	0	0	0	0

The *Percentage of U.S. RDA* columns are: Calcium, Iron, Vitamin A, Vitamin C.

Source: Jack In The Box; nutritional information provided by Foodmaker, Inc., San Diego, CA.

KENTUCKY FRIED CHICKEN

Food Item	Serving Size (g)	kcal	Protein (g)	CHO (g)	Fat (g)	Cholesterol (mg)	Vit A (mg)	Vit C (mg)	Thia (mg)	Ribo (mg)	Nia (mg)	Ca (mg)	Fe (mg)
Original Recipe Chicken													
Wing	55	178	12.2	6.0	11.7	64	<100	<1.0	0.03	0.08	3.7	47.9	1.2
Side breast	90	267	18.8	10.8	16.5	77	<100	<1.0	0.06	0.13	6.9	68.0	1.2
Center breast	115	283	27.5	8.8	15.3	93	<100	<1.0	0.09	0.17	11.5	68.0	1.0
Drumstick	57	146	13.1	4.2	8.5	67	<100	<1.0	0.05	0.12	3.2	21.2	1.1
Thigh	104	294	17.9	11.1	19.7	123	104	<1.0	0.08	0.30	5.5	65.1	1.3
Extra Tasty Crispy Chicken													
Wing	65	254	12.4	9.3	18.6	67	<100	<1.0	0.04	0.06	3.3	17.8	0.6
Side breast	110	343	21.7	14.0	22.3	81	<100	<1.0	0.09	0.10	8.5	30.4	0.8
Center breast	135	342	33.0	11.7	19.7	114	<100	<1.0	0.11	0.13	13.1	33.3	0.8
Drumstick	69	204	13.6	6.1	13.9	71	<100	<1.0	0.06	0.12	3.7	12.9	0.7
Thigh	119	406	20.0	14.4	29.8	129	131	<1.0	0.10	0.21	6.5	49.0	1.2
Kentucky Nuggets	16	46	2.8	2.2	2.9	11.9	<100	<1.0	<0.01	0.03	1.00	2.4	0.1
Barbeque sauce	28.3	35	0.3	7.1	0.6	<1.0	<370	<1.0	<0.01	0.01	0.19	6.1	0.2
Sweet 'n sour	28.3	58	0.1	13.0	0.6	<1.0	<100	<1.0	<.01	0.02	0.04	4.7	0.2
Honey	14.2	49	0.0	12.1	<0.01	<1.0	<100	<1.0	<0.01	0.00	0.04	0.6	0.1
Mustard	28.3	36	0.9	6.1	0.9	<1.0	<100	<1.0	<0.01	0.01	0.16	10.2	0.3
Chicken Littles	47	169	5.7	13.8	10.1	18	<100	<1.0	0.16	0.12	2.2	22.6	1.7
Buttermilk biscuits	65	235	4.5	28.0	11.7	1	<100	<1.0	0.24	0.19	2.6	95.0	1.6
Mashed potatoes w/gravy	98	71	2.4	11.7	1.6	<1	<100	<1.0	<0.01	0.04	1.2	21.8	0.04
French fries	77	244	3.2	31.1	11.9	2	<100	15.7	0.15	0.05	2.0	12.5	0.06
Corn on the cob	143	176	5.1	31.9	3.1	<1	272	2.3	0.14	0.11	1.8	7.2	0.08
Cole slaw	91	119	1.5	13.2	6.6	5	310	21.5	0.03	0.03	0.2	32.8	0.02
Colonel's Chicken sandwich	166	482	20.8	38.6	27.3	47	<100	<1.0	0.38	0.27	11.1	46.1	1.3

Source: Public Affairs Department, KFC Corporation, Louisville, KY.

LONG JOHN SILVER'S

Food Item	Serving Size (g)	Description	kcal	Protein (g)	Fat (g)	CHO (g)
3 Pc. Nugget dinner		6 chicken nuggets, Fryes, slaw	699	23	45	54
Apple pie	113		280	2	11	43
Barbecue sauce	34		45	0	0	11
Battered shrimp dinner		6 battered shrimp, Fryes, slaw	771	17	45	60
Bleu cheese dressing	45		225	4	23	3
Breaded clams			465	13	25	46
Breaded fish sandwich platter		Fish sandwich, Fryes, slaw	835	30	42	84
Breaded oysters		6 pieces	460	14	19	58
Breaded shrimp platter		Breaded shrimp, Fryes, slaw, 2 hush puppies	962	20	57	93
Cherry pie	113		294	3	11	46
Chicken planks		4 pieces	458	27	23	35
Clam chowder	187		128	7	5	15
Clam dinner		Clams, Fryes, slaw	955	22	58	100
Cole slaw			138	1	8	16
Cole slaw, drained on fork	98		182	1	15	11
Combo salad		4.25 oz. seafood salad, 2 oz salad shrimp, 6 oz lettuce, 2.4 oz tomato, 1 pkg crackers	397	27	29	21
Corn on the cob	150	1 ear	176	5	4	29
Fish & Chicken		1 fish, 2 tender chicken planks, Fryes, slaw	935	36	55	73
Fish & Fryes		3 fish, Fryes	853	43	48	64
Fish & Fryes		2 pc fish, Fryes	651	30	36	53
Fish & More		2 fish, Fryes, slaw, 2 hush puppies	978	34	58	92
Fish w/batter		2 pieces	319	19	19	19
Fish w/batter		3 pieces	477	28	28	28
Four nuggets and Fryes			427	16	24	39
Fryes	85		247	4	12	31
Fryes			275	4	15	32
Honey-Mustard sauce	35		56	—	—	14
Hush Puppies	47	2 pieces	145	3	7	18
Hush Puppies		3 pieces	158	1	7	20
Kitchen-breaded fish (three piece dinner)		3 kitchen breaded fish, Fryes, slaw, 2 hush puppies	940	35	52	84

LONG JOHN SILVER'S—continued

Serving Food Item	Size (g)	Description	kcal	Protein (g)	Fat (g)	CHO (g)
Kitchen–breaded (two piece dinner)		2 kitchen-breaded fish, Fryes, slaw, 2 hush puppies	818	26	46	76
Lemon Meringue pie	99		200	2	6	37
Ocean chef salad		6 oz lettuce, 1.25 oz shrimp, 2 oz seafood blend, 2 tomato wedges, ¾ oz cheese	229	27	8	13
Ocean scallops		6 pieces	257	10	12	27
One fish and Fryes			449	16	24	42
One fish, two nuggets, and Fryes			539	23	30	46
Oyster dinner		6 oysters, Fryes, slaw	789	17	45	78
Pecan pie	113		446	5	22	59
Peg leg w/batter		5 pieces 514	25	33	30	
Pumpkin pie	113		251	4	11	34
Reduced calorie Italian dressing	49		20	0	1	3
Scallop dinner		6 scallops, Fryes,	747	17	45	66
Sea salad dressing	45		220	4	21	5
Seafood platter shrimp, 2 scallops, Fryes, slaw		1 fish, 2 battered	976	29	58	85
Seafood salad		5.6 oz seafood salad, 6 oz lettuce, 2.4 oz tomato	426	19	30	22
Shrimp & Fish dinner		1 fish, 3 battered shrimp, Fryes, slaw, 2 hush puppies	917	27	55	80
Shrimp salad shrimp, 6 oz lettuce, 2.4 oz tomato		4.5 oz salad	203	28	3	16
Shrimp w/batter		5 pieces	269	9	13	31
Sweet-n-sour sauce	30		—	—	—	—
Tartar sauce	30		117	—	11	5
Tender chicken plank dinner		3 chicken planks, Fryes, slaw	885	32	51	72
Tender chicken plank dinner		4 chicken planks, Fryes, slaw	1037	41	59	82
Thousand Island dressing	48		223	—	22	8

LONG JOHN SILVER'S—continued

Food Item	Serving Size (g)	Description	kcal	Protein (g)	Fat (g)	CHO (g)
Three piece fish dinner		3 fish, Fryes, slaw, 2 hush puppies	1180	47	70	93
Treasure chest		2 pc fish, 2 peg legs	467	25	29	27
Two planks and Fryes			551	22	28	51

Source: Long John Silver's Seafood Shoppes; sampling and nutrient analysis conducted independently by the Department of Nutrition and Food Science, University of Kentucky, April 10, 1986.

MCDONALD'S

Menu Item	Serving Size	Calories	Protein (g)	Carbohydrates (g)	Total Fat (g)	Cholesterol (mg)	Sodium (mg)	Dietary Fiber (g)	Vitamin A	Vitamin C	Calcium	Iron
Sandwiches												
Hamburger	160 g	270	12	34	10	30	520	2	2	4	15	15
Cheeseburger	120 g	320	15	35	14	45	750	2	6	4	15	15
Quarter Pounder	172 g	420	23	37	21	70	690	2	4	4	15	25
Quarter Pounder with cheese	200 g	530	28	38	30	95	1160	2	10	4	15	25
McLean deluxe	214 g	350	24	38	12	60	800	3	8	15	15	25
McLean deluxe with cheese	228 g	400	27	39	17	70	1040	3	10	15	15	25
Big Mac	216 g	530	25	47	28	80	960	3	6	4	20	25
Filet-O-Fish	143 g	360	14	40	16	35	690	2	2	°	10	10
McGrilled chicken Classic	189 g	260	24	33	4	45	500	2	4	8	10	10
McChicken sandwich	190 g	510	17	44	30	50	820	2	2	2	15	15
French Fries												
Small French fries	68 g	210	3	26	10	0	135	2	°	15	°	2
Large French fries	147 g	450	6	57	22	0	290	5	°	30	2	6
Super Size French fries	176 g	540	8	68	26	0	350	6	°	35	2	8
Chicken McNuggets/Sauce												
Chicken McNuggets (4 piece)	73 g	200	12	10	12	40	350	0	°	°	°	4
Chicken McNuggets (6 piece)	109 g	300	19	16	18	65	530	0	°	°	2	6
Chicken McNuggets (9 piece)	165 g	450	28	24	27	95	800	0	°	°	2	8
Hot Mustard (1 pkg)	28 g	60	1	7	3.5	5	240	<1	°	°	°	4
Barbeque sauce (1 pkg)	28 g	45	0	10	0	0	250	0	°	6	°	°
Sweet 'n sour sauce (1 pkg)	28 g	50	0	11	0	0	140	0	6	°	°	°
Honey (1 pkg)	14 g	45	0	12	0	0	0	0	°	°	°	°
Honey mustard (1 pkg)	14 g	50	0	3	4.5	10	85	0	°	°	°	°
Salads												
Chef salad	313 g	210	19	9	11	180	730	2	90	35	16	10
Fajita chicken salad	285 g	160	20	9	6	65	400	3	160	50	4	10

Percentage of U.S. RDA (Vitamin A, Vitamin C, Calcium, Iron)

MCDONALD'S—continued

Menu Item	Serving Size	Calories	Protein (g)	Carbohydrate (g)	Total Fat (g)	Cholesterol (mg)	Sodium (mg)	Dietary Fiber (g)	Percentage of U.S. RDA			
									Vitamin A	Vitamin C	Calcium	Iron
Salads—cont'd												
Garden salad	234 g	80	6	7	4	140	60	2	60	35	6	8
Side salad	139 g	45	3	4	2	70	35	1	50	20	4	4
Croutons (1 pkg)	11 g	50	1	7	1.5	0	125	0	°	°	2	2
Bacon bits (1 pkg)	3 g	15	1	0	1	5	90	0	°	°	°	°
Salad Dressings												
Bleu cheese (1 pkg)	60 g	190	2	8	17	30	650	0	2	°	6	2
Ranch (1 pkg)	60 g	230	1	10	21	20	550	0	°	2	4	°
1000 Island	63 g	190	1	16	13	25	510	1	2	2	2	2
Lite Vinaigrette (1 pkg)	62 g	50	0	9	2	0	240	0	6	6	°	°
Red French reduced calorie (1 pkg)	68 g	160	0	23	8	0	490	0	4	6	°	°
Breakfast												
Egg McMuffin	137 g	290	17	27	13	235	730	1	10	2	15	15
Sausage McMuffin	112 g	360	13	26	23	45	750	1	4	°	15	10
Sausage McMuffin with Egg	163 g	440	19	27	29	255	820	1	10	°	15	15
English muffin	55 g	140	4	25	2	0	220	1	°	°	10	8
Sausage biscuit	119 g	430	10	32	29	35	1130	1	°	°	8	15
Sausage biscuit with egg	170 g	520	16	33	35	245	1220	1	6	°	10	15
Bacon, egg & cheese biscuit	152 g	450	17	33	27	240	1340	1	10	°	10	15
Biscuit	76 g	260	4	32	13	0	840	1	°	°	6	10
Sausage	43 g	170	6	0	16	35	290	0	°	°	°	2
Scrambled eggs (2)	102 g	170	13	1	12	425	190	0	10	°	6	6
Hash browns	53 g	130	1	14	8	0	330	1	°	4	°	2
Hotcakes (plain)	150 g	310	9	53	7	15	610	2	°	°	10	15
Hotcakes (margarine 2 pats & syrup)	222 g	580	9	100	16	15	760	2	8	°	10	15
Cheerios (1 pkg)	19 g	70	2	15	1	0	180	2	15	15	2	25
Wheaties (1 pkg)	23 g	80	2	18	0.5	0	160	2	15	15	4	30
Muffins/Danish												
Fat free apple bran muffin	70 g	170	4	38	0	0	200	1	°	°	4	6
Apple danish	105 g	360	5	51	16	40	290	1	10	°	8	6
Cheese danish	105 g	410	7	47	22	70	340	0	15	°	8	6
Cinnamon Raisin danish	105 g	430	5	56	22	50	280	1	10	°	10	8
Raspberry danish	105 g	400	5	58	16	45	300	1	10	°	8	6
Desserts/Shakes												
Vanilla lowfat frozen yogurt cone	90 g	120	4	24	0.5	5	85	0	°	2	15	2
Strawberry lowfat frozen yogurt sundae	178 g	240	6	51	1	5	115	1	°	2	20	2
Hot caramel lowfat frozen yogurt sundae	182 g	310	7	63	3	5	200	1	2	2	25	°
Hot fudge sundae	179 g	290	8	54	5	5	190	2	°	2	25	4
Nuts (sundaes)	7 g	40	2	2	3.5	0	0	0	°	°	°	°
Baked apple pie	77 g	260	3	34	13	0	200	<1	°	40	2	6
McDonaldland cookies (1 pkg)	56 g	260	4	41	9	0	270	1	°	°	°	10
Vanilla shake—small	414 mL	340	11	62	5	25	220	0	4	6	40	2

MCDONALD'S—continued

Menu Item	Serving Size	Calories	Pro-tein (g)	Carbo-hydrate (g)	Total Fat (g)	Choles-terol (mg)	Sodium (mg)	Dietary Fiber (g)	Percentage of U.S. RDA			
									Vitamin A	Vitamin C	Calcium	Iron
Desserts/Shakes—continued												
Chocolate shake—small	414 mL	340	12	64	5	25	300	1	4	6	45	4
Strawberry shake—small	414 mL	340	12	63	5	25	220	0	4	10	40	4
Milk/Juices												
1% lowfat milk (8 fl oz)	1 crtn.	100	8	13	2.5	10	115	0	10	4	30	°
Orange juice (6 fl oz)	177 mL	80	1	20	0	0	20	0	2	90	2	2
Apple juice (6 fl oz)	177 mL	80	0	20	0	0	0	0	°	°	°	2

Source: McDonald's Corporation. Oak Brook, IL 60521. (708) 575-3663. 1996.
° = less than 2% of the U.S. RDA

PIZZA HUT

Food Item (1 slice)	kcal	Protein (g)	Fat (g)	CHO (g)	Ca (mg)	Fe (mg)	Vitamin A (IU)	Vitamin C (mg)	Vitamin B₁ (mg)	Vitamin B₂ (mg)
Thick 'n' chewy, beef	620	38	20	73	400	7.2	750	<1.2	0.68	0.60
Thick 'n' chewy, cheese	560	34	14	71	500	5.4	1000	<1.2	0.68	0.68
Thick 'n' chewy, pepperoni	560	31	18	68	400	5.4	1250	3.6	0.68	0.68
Thick 'n' chewy, pork	640	36	23	71	400	7.2	750	1.2	0.90	0.77
Thick 'n' chewy, supreme	640	36	22	74	400	7.2	1000	9.0	0.75	0.85
Thin 'n' crispy, beef	490	29	19	51	350	6.3	750	<1.2	0.30	0.60
Thin 'n' crispy, cheese	450	25	15	54	450	4.5	750	<1.2	0.30	0.51
Thin 'n' crispy, pepperoni	430	23	17	45	300	4.5	1000	<1.2	0.30	0.51
Thin 'n' crispy, pork	520	27	23	51	350	6.3	1000	<1.2	0.38	0.68
Thin 'n' crispy, supreme	510	27	21	51	350	7.2	1250	2.4	0.38	0.68

Source: Research 900 and Pizza Hut, Inc., Wichita, KS.

ROY ROGERS

Food Item	Serving Size (g)	kcal	Protein (g)	Fat (g)	CHO (g)
Apple danish	71	249	4.5	11.6	31.6
Bacon cheeseburger	180	581	32.3	39.2	25.0
Biscuit	63	231	4.4	12.1	26.2
Breakfast crescent sandwich	127	401	13.3	27.3	25.3
Breakfast crescent sandwich w/bacon	133	431	15.4	29.7	25.5
Breakfast crescent sandwich w/ham	165	557	19.8	41.7	25.3
Breakfast crescent sandwich w/sausage	162	449	19.9	29.4	25.9
Breast & wing	196	604	43.5	36.5	25.4

ROY ROGERS—*continued*

Food Item	Serving Size (g)	kcal	Protein (g)	Fat (g)	CHO (g)
Brownie	64	264	3.3	11.4	37.3
Caramel sundae	145	293	7.0	8.5	51.5
Cheese danish	71	254	4.9	12.2	31.4
Cheeseburger	173	563	29.5	37.3	27.4
Cherry danish	71	271	4.4	14.4	31.7
Chicken breast	144	412	33.0	23.7	16.9
Chocolate shake	319	358	7.9	10.2	61.3
Cole slaw	99	110	1.0	6.9	11.0
Crescent roll	70	287	4.7	17.7	27.2
Egg and biscuit platter	165	394	16.9	26.5	21.9
Egg and biscuit platter w/bacon	173	435	19.7	29.6	22.1
Egg and biscuit platter w/ham	200	442	23.5	28.6	22.5
Egg and biscuit platter w/sausage	203	550	23.4	40.9	21.9
French fries	85	268	3.9	13.5	32.0
Hamburger	143	456	23.8	28.3	65.6
Hot chocolate	8 oz	123	3.0	2.0	22.0
Hot fudge sundae	151	337	6.5	12.5	53.3
Hot topped potato plain	227	211	5.9	0.2	47.9
Hot topped potato w/bacon 'n cheese	248	397	17.1	21.7	33.3
Hot topped potato w/broccoli 'n cheese	312	376	13.7	18.1	39.6
Hot topped potato w/oleo	236	274	5.9	7.3	47.9
Hot topped potato w/sour cream 'n chives	297	408	7.3	20.9	47.6
Hot topped potato w/taco beef 'n cheese	359	463	21.8	21.8	45.0
Large fries	113	357	5.3	18.4	42.7
Large roast beef	182	360	33.9	11.9	29.6
Large roast beef w/cheese	211	467	39.6	20.9	30.3
Leg	53	140	11.5	8.0	5.5
Macaroni	100	186	3.1	10.7	19.4
Milk	8 oz	150	8.0	8.2	11.4
Orange juice	8 oz	99	1.5	0.2	22.8
Orange juice	8 oz	136	2.0	0.3	31.3
Pancake platter (w/syrup, butter)	165	452	7.7	15.2	71.8
Pancake platter (w/syrup, butter) w/bacon	173	493	10.4	18.3	72.0
Pancake platter (w/syrup, butter) w/ham	200	506	14.3	17.3	72.4

ROY ROGERS—*continued*

Food Item	Serving Size (g)	kcal	Protein (g)	Fat (g)	CHO (g)
Pancake platter (w/syrup, butter) w/sausage	203	608	14.2	29.6	71.8
Potato salad	100	107	2.0	6.1	10.9
Roast beef sandwich	154	317	27.2	10.2	29.1
Roast beef sandwich w/cheese	182	424	32.9	19.2	29.9
RR bar burger	208	611	36.1	39.4	28.0
Salad bar 1,000 Island	2 T	160	NA	16.0	4.0
Salad bar bacon 'n tomato	2 T	136	NA	12.0	6.0
Salad bar bacon bits	1 T	24	4.0	1.0	38.0
Salad bar blue cheese dressing	2 T	150	2.0	16.0	2.0
Salad bar cheddar cheese	¼ cup	112	5.8	9.0	0.8
Salad bar Chinese noodles	¼ cup	55	1.5	2.8	6.5
Salad bar chopped eggs	2 T	55	4.0	4.0	0.7
Salad bar croutons	2 T	132	5.5	0	31.0
Salad bar cucumbers	5–6 slices	4	NA	0	1.0
Salad bar green peas	¼ cup	7	0.5	0	1.2
Salad bar green peppers	2 T	4	0.3	0	1.0
Salad bar lettuce	1 cup	10	NA	0	4.0
Salad bar lo-cal Italian	2 T	70	NA	6.0	2.0
Salad bar macaroni salad	2 T	60	1.0	3.6	6.2
Salad bar mushrooms	¼ cup	5	0.5	0	0.7
Salad bar potato salad	2 T	50	1.0	3.0	5.5
Salad bar ranch	2 T	155	NA	14.0	4.0
Salad bar shredded carrots	¼ cup	12	0.6	0	24.0
Salad bar sliced beets	¼ cup	16	0.5	0	3.8
Salad bar sunflower seeds	2 T	101	4.0	9.0	5.0
Salad bar tomatoes	3 slices	20	0.8	0	4.8
Strawberry shake	312	315	7.6	10.2	49.4
Strawberry shortcake	205	447	10.1	19.2	59.3
Strawberry sundae	142	216	5.7	7.1	33.1
Thigh	98	296	18.4	19.5	11.7
Thigh & leg	151	436	29.9	27.5	17.2
Vanilla shake	306	306	8.0	10.7	45.0
Wing	52	192	10.5	12.8	8.5

Source: Roy Rogers Restaurants, Marriott Corporation, Washington, DC. Nutritional data furnished by Lancaster Laboratories, 1985.

TACO BELL

Food Item	kcal	Protein (g)	Fat (g)	Calories From Fat	Saturated Fat	Cholesterol (mg)	Na (mg)	Percent U.S. RDA Ca	Fe
Tacos & Tostadas									
Chicken soft taco	223	14	10	90	4	58	553	6	8
Soft taco	223	12	11	100	5	32	539	5	10
Soft taco supreme	268	13	15	140	8	47	551	8	11
Steak soft taco	217	12	9	80	4	31	569	5	6
Taco	180	10	11	100	5	32	276	8	5
Taco supreme	225	11	15	130	7	47	287	10	6
Tostada	242	9	11	100	4	14	593	17	8
Burritos									
7 layer burrito	485	15	21	190	8	28	1115	25	25
Bean burrito	391	13	12	110	4	5	1138	19	20
Beef burrito	432	22	19	170	8	57	1303	16	22
Big beef burrito supreme	525	25	25	220	11	72	1418	20	25
Burrito supreme	443	18	19	170	9	47	1184	20	21
Chicken burrito	345	17	13	110	5	57	854	14	14
Chicken burrito supreme	520	27	23	200	9	125	1130	15	50
Chili cheese burrito	391	17	18	160	9	47	980	30	17
Combo burrito	412	17	16	140	6	32	1221	17	21
Steak burrito supreme	500	26	23	200	11	75	1350	20	15
Specialty Items									
Beef MexiMelt	262	13	14	130	7	38	711	23	8
Cinnamon twists	139	1	6	50	0	0	189	°	2
Mexican pizza	574	19	38	340	12	50	1003	31	25
Nachos	345	7	18	160	6	9	398	23	4
Nachos BellGrande	633	22	34	300	12	49	952	36	20
Nachos supreme	364	12	18	160	5	17	470	19	15
Pintos 'n cheese	190	9	9	80	4	14	640	15	7
Taco salad	838	31	55	490	16	79	1132	25	34
Side Orders & Condiments									
Green sauce	4	0	0	0	0	0	136	°	°
Guacamole	36	0	3	30	1	0	132	4	°
Hot taco sauce	2	0	0	0	0	0	91	°	°
Milk taco sauce	0	0	0	0	0	0	6	°	°
Nacho cheese sauce	51	2	4	40	2	4	196	6	°
Picante sauce	3	0	0	0	0	0	132	2	0
Pico de Gallo	6	0	0	0	0	0	65	°	°
Ranch dressing	136	1	14	130	3	20	330	2	°
Red sauce	10	0	0	0	0	0	261	°	°
Salsa	27	1	0	0	0	0	709	5	3
Seasoned rice	110	2	3	30	1	5	230	°	8
Sour cream	44	1	4	40	3	15	11	2	°

Source: Taco Bell Corporation, Irvine, CA. 1996.

° = trace

WENDY'S

Food Item	Serving Size (g)	kcal	Protein (g)	CHO (g)	Fat (g)	Cholesterol (mg)	Vit A (mg)	Vit C (mg)	Thia (mg)	Ribo (mg)	Nia (mg)	Ca (mg)	Fe (mg)
Sandwiches													
½ lb. hamburger patty	74	180	19	—	12	65	—	—	4	—	20	—	20
Plain single	126	340	24	30	15	65	—	—	25	20	30	10	30
Single with everything	210	420	25	35	21	70	5	15	25	20	30	10	30
Wendy's Big Classic	260	570	27	47	33	90	10	20	30	25	35	15	35
Jr. Hamburger	111	260	15	33	9	34	2	4	25	20	20	10	20
Jr. cheeseburger	125	310	18	33	13	34	2	4	25	50	20	10	20
Jr. bacon cheeseburger	155	430	22	32	25	50	2	15	30	50	25	10	20
Jr. Swiss deluxe	163	360	18	34	18	40	4	10	25	60	20	20	20
Kids' meal hamburger	104	260	15	32	9	35	2	2	25	20	20	10	20
Kids' meal cheeseburger	116	300	18	33	13	35	2	2	25	50	20	10	20
Grilled chicken fillet	70	100	18	—	3	55	—	—	4	4	35	—	6
Grilled chicken sandwich	175	340	24	36	13	60	2	8	30	25	50	10	20
Chicken breast fillet	99	220	21	11	10	55	—	—	8	8	60	—	70
Chicken sandwich	219	430	26	41	19	60	2	8	30	25	70	10	80
Chicken club sandwich	205	506	30	42	25	70	2	15	35	30	80	10	80
Fish fillet sandwich	170	460	18	42	25	55	2	2	40	35	20	10	15
Kaiser bun	65	200	6	37	3	10	—	—	25	20	10	10	10
White bun	56	160	5	30	3	tr	—	—	20	20	10	10	10
Sandwich Toppings													
American cheese slice	18	70	4	—	6	15	6	—	—	4	—	12	—
Bacon	6	30	2	—	3	5	—	4	4	—	2	—	—
Ketchup	14	17	—	4	—	NA	4	4	—	—	—	—	—
Lettuce	10	1	—	—	—	0	—	—	—	—	—	—	—
Mayonnaise	13	90	—	—	10	10	—	—	—	—	—	—	—
Mustard	5	4	—	—	—	0	—	—	—	—	—	—	—
Onion	10	4	—	—	—	0	—	—	—	—	—	—	—
Pickles	14	2	—	—	—	0	—	—	—	—	—	—	—
Tomatoes	21	4	—	—	—	0	—	6	—	—	—	—	—
Honey mustard	14	71	—	4	6	5	—	—	—	—	—	—	—
Tartar sauce	21	120	—	—	14	15	—	—	15	10	—	—	—
Superbar—Pasta													
Alfredo sauce	56	35	1	5	1	tr	—	—	—	—	—	6	—
Fettucini	56	190	4	27	3	10	—	—	10	6	6	—	6
Garlic toast	18.3	70	2	9	3	tr	4	—	6	2	2	2	2
Pasta medley	56	60	2	9	2	tr	6	15	6	4	4	—	4
Rotini	56	90	3	15	2	tr	—	—	6	4	6	—	4
Spaghetti sauce	56	28	—	7	0	tr	—	—	—	—	—	—	—
Spaghetti meat sauce	56	60	4	8	2	10	4	4	—	2	4	—	4
Garden Spot Salad Bar													
Alfalfa sprouts	28	8	1	1	0	0	—	4	—	2	—	—	—
Applesauce, chunky	28	22	—	6	—	0	—	—	—	—	—	—	—
Bacon bits	14	40	5	—	14	10	—	2	6	4	6	—	—
Bananas	28	26	—	7	—	0	—	4	—	2	—	—	—
Breadsticks	7.5	30	1	5	1	0	—	—	2	2	2	2	2
Broccoli	43	12	1	2	0	0	6	65	2	2	—	2	2
Cantaloupe	57	20	—	5	0	0	20	30	—	—	—	—	—
Carrots	27	12	—	2	0	0	80	4	2	—	—	—	—
Cauliflower	57	14	1	3	0	0	—	70	4	2	2	2	2
Cheddar chips	28	160	3	12	12	5	—	—	2	—	4	6	2
Cheese, shredded (imitation)	28	90	6	1	6	tr	4	—	—	15	—	20	—
Chicken salad	56	120	7	4	8	tr	—	4	—	4	6	—	2
Chives	28	71	6	18	1	0	195	313	15	25	8	25	30
Chow mein noodles	14	74	1	8	4	0	—	—	6	4	4	—	4

WENDY'S—continued

Food Item	Serving Size (g)	kcal	Protein (g)	CHO (g)	Fat (g)	Cholesterol (mg)	Percentage of U.S. RDA						
							Vit A (mg)	Vit C (mg)	Thia (mg)	Ribo (mg)	Nia (mg)	Ca (mg)	Fe (mg)
Garden Spot Salad Bar—continued													
Cole slaw	57	70	—	8	5	5	4	25	—	—	—	2	—
Cottage cheese	105	108	13	3	4	15	6	—	—	10	—	6	—
Croutons	14	60	2	8	3	—	—	—	4	4	4	—	4
Cucumbers	14	2	—	—	0	0	—	—	—	—	—	—	—
Eggs (hard cooked)	20	30	3	—	2	90	4	—	—	6	—	—	—
Garbanzo beans	28	46	3	8	1	0	—	—	2	—	—	—	6
Green peas	28	21	1	4	0	0	4	8	6	2	—	—	2
Green peppers	37	10	—	2	0	0	2	60	2	—	—	—	—
Honeydew melon	57	20	—	5	0	0	—	25	2	—	2	—	—
Jalapeno peppers	14	2	—	—	0	0	—	—	—	—	—	—	—
Lettuce—iceberg	55	8	—	1	0	0	2	4	2	—	—	—	2
Lettuce—romaine	55	9	1	1	0	0	15	20	4	4	—	2	4
Mushrooms	17	4	—	—	0	0	—	—	—	4	4	—	—
Olives, black	28	35	—	2	3	0	—	—	—	—	—	2	4
Oranges	56	26	—	7	0	0	—	50	4	—	—	2	—
Parmesan cheese	28	130	12	1	9	20	6	—	—	6	—	40	—
Parmesan cheese (imitation)	28	80	9	4	3	tr	20	—	—	—	—	50	—
Pasta salad	57	35	2	6	—	0	—	—	—	2	2	—	2
Peaches	57	31	—	8	0	0	2	2	—	—	2	—	—
Pepperoni, sliced	28	140	5	2	12	35	—	—	160	4	10	—	2
Pineapple chunks	100	60	—	16	0	0	—	15	6	—	—	—	2
Potato salad	57	125	—	6	11	10	—	10	2	—	2	—	2
Pudding—butterscotch	57	90	1	11	4	tr	—	—	—	—	—	6	2
Pudding—chocolate	57	90	—	12	4	tr	—	—	2	2	—	15	2
Red onions	9	2	—	—	0	0	—	—	—	—	—	2	—
Red peppers, crushed	28	120	5	15	4	0	200	15	10	15	20	2	15
Seafood salad	56	110	4	7	7	tr	—	2	—	2	—	20	2
Strawberries	56	17	—	4	0	0	—	50	—	2	—	—	—
Sour topping	28	58	—	2	5	0	—	—	—	—	—	—	—
Sunflower seeds & raisins	28	140	5	6	10	0	—	—	30	4	6	2	10
Three bean salad	57	60	1	13	—	—	4	—	—	—	—	—	2
Tomatoes	28	6	—	1	0	0	2	10	—	—	—	—	—
Tuna salad	56	100	8	4	6	tr	—	4	—	4	25	—	2
Turkey ham	28	35	5	—	1	15	—	—	—	4	6	—	4
Watermelon	57	18	—	4	0	0	2	10	4	—	—	—	—
Salad Dressings													
Blue cheese	15	9	—	—	10	10	—	—	—	—	—	—	—
Celery seed	15	70	—	3	6	5	—	—	—	—	—	—	—
French	15	60	—	4	6	0	—	—	—	—	—	—	—
French, sweet red	15	70	—	5	6	0	—	—	—	—	—	—	—
Hidden Valley ranch	15	50	—	—	6	5	—	—	—	—	—	—	—
Italian Caesar	15	80	—	—	9	5	—	—	—	—	—	—	—
Italian, golden	15	45	—	3	4	0	—	—	—	—	—	—	—
Salad oil	28	250	0	0	28	0	—	—	—	—	—	—	—
Thousand island	15	70	—	2	7	5	—	—	—	—	—	—	—
Wine, vinegar	15	2	—	—	0	0	—	—	—	—	—	—	—
Reduced Calorie bacon & tomato	15	45	—	3	4	—	—	—	—	—	—	—	—
Reduced calorie Italian	15	25	—	2	2	0	—	—	—	—	—	—	—
Prepared Salads													
Chef salad	331	180	15	10	9	120	110	110	15	25	6	25	15
Garden salad	277	102	7	9	5	0	110	110	10	20	6	20	10
Taco salad	791	660	40	46	37	35	80	80	30	45	25	80	35

WENDY'S—continued

Food Item	Serving Size (g)	kcal	Protein (g)	CHO (g)	Fat (g)	Cholesterol (mg)	Percentage of U.S. RDA						
							Vit A (mg)	Vit C (mg)	Thia (mg)	Ribo (mg)	Nia (mg)	Ca (mg)	Fe (mg)
Superbar—Mexican Fiesta (where available)													
Cheese sauce	56	39	1	5	2	tr	—	—	—	—	—	6	—
Picante sauce	56	18	—	4	—	NA	10	30	2	—	2	—	2
Refried beans	56	70	4	10	3	tr	—	—	4	2	—	2	6
Rice, Spanish	56	70	2	13	1	tr	6	—	45	—	8	4	10
Taco chips	40	260	4	40	10	0	—	—	2	4	—	8	4
Taco meat	56	110	10	4	7	25	—	—	8	6	10	4	10
Taco sauce	28	16	—	3	—	tr	4	2	—	—	—	—	—
Taco shells	11	45	—	6	3	0	—	—	—	—	—	—	—
Tortilla, flour	37	110	3	19	3	NA	—	—	4	2	2	8	2
French fries (small) 3.2 oz°°	91	240	3	33	12	0	—	10	10	2	10	—	4
Chili (regular) 9 oz	255	220	21	23	7	45	15	15	8	10	10	8	35
Cheddar cheese, shredded	28	110	7	1	10	30	10	—	—	6	—	20	—
Sour cream	28	60	1	1	6	10	6	—	—	2	—	4	—
Crispy chicken nuggets (6)	93	280	14	12	20	50	—	—	6	6	30	4	4
Nuggets sauces													
Barbeque	28	50	—	11	—	0	6	—	—	—	—	—	4
Honey	14	45	—	12	—	0	—	—	—	—	—	—	—
Sweet & sour	28	45	—	11	—	0	—	—	—	—	—	—	2
Sweet mustard	28	50	—	9	1	0	—	—	—	—	—	—	—
Hot Stuffed Baked Potatoes													
Plain	250	270	6	63	—	0	—	50	20	6	20	2	20
Bacon & cheese	362	520	20	70	18	20	10	60	35	15	35	8	24
Broccoli & cheese	350	400	8	58	16	tr	14	60	20	10	20	10	15
Cheese	318	420	8	66	15	10	10	50	20	100	20	6	20
Chili & cheese	403	500	15	71	18	25	15	60	20	100	25	8	28
Sour cream & chives	323	500	8	67	23	25	50	75	20	10	20	10	20
Beverages													
Frosty, small°°°	243	400	8	59	14	50	10	—	8	30	2	30	6
Cola, small	8°	100	0	25	0	0	—	—	—	—	—	—	—
Lemon-lime soft drink, small	8°	100	0	24	0	0	—	—	—	—	—	—	—
Diet cola	8°	1	0	—	0	0	—	—	—	—	—	—	—
Coffee	6°	2	0	—	0	0	—	—	—	—	—	—	—
Decaf coffee	6°	2	0	—	0	0	—	—	—	—	—	—	—
Hot chocolate	6°	110	2	22	1	tr	—	—	—	8	—	6	2
Lemonade	8°	90	0	24	0	0	—	15	—	4	—	—	2
Choc milk	8°	160	7	24	5	15	15	4	6	20	—	25	4
	8°	110	8	11	4	20	10	4	6	20	—	30	—
	6°	1	0	0	0	0	—	—	—	—	—	—	—
	64	275	3	40	13	15	2	—	8	8	6	2	8

Wendy's International, Dublin, OH.

…ormation for a large order of Fries, multiply figures by 1.3; Biggie Fries, multiply by 1.87; large Chili, multiply by …by 1.5; 20-piece Nuggets, multiply by 3.3.

…formation for a medium Frosty, multiply figures by 1.3; large Frosty, multiply by 1.7. For medium soft drink, multi-…ltiply by 2. For Biggie soft drink, multiply by 3.5.